Short Answer Questions
in Anaesthesia

Short Answer Questions in Anaesthesia

An approach to written (and oral) answers

Simon Bricker MA, MBChB, FRCA

Examiner in the Final FRCA

Consultant Anaesthetist

The Countess of Chester Hospital

Chester, UK

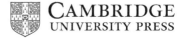

CAMBRIDGE UNIVERSITY PRESS
Cambridge, New York, Melbourne, Madrid, Cape Town, Singapore, São Paulo, Delhi
Delhi, Mexico City

Cambridge University Press
The Edinburgh Building, Cambridge CB2 8RU, UK

Published in the United States of America by Cambridge University Press, New York

www.cambridge.org
Information on this title: www.cambridge.org/9780521681001

First published 2002
Reprinted by Cambridge University Press 2005
8th printing 2013

Printed and bound in the United Kingdom by the MPG Books Group

A catalogue record for this publication is available from the British Library

ISBN-13 978-0-521-68100-1 Paperback

Contents

Preface   xiii

Preface to the 1st edition   xv

1. Advice on answering short answer questions   1

2. General Anaesthesia   13

- An adult Jehovah's witness requires surgery during which significant blood loss is probable. Describe your management.
- For what reasons should general anaesthesia for elective cases be postponed?
- What are the causes and management of hypoventilation immediately following anaesthesia?
- What are the problems of anaesthetising patients in the magnetic resonance imaging unit?
- What are the problems of monitoring patients in the magnetic resonance imaging unit?
- How may coagulation be assessed in the perioperative period?
- What causes bradycardia during general anaesthesia? What is its management?
- An adult patient develops tachycardia during general anaesthesia. Outline the causes and briefly note your management.
- How would you determine the causes of arterial hypotension (80/60 mmHg) during a transurethral prostatectomy (TURP)?
- What methods are available for the prevention of venous thromboembolism in routine surgical practice? Which patients are at particular risk?
- What factors are associated with perioperative myocardial infarction?
- What is the role of the laryngeal mask in difficult intubation?
- What problems does morbid obesity present to the anaesthetist?
- Outline the methods for detecting awareness during general anaesthesia and give a brief account of their effectiveness.
- What are the causes of awareness under general anaesthesia?
- What do you understand by the 'stress response' to surgery? Outline briefly the effects of anaesthesia on this response.
- Describe the diagnosis and management of local anaesthetic toxicity.
- Describe the complications associated with abdominal laparoscopy.
- What signs would lead you to suspect that a patient under general anaesthesia was developing malignant hyperthermia? Describe your immediate management.
- What is the pathophysiology of malignant hyperthermia? How does dantrolene affect the process? How would you investigate a patient in whom the diagnosis is suspected and who presents for non-urgent surgery?
- What features would lead you to suspect that a patient undergoing surgery had suffered venous air embolism? With what procedures may this complication be associated?

Outline the diagnosis and management of massive venous air embolism.

Describe the anaesthetic arrangements involved in a gynaecology day-case list of 15 patients.

A patient requiring surgery claims to be allergic to latex. How would you confirm the diagnosis? Outline your perioperative management.

What are the causes of heat loss during general anaesthesia? What are the effects of hypothermia in the perioperative period?

What hazards does a patient encounter when they are positioned in the lithotomy position for surgery? What additional hazards are introduced when the operating table is tilted head-down? Describe briefly how these hazards may be minimised.

What factors predispose a patient to aspirate gastric contents into the lungs during general anaesthesia? How can the risk be minimised? How should pulmonary aspiration be treated?

What factors contribute to postoperative cognitive deficits in elderly surgical patients? How may these risks be minimised?

What immunological consequences may follow homologous blood transfusion?

Outline the effects of old age upon morbidity and mortality in anaesthesia.

What are the risks associated with carotid endarterectomy? How may anaesthetic technique reduce these risks?

What is the glucocorticoid response to surgery? Describe your approach to steroid replacement both in patients who are currently receiving corticosteroids and in those who have discontinued treatment.

What are the implications of anaesthetising a patient in the prone position?

A patient presenting for total hip replacement tells you that he has a pacemaker. What further information do you require and how will this influence your anaesthetic management?

What factors would alert you to the fact that a patient might be difficult to intubate?

A patient proves impossible to intubate. What factors determine the rate of haemoglobin desaturation? What can be done to maintain oxygenation in this situation?

What safety features should be incorporated into a patient controlled anaesthesia (PCA) system for adults and what is the purpose of each? Having sent a patient to the ward with PCA what instructions would you give to the nursing staff?

You plan to anaesthetise a patient for total hip replacement under subarachnoid block with sedation. What do you understand by the term 'sedation' in this context, and what drugs and techniques are available?

Outline the causes and the physiological effects of hypercapnia. A patient has a Pa_{CO_2} of 12 kPa. How does this affect oxygenation?

What are appropriate criteria for the selection of adult patients for day-case surgery under general anaesthesia?

An 8-year-old child presents for extraction of four deciduous molar teeth in the dental chair. Describe the anaesthetic management and identify the problems that may be encountered.

What are the physiological changes that occur when a patient undergoes electro-convulsive therapy (ECT)? What are the potential complications and in which patients is ECT contra-indicated?

List the factors which may cause atrial fibrillation. How would you recognise the onset of this rhythm during anaesthesia and how would you treat it?

What are the indications for induced hypotension? What drugs may be used to achieve it? What are the problems with the technique and how can they be minimised?

What criteria are appropriate for the discharge of patients who have undergone day-case surgery? Why might overnight admission be necessary?

What place does preoperative medication (premedication) have in current adult anaesthetic practice?

An adult patient is known to be very difficult to intubate. Describe a technique of awake fibreoptic intubation. What supplemental nerve blocks may be needed?

What factors may lead to inadvertent intra-arterial injection of a drug? How would you recognise it? Describe your management of such an event.

Describe the complications of tracheal intubation.

Describe the anaesthetic management of a patient undergoing elective thyroid surgery.

A 45-year-old woman with type 1 diabetes mellitus which is controlled by insulin requires total abdominal hysterectomy. Describe the anaesthetic management.

What is the anaesthetist's contribution to safe intraocular surgery under general anaesthesia?

3. Anaesthesia and Medical Disease 99

- A patient who has undergone heart transplantation requires non-cardiac surgery. What problems may this present for the anaesthetist?
- What are the anaesthetic implications of dystrophia myotonica?
- What are the anaesthetic considerations in a patient with autonomic neuropathy?
- Describe your management of a patient who requires surgical removal of a phaeochromocytoma.
- A patient who is HIV sero-positive is scheduled for laparotomy. What factors determine the risks of transmission to anaesthetic staff? How may this risk be minimised?
- A 20-year-old patient requires open reduction and fixation of a forearm fracture sustained 12 hours previously. He has sickle cell disease. Describe the anaesthetic management.
- A 38-year-old woman requires total abdominal hysterectomy. She has multiple sclerosis. How does this influence your anaesthetic management?
- A 75-year-old man with chronic obstructive airways disease requires a transurethral resection of the prostate. Outline the advantages and disadvantages of subarachnoid anaesthesia for this patient.
- A 25-year-old intravenous drug abuser requires surgery for a compound tibial fracture. What problems may this present for the anaesthetist?
- What features are important in the anaesthetic management of a patient with myasthenia gravis?
- A patient with hepatic porphyria requires general anaesthesia. Why may this be significant?
- A patient presenting for elective surgery is found to be anaemic. What are the implications for anaesthetic management?
- How would you assess a patient with chronic obstructive pulmonary disease (COPD) who presents for laparotomy? What are the major perioperative risks and how may they be reduced?
- A surgical patient smokes 20–30 cigarettes a day and requires a general anaesthetic. Does this have any significance?
- A patient in chronic renal failure requires a laparotomy. What are the anaesthetic implications?
- Outline the anaesthetic implications of managing patients with thyroid disease who require non-thyroid surgery.
- Describe the assessment of a patient with arterial hypertension. Why is it important that it should be treated preoperatively?
- A patient has a history of chronic alcohol abuse. What are the anaesthetic implications?

4. Medicine and Intensive Care 131

- Describe the diagnosis and management of Guillain–Barré syndrome.
- Outline your management of a patient with status asthmaticus whom you are asked to see in the A&E department.
- What are the indications for tracheostomy in adults?
- Classify each type of heart block and describe the appropriate treatment in the perioperative period.
- What are the causes of muscle weakness in the intensive care patient?
- List the indications for renal support in intensive care patients? What are the principles of haemofiltration? What complications may be associated with the technique?
- What factors influence your decision to wean an intensive care patient from mechanical ventilation?
- What are the indications for nutritional support in the critically ill? Outline the advantages and disadvantages both of parenteral and of enteral nutrition.
- What can be measured directly and what can be derived from pulmonary artery catheters? What is the clinical value of these measurements?
- What is the aetiology and pathogenesis of Acute Lung Injury (ARDS)? How is it diagnosed? Outline its management.
- What factors determine oxygen delivery? How might you optimise this prior to major surgery?
- Under what circumstances does oxygen have adverse effects? What are the symptoms of toxicity? Outline the underlying mechanisms.
- What are the indications for cricothyroidotomy and for percutaneous

tracheostomy? Describe a technique for performing these procedures with
reference to the anatomy involved. List the main complications.

5. Obstetric Anaesthesia and Analgesia 155

- A woman complains of persistent headache following a regional anaesthetic for
  obstetric delivery. What are the distinguishing clinical features of the likely
  causes?
- What are the anaesthetic options for manual removal of retained placenta?
- A fit primigravida suffers inadvertent dural puncture with a 16G Tuohy needle
  during attempted epidural insertion for analgesia in the first stage of labour
  (cervix 4 cm dilated). What is your management?
- A fit multigravida complains of a typical post dural puncture headache 24 hours
  after inadvertent dural puncture with a 16G Tuohy needle during attempted
  epidural insertion for analgesia. What is your management?
- What are the advantages of retaining motor power in a woman having an
  epidural for normal labour? How can this be achieved? What checks should be
  made before allowing the woman to get out of bed?
- A fit primigravida is undergoing elective caesarean section for breech
  presentation under subarachnoid anaesthesia and suffers amniotic fluid
  embolism. What is the pathophysiology? How may it present and what is the
  differential diagnosis?
- What is the aetiology of pre-eclampsia? List the clinical features of severe pre-
  eclampsia and outline the relevance of the condition for anaesthesia.
- You have sited a lumbar epidural catheter for pain relief in the first stage of labour
  but the midwife tells you that it is ineffective. Why might it have failed and what
  is your management?
- What clinical features would alert you to the fact that a woman undergoing
  caesarean section under subarachnoid anaesthesia was developing a high block?
  Describe your management.
- A woman undergoing caesarean section under subarachnoid anaesthesia
  complains of pain. Describe your management. How may this situation be
  prevented?
- What are the pathophysiological and clinical features of HELLP syndrome? What
  are the diagnostic laboratory findings and the priorities in management?
- Describe the anaesthetic management of major intrapartum haemorrhage
  requiring emergency operation.
- Describe the management of emergency caesarean section for cord prolapse in a
  fit 21-year-old primagravida.

6. Paediatric Anaesthesia 177

- How does the physiology of an infant aged 6 months differ from that of an adult?
- What are the anatomical differences of relevance to the anaesthetist between an
  infant aged 6 months and an adult?
- Describe the anaesthetic management for a 5-year-old patient who requires re-
  operation for haemorrhage an hour after tonsillectomy.
- A 6-week old child presents for pyloromyotomy (for pyloric stenosis). Describe
  the management of this case.
- What are the problems associated with anaesthetising patients with Down
  syndrome?
- Describe your procedure for cardiac life support of a child aged 5 years.
- You are called to A&E to see a 3-year-old child with stridor. What are the principal
  differential diagnoses?
- A 3-year-old child presents to A&E with a presumptive diagnosis of acute
  epiglottitis. List the differential diagnoses. How would you manage this
  condition?
- A 10-year-old boy is brought into A&E unconscious, having been found at the
  bottom of an outdoor swimming pool. His rectal temperature is 30°C and his
  heart rate is 25 b.p.m. Describe your management.
- A 5-year-old girl is brought into A&E, having been rescued from a house fire. An
  estimated 20% of her body surface area has been affected and she has burns to
  face, neck and torso. Describe your management.
- A 2-year-old child is believed to have inhaled a foreign body two days ago,
  although there are no signs of upper airway obstruction. The child requires
  bronchoscopy: outline your anaesthetic management.

- What are the choices for postoperative analgesia for a child aged 4 years presenting for repair of inguinal hernia as a day case? State briefly the advantages and disadvantages of each method.
- Outline the circulatory changes that take place at birth. What problems may congenital heart disease present to the anaesthetist?
- An 8-week-old male infant weighing 3.0 kg is scheduled for inguinal hernia repair. He was delivered prematurely at 34 weeks. List the risk factors and state how these can be minimised.
- How does the common cold influence fitness for anaesthesia in children?

7. Neuroanaesthesia 203

- What are the causes of raised intracranial pressure? Describe the clinical features and explain the underlying pathophysiological mechanisms.
- A young adult requires intramedullary nailing of a femoral fracture 18 hours after an accident in which he was knocked unconscious. What are the anaesthetic options in this case?
- A young adult is admitted with an acute head injury. What are the indications for tracheal intubation, ventilation and transfer to a neurosurgical unit.
- How would you manage the transfer of a patient to a regional neurosurgical unit for evacuation of an extradural haematoma?
- A patient is admitted to the ITU with a severe closed head injury. There is no focal lesion requiring neurosurgical intervention. What principles govern your management during the first 24 hours?
- What are the pathophysiological insults which exacerbate the primary brain injury following head trauma? How can these effects be minimised?
- What particular problems may occur during lower abdominal surgery in a patient who suffered a traumatic transection of the spinal cord at the level of C6 four weeks previously? How would you minimise them?
- Describe how cerebral blood flow is regulated. How may it be influenced by general anaesthesia?
- What are the pathophysiological insults which exacerbate the primary brain injury following head trauma? How can these effects be minimised?

8. Acute and Chronic Pain 215

- What methods of pain relief are available following abdominal hysterectomy?
- What is meant by 'neuropathic' pain? What symptoms does it produce? Outline with brief examples the major causes.
- List with brief examples the causes of neuropathic pain. What treatments are available?
- What are the clinical features of post-herpetic neuralgia? How may it be treated?
- A 62-year-old man is to undergo an above-knee amputation. What can be done to relieve any pain he may experience thereafter?
- What are the clinical features of trigeminal neuralgia and what is its pathogenesis? Describe the main treatments that are available.
- Outline the causes and the clinical features of the 'Complex Regional Pain Syndrome'? How is it managed?
- What are the principles of the management of cancer pain?
- A 62-year-old man presents for major gastrointestinal surgery. How may the choice of pain management influence his recovery from surgery?

9. Trauma and Emergency Anaesthesia 231

- What fluids are available for the restoration of circulating volume in a patient suffering from acute blood loss? Discuss the advantages and disadvantages of each.
- A 25-year-old man is admitted with a fracture of the cervical spine at C5/6 with spinal cord trauma. There are no other injuries. Describe the management of this patient in the first 48 hours after injury.
- Describe the anaesthetic management of a patient with a perforating eye injury who had a large meal about an hour before the accident.
- Describe the diagnosis and immediate assessment of a patient with smoke inhalation injury.
- Outline the key points in the management of a patient with massive haemorrhage.

- What is the physiological response to the rapid loss of 1 litre of blood in the adult?
- Explain, with examples, the mechanisms by which a pneumothorax may occur.
- List the important causes of pneumothorax. What are the diagnostic features and what is the immediate management?
- For what reasons may a central venous catheter be inserted? Describe the normal pressure waveform and outline the value of central venous pressure monitoring. List the factors that may decrease and increase central venous pressure.

10. Anatomy, Applied Anatomy and Regional Anaesthesia 247

- Describe the anatomy of the coeliac plexus. What are the indications for its therapeutic blockade?
- Describe the innervation of the larynx. What are the clinical consequences of damage to motor nerves?
- Describe the arterial blood supply of the myocardium. What are the consequences of occlusion in the main parts of this arterial supply?
- Describe the anatomy of the nerves at the ankle which supply the foot. List the techniques that can be used to provide analgesia for surgery on the forefoot.
- Describe the anatomy of the femoral nerve relevant for the performance of a femoral nerve block. What is a 'three-in-one block' and for what may it be used?
- Describe, with reference to the anatomical landmarks, the different approaches which are used commonly for local anaesthetic block of the sciatic nerve. Why is this block performed?
- Describe how the main nerves which innervate the upper limb are formed from the brachial plexus. List the common approaches to local anaesthetic block of the plexus together with the main indications for their use.
- Describe the anatomy of the internal jugular vein. List the complications of cannulation of this vessel and outline how each may be avoided.
- Prior to subarachnoid or extradural block what landmarks are guides to the vertebral level? What are the main determinants of block height following subarachnoid injection of local anaesthetic solution?
- Describe the anatomy of the sacrum. What are the clinical differences between sacral extradural (caudal) block in adults and in children?
- Describe the anatomy of the epidural space at the level of the fourth lumbar vertebra. What are the main complications of extradural analgesia?
- Describe the anatomy of the stellate ganglion and outline how you would perform a block. What are the indications for stellate ganglion block? List the main complications.
- Describe how you would perform an interscalene block. What are the main indications and advantages? What are its disadvantages and specific complications?
- A patient requires open reduction and internal fixation (ORIF) of fractured radius and ulna, but refuses general anaesthesia. Compare the local anaesthetic blocks that might be considered suitable for this procedure.
- What are the advantages of subarachnoid (spinal) anaesthesia compared with general anaesthesia? Outline the contraindications and list the main complications.

11. Pharmacology and Applied Pharmacology 273

- Compare and contrast 'Ametop' (amethocaine gel) and EMLA cream. Are there any dangers associated with their use?
- A patient with a history of depression requires a hemicolectomy for likely carcinoma. He is taking a monoamine oxidase inhibitor (MAOI). What is your anaesthetic management?
- Describe the advantages and disadvantages of nitrous oxide in modern anaesthetic practice.
- Give an account of the mechanisms of action of nitrous oxide. Explain why it is a potentially toxic agent.
- What drugs are used to treat hypotension caused by subarachnoid block? What factors influence your choice of agent in this situation?
- Compare the pharmacology of atropine, hyoscine and glycopyrrolate. Outline their main uses in anaesthetic practice.
- Outline the pathways which mediate nausea and vomiting. Which groups of patients are particularly at risk in the perioperative period? Where do the commonly used anti-emetic drugs exert their actions?

- Describe the effects of magnesium sulphate. What are its uses in the acutely ill?
- Describe the pharmacology of propofol.
- Describe the pharmacology of ketamine.
- What drugs may be used for the immediate control of acute hypertension or to induce deliberate hypotension? What is their mechanism of action?
- What is meant by 'chirality'? What is its relevance for anaesthetic drugs?

12. Clinical Measurement and Equipment 297

- Describe the physical principles of the pulse oximeter. What are the limitations of the technique?
- Describe the physical principles which underlie the function of a 'Rotameter' flowmeter. What factors may lead to inaccuracies in its use?
- How does a capnometer or capnograph measure CO_2 concentration? What useful information is conveyed by the capnogram (the graph of CO_2 against time)?
- How can jugular venous bulb oxygen saturation be measured? What is the purpose of this investigation? What factors cause it to increase or decrease?
- Explain the basic principles of surgical diathermy. What are its potential problems?
- Outline ways of measuring humidity and evaluate the methods by which gases can be humidified in clinical practice. Why is this important?
- Describe the features of a modern anaesthetic machine that contribute to the safety of a patient undergoing general anaesthesia.
- Classify the common types of hypoxia. What are the features of an anaesthetic machine which are designed to minimise the risk of delivering hypoxic gas mixtures?
- What factors associated with the anaesthetic machine and patient breathing system may cause barotrauma? How is the risk reduced? Why is a high airway pressure alarm system important during general anaesthesia?

13. Cardiac and Thoracic Anaesthesia 313

- What are the main postoperative problems which occur in the first 24 hours following a coronary artery by-pass graft? Outline their management
- What are the principles of cardiopulmonary bypass in the adult? What are the main complications of this technique?
- What are the anaesthetic implications of mitral stenosis?
- What are the anaesthetic implications of aortic stenosis?
- How do you confirm that a double-lumen endobronchial tube has been placed correctly? Outline the possible complications associated with this procedure.
- What physiological changes are associated with one-lung anaesthesia? Describe the management of a patient in this situation who becomes hypoxic.

Index 325

Preface

The syllabus for the Final FRCA is wide, and it is tested in different ways: by multiple choice questions, by orals in anaesthesia and clinical science, and by written short answer questions. The aim of this book is to give you some insight into the short answer section and some guidance as to how best you might succeed. The introduction explains the paper and offers advice about technique, and the 180 questions that follow comprise topics that are typical of those that might appear. Each title is followed by a short preamble which is intended to establish the relevance of the subject that is being asked, and by a specimen introduction to the answer. It is not intended that you necessarily should reproduce these introductions in your own papers, but they are included as examples of ways in which answers could begin. There follows the body of the text which is presented mainly in the form of bulleted lists accompanied by supporting information and explanation, a format whose purpose is to make the significant details clear and accessible. At the end of each topic a section entitled 'Marking points' attempts to reinforce the objective of the question and to clarify any particular aspects that may be important for a pass.

Although the questions are structured as if for a written answer, it is worth emphasising that many of the subjects could appear in a slightly different form in one or other part of the oral examination. It is for this reason that many of the topics include substantially more detail than would be needed to pass a written question, but enough to allow you to give a reasonable account of yourself in the vivas.

This is not a textbook of anaesthesia but an exam-orientated guide. Yet it would be disappointing were the practice of clinical anaesthesia to bear no relation whatever to the examination syllabus. So although the questions in this book are constructed primarily for the convenience of examination candidates, I would hope also that they comprise a succinct summary of information, albeit unreferenced, that would be of interest to other practising clinicians.

I had always wondered why the authors of medical textbooks, however modest, paid tribute to the forbearance of their families. Now we know!

Simon Bricker
2002

Preface to the 1st Edition

The guidelines provided in this book include the main elements of each answer in note form. These answer notes are composed of simple and basic knowledge in the field of anaesthesia.

They do, however, introduce the reader to methods and systems of answering, which would enable any examination candidate to encapsulate the relevant material in the brief time available in a short answer question exam. It is also worth noting that the same questions could be asked in a *viva voce* examination. It would be immensely helpful to any candidate to have ready-organised answers in mind, in the style of the ones in this book. Such an organised approach would impress any examiner.

Reading this book is about learning the skills of succinct, accurate and comprehensive communication. This is a fundamental skill of medical practice, which is usually learned by copying the talents of senior colleagues. This 'apprenticeship' method has stood the test of time for the medical profession for many centuries.

It is hoped that those who read this book will find answering examination questions easier as a result. This is very worthwhile for you, the reader. If it also improves communication between doctors (and others), then it will have exceeded its primary purpose and achieved something important for our profession.

G.B. Rushman
1997

Abbreviations

$(A-a)DO_2$	Alveolar-arterial oxygen difference	CVP	Central venous pressure
ACE	Angiotensin converting enzyme	CVA	Cerebrovascular accident
		CVS	Cardiovascular system
ACT	Activated clotting time	CXR	Chest X-ray
ACTH	Adrenocorticotrophic hormone	DBP	Diastolic blood pressure
		DC	Direct current
AF	Atrial Fibrillation	DIC	Disseminated intravascular coagulation
APPT	Activated partial thromboplastin time	DVT	Deep venous thrombosis
		ECF	Extracellular fluid
ARDS	Adult respiratory distress syndrome	ECG	Electrocardiogram
		EEG	Electroencephalogram
ASD	Atrial septal defect	EMG	Electromyogram
ATP	Adenosine triphosphate	$ETCO_2$	End-tidal carbon dioxide
AV	Atrio-ventricular	ETT	Endotracheal tube
A-V	Arterio-venous	FBC	Full blood count
BMI	Body mass index	FEV_1	Forced expiratory volume in 1 second
BP	Blood pressure		
BT	Bleeding time	F_1O_2	Inspired fraction of oxygen
CBF	Cerebral blood flow	FRC	Functional residual capacity
CEPOD	Confidential enquiry into peri-operative deaths	FVC	Forced vital capacity
		GA	General anaesthesia
CFAM	Cerebral function analysing monitor	GFR	Glomerular filtration rate
$CMRO_2$	Cerebral metabolic rate for oxygen	HPA	Hypothalamo-pituitary-adrenal
		HR	Heart rate
CN	Cyanide	HDU	High dependency unit
CNS	Central nervous system	IABP	Intra-arterial blood pressure
CO	Cardiac output, or Carbon Monoxide	ICP	Intracranial pressure
		IHD	Ischaemic heart disease
CO_2	Carbon Dioxide	IOP	Intraocular pressure
COPD	Chronic obstructive pulmonary disease	IPPV	Intermittent positive pressure ventilation
CPAP	Continuous positive airways pressure	ITU	Intensive Care Unit
		kPA	Kilopascal
CPP	Cerebral perfusion pressure	LMA	Laryngeal mask airway
CRF	Chronic renal failure	LOR	Loss of Resistance
C-spine	Cervical spine	LVEDP	Left ventricular end-diastolic pressure
CT	Computerised tomography		
CTG	Cardiotocogram		

LVEDV	Left ventricular end-diastolic volume	PE	Pulmonary embolus
LVH	Left ventricular hypertrophy	PEEP	Positive end-expiratory pressure
MAC	Minimum alveolar concentration	PICU	Paediatric intensive care unit
MAO	Monoamine oxidase	PIH	Pregnancy-induced hypertension
MAP	Mean arterial pressure	PONV	Post-operative nausea and vomiting
MCV	Mean corpuscular volume		
$MgSO_4$	Magnesium sulphate	PORM	Post-operative respiratory morbidity
MI	Myocardial infraction		
MR	Magnetic	PPF	Plasma protein fraction
MRI	Magnetic resonance imaging	PT	Prothrombin time
NG	Naso-gastric	PVR	Pulmonary vascular resistance
NIBP	Non-invasive blood pressure	RBF	Renal blood flow
N_2O	Nitrous oxide	RSI	Rapid sequence induction
NSAID	Non-steroidal anti-inflammatory drug	RUQ	Right upper quadrant
		RVH	Right ventricular hypertrophy
O_2	Oxygen	SA	Sino-atrial
OHDC	Oxygen-haemoglobin dissociation curve	SAB	Subarachnoid block
		SAG-M	Saline, Adenine, Glucose-Mannitol
ORIF	Open reduction and internal fixation	SBP	Systolic blood pressure
PA	Pulmonary artery	SGB	Stellate ganglion block
P_aCO_2	Partial pressure of arterial carbon dioxide	SpO_2	Oxygen saturation (plethysmographic)
P_aO_2	Partial pressure of arterial Oxygen	SVR	Systemic vascular resistance
		SVT	Supra-ventricular tachycardia
PAOP	Pulmonary artery occlusion pressure	TAH	Total abdominal hysterectomy
		TAPVD	Total anomalous pulmonary venous drainage
PCA	Patient controlled analgesia		
PCEA	Patient controlled epidural analgesia	TENS	Transcutaneous electrical nerve stimulation
PCOP	Pulmonary capillary occlusion pressure	TURP	Trans-urethral resection of prostate
PCWP	Pulmonary capillary wedge pressure	URTI	Upper respiratory tract infection
PCV	Packed cell volume	VR	Venous Return
PDA	Patent ducts arteriosus	VSD	Ventricular septal defect
PDPH	Post-dural puncture headache	VT	Ventricular

Advice on answering short answer questions

Postgraduate examinations evolve in mysterious ways, and so when puzzled candidates for the Final FRCA query the rationale for a twelve-question short answer paper they may find the answer opaque. The 'educationalists', they are told, believe that the paper should contain not just twelve questions, but should have as many as twenty, if not more. It is as if the invocation of this higher educational authority is meant to explain everything about the science of examinations: despairing candidates meanwhile have to count themselves lucky that they only have to answer a mere 12 questions in 3 hours. You may be surprised to know that at least some of the Final examiners share this unease about the current format. There are concerns that the pressure imposed by having to complete an answer in less than 15 minutes militates against the original purpose of this part of the examination, which was '*to assess the understanding of facts, and judgement, understanding and communication skills.*' Examiners are aware that you face a significant challenge and you may even start this part of the examination with their sympathy.

The composition of the paper

The Final FRCA in its current format dates from November 1996 and the initial information from the College about the short answer section stated that, in this new part of the examination '*...questions will tend to follow the pattern of including a question which relates to the following areas: paediatric, neurosurgical, obstetric, cardiothoracic, trauma and emergency, acute and chronic pain, medicine and surgery, clinical measurement, regional and local anaesthesia, dental and maxillo-facial anaesthesia, ENT and ophthalmic anaesthesia, and intensive care medicine.*' This rubric no longer appears in College documents and a review of the papers since that time shows that the questions do not necessarily follow this topic list. The list does however form a broad template for the construction of each successive paper and these tend to comprise a mixture of questions that are newly set and some that have appeared previously. A new question is an unknown quantity: whether it is a good discriminator will not become clear until a large number of candidates have attempted it. Questions that appear more than once have proved themselves to be satisfactory. They allow a degree of quality control and audit and they also permit some comparison of standards of performance. It would be most unusual, therefore, were a paper to contain 12 entirely new questions, and so it makes sense for you to review the past papers because it is certain that some of the questions will reappear. An important source of new questions is the review articles that will have been published in the last 6–12 months in the major anaesthesia journals.

As far as possible the examination aims to test both knowledge and judgement which, broadly speaking, is the way that an individual uses that knowledge. The first may be more readily acquired than the second, but it is judgement which is the more important. It is vital, therefore, for you to have confidence in your clinical experience. If, for example, the question asks about the immediate management of status asthmaticus, carbon monoxide poisoning, head injury or some other condition which recently you have encountered, then be confident in describing what you actually did. It is much better to take this approach rather than struggle to recall the small print theory or the minutiae of drug doses with which you are unfamiliar. Remember that you are aiming to persuade the examiners that your clinical practice is credible.

Because examiners are aware of the difficulty in condensing into two or three sides your knowledge about large topics such as 'anaesthesia for aortic aneurysm repair', the recent tendency is for some questions to have a more narrow focus. A question, for instance, will ask not about the general difficulties of *anaesthetising* patients in a magnetic resonance scanner but about the specific problems of *monitoring* patients in such a unit.

The marking system

All parts of the FRCA examination employ what is known as 'close marking'. This means that instead of being given a numerical mark a candidate is awarded one of four grades which range from '1' to '2+'. A '1' represents a poor fail and '1+' a fail; a '2' is a pass and a '2+' is an outstanding pass. Each of the 12 separate written answers receives one of these marks, which then, unusually for the FRCA examination, is converted into a numerical value. A '1' grade is given 1 mark, a '1+' receives 1.5 marks, a '2' receives 2 marks and a '2+' receives 2.5 marks. The total achieved determines into which final band the candidate will fall. A total of 18 or less results in an overall '1' mark for the paper, 18.5–20.5 converts to a '1+' mark, 21–24.5 marks converts to a '2' and 25 or more will receive a '2+'. You will see, therefore, that this section of the examination can be passed if a candidate gets '2's for six questions and only '1+'s for the remaining six. In other words you can pass even if you fail half of the questions. Given this marking system it is even possible to pass, in theory at least, by receiving a '2+' on three answers and by failing the remaining nine (75% of the paper) with a '1+'. This information is important because it means that the short answer paper is the only part of the Final FRCA examination in which a '2+' in one section of the test can redeem a poor performance in another. It is important to stress, however, that candidates should not aim to pass by concentrating so hard on those questions that they believe they can answer well that they omit some others. The omission of a question, or failure to make a genuine attempt to answer the question will result in an automatic '0' mark for the paper and overall failure. A candidate with a '0' (veto) mark cannot proceed to the vivas.

How the questions are marked

The FRCA is a structured examination. This means, for example, that during the oral part of the examination all the candidates during a particular session are asked the same question. It is obvious that each candidate receives the same written papers but in order to standardise the marking the examiners also use guidance answers which outline the major points which a candidate is expected to have covered. This approach certainly makes the FRCA fairer and more objective, but it would be unrealistic to assume that all subjective opinion is removed. At each sitting of the examination every examiner marks a set of the same anonymous papers and the results are audited. There is always a spread of marks around the mode which demonstrates simply that some examiners are less severe than others. This is inevitable in any system in which human judgements are involved, but your consolation is that the number of examiners who are harsh is matched by the number who are lenient and you will never encounter the same examiners twice. The system does not allow those who marked your short answer paper to examine you in any other part of the examination.

Presentation, layout and legibility

Each examiner will receive between 180 and 200 answers to mark and will have 10 days or less in which to complete the task. If each answer is given 5 minutes' consideration then the examiner, who by the way has to be a full-time clinician, will have to find over 15 hours during their normal working week in which to mark the papers. Given the number of questions and the time constraints it is obvious that judicious presentation of your answers will help.

You do not have very long, so unless it helps you to focus on the question do not waste time by writing it out at the top of the answer. Some candidates abbreviate the full question to, for example, *'Paediatric resus.'*, *'Awareness'* or *'Day case'*. This may help the examiner to identify the question but it is not necessary for your success.

These are not essays but are short answers, and some of the questions suggest their own layout by asking you, for example, to *'List the common causes of, or the predisposing factors for....'* a particular condition, or to *'classify the types of...'*. Such questions clearly invite you to produce a bulleted list. Similarly it is appropriate to deal with questions which ask you to outline the advantages and disadvantages of a technique, or its indications and contraindications, by constructing two lists. This approach is also appropriate for all the questions which require you to present discrete pieces of information; when you are asked for instance *'What are the problems of...'*, *'What is the differential diagnosis of...'*, *'What are the risks of...'*, *'What factors contribute to...'*. A list should not, however, comprise one-word answers. If the question asks you to classify the types of heart block, the examiner will expect to read more than bullet points with '1st degree', '2nd degree', and '3rd degree'. Some expansion will be required. It is helpful to fill out your answers with brief examples. If a drug has cardiac side-effects and you simply write *'....may be associated with arrhythmias'*, an examiner may think that you are simply guessing and overall your answer is likely to lack depth and focus. If, on the other hand, you were to write *'...may be associated with a number of different cardiac arrhythmias of which the most important is supraventricular tachycardia'*, your answer will appear more considered and more impressive, even though it may not actually contain that much more information.

If a question asks you to describe your anaesthetic management of a specific condition the use of lists is less appropriate, but your answer will appear more lucid if it is broken down into headings such as *'Preoperative assessment, investigation and preparation; Intra-operative management; Recovery and Postoperative Care.'* If you are considering a particular anaesthetic technique remember to consider all the possible alternatives: general anaesthesia, regional anaesthesia, sedation plus analgesia and so on. Do not list all the alternatives when some are wholly inappropriate. It is, however, worth discussing potential techniques even if subsequently you discard them after reasoned consideration.

You can create your own structured templates for a variety of possible questions, and this is useful for two reasons. Not only does it allow you to produce a clear and thorough answer to a question about which you are confident, but also it can help you with those questions in which you feel your knowledge is limited.

Many of the questions can be answered using headings and subheadings. This works well if you have a good grasp of the topic. It is worth spacing the headings out so that you can incorporate extra information should it occur to you. If you are struggling then your list will be a short one and the deficiencies will be very obvious. If you revert to blocks of written text your answer may appear more substantial and may even persuade the examiner that you know more than actually is the case. Some candidates may have been advised to present their headings in a different colour, and to underline key points. This is all very decorative but it can be overdone: when the underlining is excessive the identification of key points appears haphazard. It may indeed emphasise the fact that a candidate has no sense of priority. If you are asked a question which begins with '*What are the main factors in...*', you should outline the important or common details first. The examiner is likely to doubt your clinical judgement if your first heading in response to the question '*What are the significant complications of lumbar extradural analgesia...*' is '*Horner's syndrome*'.

Some candidates take too literally the advice that these are short answer questions rather than essays by filling their answers with abbreviations. Given the time constraints it is certainly acceptable to use common abbreviations such as 'ICP' (intracranial pressure), 'BP' (blood pressure), 'HR' (heart rate) or 'PCWP' (pulmonary capillary wedge pressure). The use of ambiguous or uncommon abbreviations will do you no favours, particularly if they are incorporated into a sentence such as this one: '*The eff on pt = pred. Thio idem as steroids. Pt may c/o CP*'. You will not pass a question if you are unable to make your meaning clear. This will also apply if your answers are illegible. Examiners do make every effort to allow for the fact that some candidates have poor handwriting, but it is obvious that some of their points may be missed. You will be unable to change your writing style very much, but if you do have this problem then it is at least worth spacing out your answers and putting some of your main headings in block capitals. You may not be a calligrapher but you may be an artist, in which case diagrams may be useful. Drawings are sometimes requested in questions about anatomy, but this is to prevent you from spending a lot of time in laborious description. A broad outline is usually all that is required and not a detailed line drawing that will take up excessive time.

Some general points

Given the time pressure that you are under it is worth developing some structured approaches to questions. You may be asked, for example, about '*problems associated with....*', which may include anything from hypercapnia to obesity. Rather than launch into the first thing that occurs to you, start with a definition:

- **Hypercapnia:** 'The normal partial pressure of carbon dioxide in arterial blood is between 4.5 and 6.0 kPa depending on the reference laboratory, and so hypercapnia may be defined as a Pa_{CO_2} of greater than 6.0 kPa. It may further be classified into 'moderate' and 'severe' hypercapnia with clinical features which vary accordingly.'

- **Obesity:** 'Obesity, typically, is defined by the body mass index (kg m^{-2}) which allows classification of patients as being overweight", obese" and morbidly obese". It is the morbidly obese, as defined by a BMI (body mass index) of over 35 in whom anaesthesia is most problematic.'

Chronic medical problems are a popular topic in the examination and this approach can work equally well:

- **Rheumatoid arthritis:** 'Rheumatoid arthritis is a chronic autoimmune disease characterised by a destructive polyarthritis and which has systemic features of importance to the anaesthetist which can be outlined as follows....'

- **Diabetes mellitus:** 'Diabetes mellitus is a heterogeneous group of endocrine disorders in which the common feature is a relative or absolute absence of insulin. The resulting disorder of glucose metabolism affects all body systems, the most important of which from the anaesthetist's point of view are the cardiovascular, renal....'

Starting a written, or indeed an oral answer in this way, gives it a degree of authority which is more likely to impress the examiner that a candidate is orderly, well informed and clear thinking.

Some structured responses can be wide ranging. If, for instance, you are asked about the contraindications to a particular procedure you could begin with the statement that:

- 'There are relative and absolute contraindications to this procedure, but arguably' – (the use of this word suggests that you are well read enough to know that it may be controversial) – 'the only absolute contraindication is patient refusal. Other contraindications require a risk–benefit analysis which should almost certainly involve discussion with the patient, and which include…'

You will see, therefore, that you can construct some set responses which are accurate and appropriate but which can apply to a fairly wide range of questions and which will allow you further time to order your thoughts.

But beware. Although it is very useful to use a structured approach to questions you should be careful lest this leads you into the production of what can be called 'generic' answers. If, for example, a question asks about the relief of acute pain following a particular surgical procedure, it is very easy to produce a standard answer which includes methods of pain assessment and treatment using the WHO analgesic ladder. This, of course, could apply to all forms of acute pain after any injury or surgical operation. These are certainly valid points which might form part of a short introduction, but the examiners will expect the answer to be much more sharply focussed on the particular patient and the specific surgical procedure. Another example comes from the advanced life support courses which have encouraged the 'Airway', 'Breathing', 'Circulation' approach to a variety of acute emergencies. Some candidates have been known to extend this approach to the management, for instance, of chronic pain problems for which it is ludicrously inappropriate. Non-specific answers will fail.

At the examination

The advice that follows may seem banal but the evidence from candidates' papers confirms, unfortunately, that it is still required.

Read the instructions carefully. There is no choice of questions and at present the examination requires that you answer all 12 questions within 3 hours. This allows you only 15 minutes per question and conventional advice has it that you should give each one approximately the same time. If you plan to spend longer on those questions with which you are familiar at the expense of some others then you do need to remember how the marking system operates. You may well achieve a '2+' in a subject about which you know a good deal, but unless you cover all the major points and most of the minor ones you may just fall short despite your best efforts and end up with a creditable '2'. The nature of the marking system, however, means that a half page answer which is almost totally inaccurate will still receive a '1', because there is no lower mark for an examiner to give. So with some thought, when faced with a question about which you feel you know little, it may be possible for you to raise the '1' to a '1+' with much less effort than you expended in trying to achieve that '2+'. In the end you must choose your own strategy, but keep these thoughts in mind.

When you read some questions it may occur to you that you know little or nothing about the subject that is asked. You almost certainly know more than you think. Take, for example, the anaesthetic management of a patient undergoing correction of kyphoscoliosis. You may never have seen major spinal surgery, but you would probably realise that these operations are prolonged, may involve substantial blood loss, will be undertaken in the prone position, and may well need high dependency care in the immediate postoperative period. Thereafter you may have to think a bit more laterally, by considering, for instance, why scoliosis requires correction. If the answer is not obvious to you then consider what problems beset any adult patients who you may have seen with this condition. Typically the adult with longstanding uncorrected spinal deformity will have pulmonary function tests which demonstrate a restrictive pattern. You can surmise, therefore, that corrective surgery is aimed both at reducing skeletal deformity and preventing any deterioration in respiratory function. Preoperative assessment should include pulmonary function tests and their result may determine where the patient should be nursed postoperatively. Ask yourself what is the typical age of these patients (they are usually teenagers) and are there any problems associated with this age group. Ask yourself whether or not this condition is usually associated with other diseases or congenital abnormalities. Consider the worst case scenario: this suggests to the examiner that you are prepared for every eventuality and it may prevent you from missing something important. With kyphoscoliosis what is the worst that could happen preoperatively? (Respiratory failure and possible cardiac problems.) What is the worst intraoperatively? (Prolonged surgery, hypothermia, massive blood loss, pneumothorax, problems with spinal distraction.) What is the worst case scenario in the postoperative period? (Respiratory compromise, severe pain, spinal cord ischaemia.)

Read the question properly. If it asks for the indications for a regional technique then the examiner will neither expect nor wish to read a detailed account of how to perform the block. Examiners can be irked by the answer which is cluttered with details such as the need for trained assistance, venous access after full explanation, a thorough machine and equipment check, full monitoring, all resuscitation drugs to hand, the cardiac arrest team primed and the intensive care bed booked. Similarly, if, to take the example already cited, the question asks about the problems of monitoring patients in the magnetic resonance scanner you cannot pass if you devote your answer to the problems of *anaesthetising* patients in that environment. Most of the questions have been worded carefully, not in any attempt to trick, but so as to ensure that they are not ambiguous or do not tempt candidates into a much fuller answer than is necessary. Some topics require a fuller account than others, but you are not expected to fill more than two or three pages of the examination booklet on any one question. Some answers can be completed satisfactorily in less.

Do not give a list of complications and side effects unless the question specifically asks you so to do. You may end up writing copiously in the belief that you are doing well, whereas the reality is that you will just be wasting time.

Each paper usually contains one question on equipment or clinical measurement. In these questions there is no substitute for knowledge, but even if the scientific details elude you, it may be possible to salvage something by reverting to your clinical experience of the matter in question. The same applies to questions about anatomy. There are usually two parts to the question: anatomical details and their application. A question may ask you, for example, to describe the anatomy of the coeliac plexus and to list the indications for its block. If the anatomy is unfamiliar then a broad, if sketchy, description of the anatomy accompanied by a reasonable account of the clinical application may get you a 1+ mark for an answer which you might have given up as hopeless.

People have different strategies for the short answer paper and those who run the various FRCA preparation courses may offer conflicting advice. Some recommend that first you should scan all the questions, identify the topics on which you feel confident and allocate your time accordingly. They may suggest that you make rough notes for all the questions on a blank sheet of paper, to which you can add further points if and when they occur to you. Others believe that it is better to open the paper and to look at only one question at a time. You then answer this question within the allocated time before moving on to look at the next. Those who advocate this approach believe that the candidate is able to focus directly on the topic, easy or difficult, without being distracted by worries about some or all of the remaining questions. None of these methods is either right or wrong. What is important is that one is successful for you. The only way of identifying which of them is the best is to try them all and see which works. Practice is vital, not only to identify your best tactic, but to familiarise yourself with a format of examination which previously you may never have encountered.

What the words in examination questions mean

Traditional examination essay questions invited candidates to 'Discuss...' or to 'Describe...' a particular topic. The meaning of these words is actually very straight-forward: but they seemed always to cause disproportionate confusion. Their use was supposed to have been abandoned, but in a recent paper the word 'describe' appeared twice and the word 'discuss' once. The glossary below aims to define within the context of this examination what is meant by the various terms that may appear.

'Outline the advantages and disadvantages of...'
As in: 'Outline the advantages and disadvantages of intrathecal block in...'
To 'outline' is to give the main features of, or general principles about a subject. A large amount of detail is not required. In this example you would be expected to list each factor and give a small amount of additional information.

'List the.....'
As in: 'List the predisposing factors for gastric aspiration in...'
To 'list' is to write down a number of connected items. In some respects this is similar to 'outline', but less detail is required.

'What **factors** contribute...'
As in: 'What factors contribute to postoperative cognitive defects in the elderly...'
A 'factor' is a circumstance, fact or influence which contributes to an end result. In the above example factors could therefore be social, pharmacological, surgical, etc.

'Classify the...'
As in: 'Classify the types of heart block...'
To 'classify' is to arrange in, or to assign to, classes or categories. This kind of question is only asked about topics which have already been formally classified in this way. You will not be expected to construct your own classification.

'What are the **problems** of...'
As in: 'What are the problems of monitoring a patient in the MRI (magnetic resonance imaging) unit...'
A 'problem' is a difficult matter requiring a solution. In this example and others it is almost a synonym for the word 'difficulty'.

'Describe the...'
As in: 'Describe your procedure for cardiac life support of a child...'
To 'describe' is to state the characteristic(s) of, or the appearance of, a particular subject. In most questions the word is used to mean the same as to 'state'.

'Discuss the...'
As in: 'Discuss the factors which...'
To 'discuss' is to examine by argument. If, therefore, you were asked to discuss a particular technique, you would be expected to consider the risks and benefits in comparison with others and to come to a considered conclusion.

'*What is the **aetiology** of...*'
As in: 'What is the aetiology of the systemic inflammatory response syndrome.'
The 'aetiology' is the assignment of a cause or reason for a particular condition or event.

'*What is the **significance** of...*'
As in: 'What is the significance of a raised preoperative creatinine and urea?'
'Significance' is in effect a synonym for 'importance'. In this example the question is asking 'what are the important reasons for..' impaired renal function preoperatively.

'*Outline your **management** of...*'
As in: 'Outline your management of a head injury prior to transfer...'
'Management' is the technique of treating a disease or condition. In this example you would be expected to include aspects of all medical treatment, including anaesthetic, as appropriate.

'*Describe the **anaesthetic management** of...*'
As in: 'Describe the anaesthetic management of pyloric stenosis...'
'Anaesthetic management' means all the anaesthetic aspects of treating a particular condition. In the above example, therefore, you would not be expected to give details about the initial resuscitation and rehydration of the baby. Remember, however, that anaesthetic management should always include immediate preoperative and post-operative care.

'*Describe the **principles** of...*'
As in: 'What are the principles involved in pulse oximetry...'
A 'principle' (in this context a physical principle) is a natural law which forms the basis of the working of a machine. In other words you are being asked to explain how a particular piece of apparatus works.

'*How would you **determine**...?*'
As in: 'How would you determine a patient's fitness for anaesthesia?'
To 'determine' means to find out or to establish precisely. In this example the word implies that there are some precise physical indices that should be identified.

'*How would you **assess**...?*'
As in: 'How would you assess a patient's fitness for anaesthesia?'
To 'assess' means to estimate the size or the quality of a particular subject. The use of 'assess' rather than 'determine' implies that there may be qualitative as well as quantitative indices involved.

The outline answers

All examinations include some questions which by common agreement are idiotic. This even may be your view of some of the examples which are found in this book. If such is the case then the examples should still provide useful practice for the real thing. Each is prefaced with a comment about the topic which attempts to place it in context, to suggest the underlying rationale and to indicate its importance. When you encounter the short answer paper itself it may help focus your answer if you ask yourself what you believe to be the aim of any particular question.

There follows an 'introduction' to the answer. These are not intended to be right or wrong. They are simply examples to indicate how you might engage the examiner's interest by offering, for instance, an overview of the importance of the subject, or by giving a succinct definition of the topic to focus attention on the answer that is to follow.

The notes in this book are not intended to represent complete and perfect answers. Well-informed readers may take issue with some of the statements and will doubtless identify omissions. This should come as no surprise because this is not a textbook of anaesthesia, but is an exam-orientated aid. Most of the answers are presented in the form of bulleted lists with explanations; a format whose purpose is to make the information clear and more accessible. Your answers need not necessarily follow this format although in many cases it would be appropriate for them so to do. Many of the specimen answers do, however, contain substantially more detail than is required for a short written answer. Were you to reproduce them faithfully without further embellishment then you would pass comfortably. In many instances the key points alone would prove sufficient to gain you a '2'. The additional information is also intended to provide a structure on which to base your answers were the question, or a variation of it, to appear in the oral part of the examination, and to allow you to discuss the topic with some confidence.

The 'Marking points' which appear at the bottom of each question clarify the overall objective of the question and emphasise particular aspects that you should expect to cover.

Pharmacology topics

A chapter on pharmacology has been included, although you are more likely to encounter direct questions about anaesthetic drugs in the applied science part of the oral examination. The subject lends itself well to a structured answer which will help to ensure that you do not omit important information. One such template is outlined below. It is offered as one example of several ways in which pharmacology questions can be approached.

Introduction
Definition of the essential nature of the agent in question. For example:

> Propofol is a substituted phenol which is used primarily for the induction of anaesthesia in both adults and children.

Chemistry
More information (if you know it) about the chemistry of the drug. For example:

> Propofol is a substituted stable phenolic compound: 2,6 di-isopropylphenol. It is highly lipid soluble and water insoluble and is presented as either a 1% or 2% emulsion in soya bean oil. Other constituents include egg phosphatide and glycerol. It is a weak organic acid with a pK_a of 11.

Mechanism of action
Outline the main action of the agent. For example:

> In common with many other drugs which produce general anaesthesia the mechanism of action is not wholly clear. It may enhance inhibitory synaptic transmission by activation the Cl^- channel on the β_1 subunit of the GABA receptor. It also inhibits the NMDA subtype of glutamate receptor.

Uses
Describe the main uses of the drug. For example:

> Propofol is used for the induction of anaesthesia, for the maintenance of anaesthesia, for sedation in intensive care, and for sedation during procedures under local or regional anaesthesia. It has an anti-emetic action and is sometimes given by very low dose infusion to chemotherapy patients.

Dose and routes of administration

Give a brief account. For example:

> The drug is only used intravenously. A dose of 1–2 mg kg^{-1} will usually induce anaesthesia in adults. Children may require twice as much.

Onset and duration of action

Make a brief comment. Quote the half-life if you know it. For example:

> An induction dose of propofol will lead to rapid loss of consciousness (within a minute). Rapid redistribution to peripheral tissues (distribution half-life is 1–2 minutes) leads to rapid awakening. The elimination half-life is quoted at between 5 and 12 hours.

Main effects and side effects

Use a systems approach, but begin with the main system which the drug affects. Do not begin a description of a neuromuscular blocker with an account of its effect on the gravid uterus. List important side effects before trivial ones. To do otherwise may persuade the examiner that you have simply learned everything by rote without applying any sense of priority to the information. For example:

> Propofol has the following effects: CNS – depression and induction of anaesthesia. May be associated with excitatory effects and dystonic movements, particularly in children. The EEG displays initial activation followed by dose-related depression. The data sheet states that it is contraindicated in patients with epilepsy, although this has been disputed. CVS – systemic vascular resistance falls and it is unusual to see compensatory tachycardia. A relative bradycardia is common and the blood pressure will fall. Propofol is a myocardial depressant. RS – propofol is a respiratory depressant which also suppresses laryngeal reflexes. GIT – the drug is anti-emetic. Other specific problems include pain on injection and the risk of hyperlipidaemia in intensive care patients on prolonged infusions.

Pharmacokinetics

Large quantities of pharmacokinetic information relating to clearance and volume of distribution and so on are not strictly necessary. Moreover it is unlikely to be information which most examiners themselves will have readily to mind. It is, however, worth citing a particular detail if it has clinical relevance. The pK_a of local anaesthetic drugs is one example. In respect of metabolism and elimination, lipid-soluble drugs will cross lipid membranes such as the blood–brain barrier and the placenta, and will undergo metabolism in the liver. Water-soluble drugs do not cross such membranes and are eliminated renally. Details of metabolites are important only if they are potentially toxic (halothane) or pharmacologically active (morphine). For example:

> Propofol is highly protein bound (98%) and has a large volume of distribution (4 L kg^{-1}). Distribution half-life is 1–2 minutes and elimination half-life 5–12 hours. Metabolism is mainly hepatic with the production of inactive metabolites and conjugates which are excreted in urine.

Miscellaneous

For completeness it is worth citing information that is of specific relevance to anaesthetic practice. For example:

> Propofol is not a trigger for malignant hyperpyrexia and it may also be used safely in patients with porphyria. It does not release histamine and adverse reactions are very rare.

Oral questions

This book is primarily about the short written answer section of the examination. It is worth remembering, however, that many of these topics may also appear in the oral parts of the examination. The clinically orientated questions may form part of the second half of the morning vivas, while some of the anatomy, measurement and pharmacology questions may arise in the afternoon science vivas. The information that is presented in these outline answers would be sufficient in most instances to get you through. On average you will have about 7 minutes on the topic. Should a question have somewhat limited scope you may spend only 5 minutes or so discussing it before moving on for the final 10 minutes to a more substantial subject. The vivas are structured and the examiners have no choice of question. This does mean that they cannot be criticised as they sometimes have been in the past for examining in excessive depth on their own specialist subject. It does also mean, however, that they may be examining in a subject in which they do not even have a current generalist interest. A paediatric cardiac anaesthetist may find himself asking questions about chronic pain in adults, or a chronic pain specialist questions about the implications for the anaesthetists of congenital heart disease. That is not to imply that examiners are ignorant on these topics, but it may be that your clinical experience is more recent than theirs, and you should let that give you confidence. If you have recently seen an innovative technique used in a pain clinic or in intensive care then cite it in discussion. It will give you credibility and if you are very lucky it may dent theirs. You should recognise, however, that you will have little scope for manipulating the viva. Some candidates try to divert the questioning towards an area that they have prepared, such as the 'pressor response to laryngoscopy and intubation', and try to use up time by embarking on a mini lecture on the topic. It will not work. The examiners are following a script, albeit loosely, which relates to the structured question in hand and they will not allow you your excursion. You will, however, be able to use some of your own responses, structured along the lines suggested above. Start the answer with a capable definition, use a logical and ordered approach, and have confidence in your clinical experience.

General anaesthesia

An adult Jehovah's witness requires surgery during which significant blood loss is probable. Describe your management.

This is a not uncommon problem which influences preoperative preparation, requires some modification of anaesthetic management and includes an ethical dimension. This situation can be far from easy and the question seeks both a mature overview and a rational anaesthetic plan.

Introduction
Jehovah's Witnesses, of whom there are an estimated 150 000 in the UK, interpret the scriptures in a literal way, which means that they extrapolate to blood transfusion the biblical prohibition about eating blood. Perioperative management requires elucidation of their precise beliefs before introduction of the various options for optimising their surgical outcome.

Religious beliefs
- Witnesses have a range of attitudes. The strictest individuals will accept neither blood, blood products, platelets, albumin, immunoglobulins nor clotting factors. They will not accept autologous transfusion (because the blood has lost contact with the body), nor cell savers, but may accept cardiopulmonary bypass.
- The anaesthetist must establish precisely what is acceptable to the patient and must treat accordingly. The patient has the absolute right as an adult to refuse treatment. If the anaesthetist finds the demands difficult then the patient should be referred on to other colleagues as appropriate.

Preoperative assessment
- Management will depend on the patient's condition:
  - Check haemoglobin and optimise if necessary: haematinics, stop NSAIDs (non-steroidal anti-inflammatory drugs) (occult bleeding and antiplatelet action), consider recombinant erythropoietin (increases PCV (packed cell volume) by 2% daily).

Operative management
- Goal is to minimise blood loss while maintaining tissue oxygenation:
  - Regional anaesthesia where appropriate.
  - Careful positioning to reduce venous pressure.

— Scrupulous surgical technique.
— Hypotensive anaesthesia (some dispute its value).
— Hypothermic anaesthesia (reduces oxygen consumption).
— Haemodilution so that net volume of blood lost is reduced.
— Drugs: desmopressin (increases Factor VIII), tranexamic acid (inhibits plasminogen activation and fibrinolysis), ethamsylate (reduces capillary bleeding), aprotinin (inhibits the fibrinolysis).

Postoperative care
- Goals are to maximise oxygen delivery, minimise oxygen consumption and minimise continued blood loss: in the worst case scenario this may entail:
  — ITU admission: IPPV with 100% (+/– hyperbaric oxygen in extremis); sedation, analgesia.
  — Hypothermia (moderate) plus neuromuscular blockade.
  — Pre- and perioperative drug therapy as above to continue.

Marking points: Potentially this is a large subject. Main points should include full discussion with the patient and their right to refuse treatment, together with a sensible account of how to optimise their condition in the perioperative period.

For what reasons should general anaesthesia for elective cases be postponed?

Preoperative assessment is fundamental to anaesthetic practice. In the face of pressure to proceed with surgical cases anaesthetists must stand firm as advocates of patient safety.

Introduction

All anaesthesia and surgery poses some risk and the decision to proceed with either rests on a risk–benefit analysis, albeit crude. The overriding criterion for the decision whether to proceed should be whether the patient's condition could in any way be improved. If the patient is not in optimal condition then ideally surgery should be deferred. Some of the more significant causes are outlined below.

Cardiovascular

- Recent myocardial infarction (depends on timing and the nature of the surgery).
- Ischaemic heart disease causing crescendo or unstable angina pectoris.
- Heart failure: one of the single most important risk factors for anaesthesia (Goldman).
- Untreated or inadequately treated hypertension. Systolic hypertension is as important as diastolic.
- Uncontrolled cardiac arrhythmia – commonly fast atrial fibrillation.
- Anaemia. Depends on level of anaemia and proposed surgery – but the ideal would be to restore haemoglobin to normal levels before proceeding.

Respiratory

- Acute chest infection or upper respiratory tract infection. Recent coryza may deter some anaesthetists. Some recommend deferring paediatric elective surgery for 4–6 weeks. Others believe this to be impractical.
- Inadequately treated asthma or other chronic airways disease.

Gastrointestinal

- Acute disorder not related to the surgery.

Systemic and metabolic

- Acute or recent viraemia (risk of myocarditis).
- Serious electrolyte abnormality, particularly hyper- or hypokalaemia.

Investigations

- Inadequate for the clinical history – e.g. ECG and CXR in appropriate patients.

Preoperative preparation

- Adequate fasting (protocols vary between hospitals), appropriate bowel preparation, appropriate antacid, e.g. elective caesarean section.
- Morbid obesity: the patient is twice as likely to die after surgery (of any type) than a patient of normal weight. It may not be realistic, however, to insist on significant weight loss before elective surgery.
- Smoking: smokers may fare worse postoperatively than non-smokers. It may, however, be unrealistic to expect patients to make major lifestyle changes immediately before surgery.

Marking points: This is a core area of anaesthetic practice and would be marked accordingly.

What are the causes and management of hypoventilation immediately following anaesthesia?

Postoperative respiratory insufficiency is an important complication of anaesthesia (and surgery) which all anaesthetists should be able to recognise, to diagnose and to treat.

Introduction

Hypoventilation may be defined, strictly, as the inability of a patient to maintain respiration adequate to eliminate carbon dioxide. It may be an acute problem or a pre-existing medical problem which is exacerbated by the effects of anaesthesia and surgery.

- **Pre-morbid state.** Pre-existing conditions which increase the likelihood of postoperative hypoventilation include: chronic respiratory disease, particularly COPD (Chronic obstructive pulmonary disease); neurological disorders such as motor neurone disease, autonomic neuropathies (e.g. Shy–Drager syndrome), morbid obesity, muscular dystrophy, myasthenia, myotonic syndromes, hypothyroidism, raised intracranial pressure. These and other conditions are rare, but collectively there are many.
- **Anaesthetic drugs.** Benzodiazepine and other anxiolytics, induction agents, opioid analgesics, volatile anaesthetic agents and nitrous oxide are all respiratory depressants whose effects may persist into the postoperative period.
- **Neuromuscular blocking drugs.** Incomplete reversal of action or enzyme deficiency (suxamethonium and mivacurium).
- **Hypercarbia.** At a $P_a\text{CO}_2$ greater than ~12 kPa CO_2 narcosis may supervene. Clinical signs of CO_2 retention (sympathetic stimulation) may not always be apparent. It is caused by and is also a cause of hypoventilation.
- **Hypocarbia.** Anaesthetic drugs raise the threshold of sensitivity to CO_2 and over-ventilation may suppress the stimulus to breathe.
- **Airway obstruction.**
- **Pain.** Restriction of adequate respiratory excursion due to the pain, e.g. of an upper abdominal incision.
- **Circulatory inadequacy.** Cardiovascular insufficiency. Shock.

Management

- **Airway:** relieve obstruction if any.
- **Breathing:** ventilation of lungs (remember that CO_2 elimination is the main priority; oxygenation commonly is not a problem).
- **Circulation:** assessment and maintenance as appropriate.
- **Diagnosis.**
- **Eliminate cause** (if possible): supportive therapy meanwhile.

> **Marking points:** This is a question about routine anaesthetic practice and all the common causes should be mentioned, as well as the first line management.

What are the problems of anaesthetising patients in the magnetic resonance imaging unit?

General anaesthesia within an MRI scanner should be avoided wherever possible, but there are always patients, particularly children, in whom there is no choice. The consequences of ignorance are more likely to be disastrous than in the CT (Computerised tomography) scanner or in X-ray and so knowledge of this area is important.

Introduction

Magnetic resonance imaging is an investigation which complements computerised tomography in providing high quality images of soft tissue. The technique is based on the principle that when a cell nucleus with an unpaired proton is exposed to an electromagnetic field it becomes aligned along the axis of that field. When the electromagnetic field is removed the nucleus resumes its original position and as it does so it emits low radiofrequency radiation. MRI requires the generation of very strong magnetic fields (typically 1.5 Tesla) and it is these which present the main problems for the anaesthetist.

- **Generic problems.** There are the generic problems of anaesthetising patients in remote, unfamiliar and isolated areas. Patients commonly are children.
- **Practical problems.** There are practical difficulties in relation to the physical environment. The patient is enclosed within a narrow tube to which access is limited. The scanner is noisy and some patients may be very claustrophobic. Scanning may be prolonged.
- **Magnetic field.** All ferromagnetic items within the 50 Gauss line will be subject to movement and will also interfere with the generated image. Items typically affected include needles, watches, pagers, stethoscopes, anaesthetic gas cylinders, ECG electrodes. If these items are close to the field they will become projectile objects.
- **Anaesthesia delivery.** Anaesthetic machines which contain ferrous metals (there are some non-magnetic machines and cylinders available) must remain outside the 50 Gauss line. The machine requires very long anaesthetic tubing and long leads.
- **Infusion pumps.** May fail if the field strength exceeds 100 Gauss.
- **Monitoring.** The field may induce current within electric cabling. The consequent heating may lead to thermal injury. Long sampling leads for gas analysis extends delay. Standard ECG electrodes cannot be used.
- **Pacemakers.** Cardiac pacemakers require special consideration as they will malfunction in fields over 5 Gauss.
- **Implants and foreign bodies.** Most patient implants (metal prostheses, etc.) are non-ferrous, although some surgical clips and wires may be magnetic. Metal foreign bodies are likely to be ferrous.

Marking points: Safe anaesthesia for MR (magnetic) scanning requires scrupulous attention to detail and some detailed knowledge of the force fields and their effects. Your answer should make clear that you cannot be too thorough.

What are the problems of monitoring patients in the magnetic resonance imaging unit?

This is a more focused question which deals with monitoring rather than anaesthetising patients within an MRI scanner. As in the previous question knowledge of this area is important because the consequences of ignorance are more likely to be disastrous than in the CT scanner or in X-ray.

Introduction

Magnetic resonance imaging is an investigation which complements computerised tomography in providing high quality images of soft tissue. The technique is based on the principle that when a cell nucleus with an unpaired proton is exposed to an electromagnetic field it becomes aligned along the axis of that field. When the electromagnetic field is removed the nucleus resumes its original position and as it does so it emits low radiofrequency radiation. MRI requires the generation of very strong magnetic fields (typically 1.5 Tesla) and it is these which present the main problems for the anaesthetist who is monitoring a patient within the scanning tube.

- **Practical problems.** There are practical difficulties which relate to the physical environment. The patient is enclosed within a narrow tube to which access is limited. The scanner is noisy and so respiratory noises and alarm signals may not be audible.
- **Magnetic field.** All ferromagnetic items within the 50 Gauss line will be subject to movement. Monitoring items typically affected include stethoscopes and ECG electrodes. If these items are close to the field they will become projectile objects.
- **Current induction.** The field may induce current within electric cabling. The consequent heating may lead to thermal injury. Long sampling leads for gas analysis extends delay. Standard ECG electrodes cannot be used. An oesophageal stethoscope is useful.
- Dedicated non-magnetic equipment is now available in some units. If it is not available then precautions should be taken as follows:
  - **Pulse oximetry.** Probes are non-ferrous but a distal site should be used and cable should be insulated.
  - **Blood pressure.** Direct intra-arterial measurement is suitable from a distal site such as the dorsalis pedis or posterior tibial arteries. Non-invasive cuffs must have plastic connections as well as long leads to the machines which must be outside the 50 Gauss line.
  - **ECG.** Only non-ferrous electrodes can be used.
  - **Gas analysis.** Main problem is with the delayed sampling time due to long tubing.
  - **Airways pressures, respiratory indices.** Usually displayed at the anaesthetic machine. Again the problems are those associated with long anaesthetic tubing.

Marking points: Safe anaesthesia, which includes monitoring, for MR scanning requires scrupulous attention to detail. Your answer should make this clear.

How may coagulation be assessed in the perioperative period?

This question aims to examine your understanding of the available tests. The topic is important both in the context of acute derangement and also for the many patients who are taking aspirin or who present for surgery while receiving anticoagulant medication.

Introduction

Disorders of coagulation, both congenital and acquired, are important for the anaesthetist not only because of their consequences for surgery, but also because of their impact on anaesthetic techniques, particularly neuraxial blockade. Assessment of coagulation is usually made by laboratory tests, although there are some simple indicators which can be helpful. Primary haemostasis results from platelet aggregation. Coagulation factors; intrinsic (which circulate within the intravascular compartment) and extrinsic (which are found in tissues), act to stabilise the clot. Tests of coagulation look at all these areas.

- **Clinical history.** May be useful if patient describes prolonged bleeding, e.g. after dental extractions, or easy or spontaneous bruising. Family history is of obvious importance.
- **Platelet numbers.** A platelet count is simple and reliable if it is low. A normal count does not exclude abnormalities of platelet function; tests for which are not readily available.
- **Thromboelastography.** Gives information about the speed of formation and the quality of a clot.
- **Bleeding time (BT).** Unhelpful. Even when the performance of the test is standardised, there is a wide normal range. A normal BT does not exclude potential problems, nor an abnormal one predict them.
- **Whole blood clotting.** Clinical observation in theatre can confirm that a patient is oozing abnormally or that blood appears to be clotting. A sample can be placed in a plain glass tube and observed to see whether or not it clots.
- **Prothrombin time (PT).** Assesses the extrinsic coagulation pathway.
- **Activated partial thromboplastin time (APTT).** Assesses the intrinsic pathway.
- **Activated clotting time (ACT).** Most commonly used in cardiopulmonary bypass to assess the effects of complete anticoagulation with heparin and its reversal by protamine.
- **Blood haemoglobin photometer** ('Hemocue'). Very useful for rapid ward/theatre estimation.
- **Fibrinogen.** Depleted fibrinogen occurs, e.g. during massive transfusion.

Marking points: Examiners expect the standard list of laboratory tests, but also want to see a commonsense clinical approach and a balanced view of an important problem.

What causes bradycardia during general anaesthesia? What is its management?

This is a common perioperative problem, the management of which should be routine.

Introduction

In an adult patient and in older children a bradycardia is usually defined as a pulse rate of less than 60 beats per minute. In young children the threshold rate is higher: 100 per minute in neonates and 80 per minute in infants.

Causes

- **Hypoxia.** The most important cause. A bradycardia may be a late, if not preterminal sign, but hypoxia must be the first factor to be considered.
- **Vagally mediated.** Common stimuli include traction on extraocular muscles, anal or cervical dilatation, visceral traction, and sometimes, instrumentation of the airway.
- **Drug induced.** Pre-existing medication may contribute, e.g. beta-adrenoceptor blockers and digoxin, as may drugs used by the anaesthetist: volatile agents in high concentrations, or halothane in normal concentrations, suxamethonium, opioids, anticholinesterases. Low doses of atropine may provoke a paradoxical bradycardia (the Bezold–Jarisch reflex).
- **Cardiac disease.** Most commonly ischaemic change which affects the conducting system.
- **Cardiovascular fitness.** Highly trained athletic individuals have both a greater stroke volume and a higher degree of resting vagal tone.
- **Endocrine disease.** Typically hypothyroidism.
- **Metabolic.** Hyperkalaemia.
- **Spinal anaesthesia** which affects the cardiac accelerator fibres from T1 to T4. Theoretically. Many anaesthetists who are very experienced in spinal anaesthesia do not believe that this occurs very often in practice.
- **Neurological.** Raised intracranial pressure.

Management

- First of all diagnose the cause, and if it is amenable to treatment then act accordingly. Is it hypoxia? Treat immediately. Is it surgical stimulus? If so then stop traction on the extraocular muscles or the mesentery.
- Is it compromising the circulation? If blood pressure and oxygenation are being maintained then treatment may not immediately be necessary.
- If treatment is required the most effective immediate first line drug is an anticholinergic agent; atropine, hyoscine, glycopyrrolate. Atropine works quickest. Atopine is not a treatment for hypoxia.

Marking points: Candidates must emphasise that the most important, although by no means the commonest, cause is hypoxia. A reasoned response to the problem rather than simply the reflex use of atropine will give your answer, and your clinical practice, more credibility.

An adult patient develops tachycardia during general anaesthesia. Outline the causes and briefly note your management.

This is another common perioperative problem, the management of which should be routine.

Introduction

In an adult patient a tachycardia is usually defined as a pulse rate of greater than 100 beats per minute. It may be primary or compensatory and so there are a large number of potential causes, the broad classes of which are outlined below. Diagnosis will depend on the clinical context.

Causes and management

- **Inadequate anaesthesia:** there may be other clinical signs such as hypertension; reactive pupils; sweating; movement; lachrymation. It is treated by deepening anaesthesia as appropriate.
- **Inadequate muscle relaxation.** Similar to the first point, but an anaesthetised patient who is breathing against a ventilator may develop a tachycardia. Treat by giving a further dose. Muscle relaxant drugs are not anaesthetics, but they do cause some deafferentation and reduce input to the reticular activating system.
- **Inadequate analgesia:** this may also manifest as signs of sympathetic overactivity as above. The most appopriate management is to give further analgesia. Anaesthesia may also be deepened.
- **Hypovolaemia:** actual (fluid loss) or effective (vasodilatation). Replace fluid. If this is due to pharmacological vasodilatation then it is preferable to treat with a vasopressor. (Alpha$_1$ agonists are more immediately effective than ephedrine.)
- **Hypercarbia.** Is this a manifestation of malignant hyperpyrexia? Almost certainly not, but the question should be asked. Check CO_2 absorber. Increase minute ventilation if appropriate.
- **Hypoxia.** (The initial response is tachycardia.) Seek the cause and treat immediately.
- **Sepsis.** Clinical context will indicate whether this is likely (e.g. laparotomy for intestinal perforation). Will need full supportive therapy after immediate resuscitation.
- **Cardiac arrhythmia.** SVT or VT (Ventricular). May be primary or secondary. May need synchronised DC shock if hypotensive. Other measures include drugs: e.g. adenosine for SVT, verapamil, amiodarone, digoxin as appropriate. Carotid sinus massage may abort an SVT.
- **Drugs:** e.g. anticholinergic drugs, catecholamines, oxytocin.
- **Endocrine problems:** phaeochromocytoma, thyroid storm. The management of such problems is complex, but will include beta-adrenoceptor blockers.
- **Malignant hyperpyrexia.** Initiate immediate management according to standard guidelines.

Marking points: This is a common occurrence in anaesthesia and the account should incorporate all of the major factors which may lead to a tachycardia.

How would you determine the causes of arterial hypotension (80/60 mmHg) during a transurethral prostatectomy (TURP)?

The operation of TURP (Trans-urethral resection of prostate) has been chosen because of the additional diagnostic problems that it poses. A logical approach that is based on first principles and which incorporates those particular problems is an impressive way to deal with the question.

Introduction

Arterial hypotension during TURP has several causes, diagnosis of which is best based upon a logical approach to the prime determinants of systemic blood pressure. Blood pressure is a function of cardiac output (itself determined by the product of heart rate and stroke volume) × systemic vascular resistance. Anaesthesia for and the operation of TURP can influence several parts of this equation.

Generic causes

- **Regional anaesthesia.** Subarachnoid block (SAB), extradural block and sacral extradural (caudal) block for supplementary analgesia are all used for TURP. All (caudal less so) may drop blood pressure by sympathetic blockade and vasodilatation.
- **General anaesthesia.** Excessive depth of anaesthesia, or hypocapnia due to overventilation may decrease cardiac output.
- **Co-morbidity** in an elderly male population. Ischaemic heart disease and hypertension.

Specific causes

- **Blood loss** associated with TURP. Estimates place this at between 10 and 20 ml per gram of prostate resected. This is hard to assess prospectively, but may help assessment of blood loss retrospectively. Blood loss is difficult to quantify accurately: it requires collection of all fluids (large volumes) into a single container and a photocolorimetric assessment. Concerns about blood-borne diseases make theatre staff reluctant to handle large volumes of fluids in this way.
- **Bradycardia.** May be associated with distension of the bladder. May also follow bladder rupture with intra-abdominal leakage of fluid.
- **Cardiac failure** associated with fluid overload. Irrigation fluid in a bag 1 m above the patient may infuse into venous sinuses in the prostatic bed at a rate of at least 20 ml min^{-1}. (Some studies have identified absorption rates much higher: at >80 ml min^{-1}).
- **TUR syndrome.** More commonly this fluid (usually glycine 1.5%) will lead to the TUR syndrome. Characteristic features include hypotension and bradycardia, cerebral oedema leading to confusion, and convulsions due to hyponatraemia.

Marking points: This question asks for an overview of possible causes. It does expect mention of the factors specific to TURP (occult blood loss, fluid overload and the TUR syndrome) but do not assume that it expects a detailed account of the latter.

What methods are available for the prevention of venous thromboembolism in routine surgical practice? Which patients are at particular risk?

This is an important problem which some authorities claim is responsible for 10% of hospital deaths. Although anaesthetists do not always get involved in initiating prophylaxis, they should be aware of both risk factors and prevention.

Introduction

Pulmonary thromboembolism caused by deep venous thrombosis is an important cause of mortality in hospital patients. Many of these deaths are preventable, and all patients at risk should be assessed for one or more of the methods of prophylaxis which are outlined below.

- **Physical methods** (simple and safe; limited efficacy in high risk cases)
  — Early mobilisation.
  — Physiotherapy (encourages mobilisation).
  — Graduated compression (TED) stockings.
- **Complex physical methods**
  — Intermittent pneumatic compression boots (e.g. 'Flotron'): should be started before surgery (thrombus may start to form as soon as the calf is immobile against an operating table) and continue for at least 16 hours thereafter.
  — Foot pumps: aim to mimic action of muscle pump of lower leg.
- **Pharmacological methods**
  — Heparin: unfractionated, low dose (5000 units sc) started before surgery and continued 8–12 hourly until discharge (longer in high risk patients).
  — Heparin: low molecular weight, e.g. enoxaparin, dalteparin or tinzaparin. Longer duration of action and once daily dose.
  — Warfarin: usually long-term administration in high risk non-surgical patient.
  — Dextran 70: some evidence of benefit, but its use goes in and out of fashion.
  — Cyclo-oxygenase inhibitors: aspirin and NSAIDs – usually coincidental treatment rather than deliberate prescribing preoperatively.
- **Anaesthetic technique**
  — Regional anaesthesia (central neuraxial): reduces DVT (deep venous thrombosis) risk by increasing lower limb blood flow.

Risk factors

- **Patient factors: congenital**
  — Hypercoagulable states: antithrombin III deficiency, protein C and protein S deficiency, antiphospholipid syndrome (especially in pregnancy), thrombophilia, Factor V Leiden mutation and other syndromes (very rare).
- **Patient factors: acquired**
  — History of previous DVT or PE (Pulmonary embolus), family history.
  — Obesity.
  — Age >60.
  — Drugs: oestrogen oral contraceptives.
  — Immobility.
  — Pelvic and lower limb surgery.
  — Prolonged surgery.
  — Burns.
  — Inflammatory bowel disease.
  — Varicose veins.
  — Malignancy.

Marking points: This is a common and important clinical problem to which the anaesthetist can make a contribution. This question tests whether or not this is clear to the candidate.

What factors are associated with perioperative myocardial infarction?

Ischaemic heart disease is pandemic in the developed world and an understanding of its significance in the perioperative period is essential for all anaesthetists.

Introduction

Up to a third of all deaths in the UK are caused by ischaemic heart disease, and given that anaesthesia and surgery may have profound effects on the cardiovascular system, anaesthetists have to be aware of the key risk factors for myocardial infarction in the perioperative period.

- **Myocardial oxygen supply and demand**
  - If demand exceeds supply myocardial ischaemia will result.
  - Prime determinants of demand include: systolic wall tension (systolic BP, afterload; LVEDP (Left ventricular end-diastolic pressure), preload; ventricular volume), contractility, heart rate.
  - Prime determinants of supply include: coronary artery patency, oxygenation, effective cardiac output (adequate blood volume; normal heart rate to allow diastolic perfusion and ventricular filling; good contractile state).
  - HR and LVEDP are important: affect demand and supply simultaneously – as both rise so demand increases and supply decreases.

These factors allow a summary of the main risks:

- **Patients who have cardiac risk factors in general, in which some of the determinants above are already affected (mainly coronary artery patency)**
  - Increasing age: about 20% of patients >60 years will have coronary artery disease.
  - Gender: males have 2× the chance of having ischaemic heart disease (IHD) at 65 years than females.
  - Family history: first degree male relatives of those with fatal myocardial infarction (MI) have 5× the risk.
  - Smoking: risk at least 2×.
  - Hypercholesterolaemia and hyperlipidaemia: risk increases at least 10×.
  - Diabetes mellitus: risk at least 2×.
  - Hypertension: systolic hypertension increases risk 5×.
  - Combined factors increase the risk several fold.
- **Specific risk factors (supply and demand factors)**
  - Previous MI, and particularly a recent MI. Incidence in patients with no prior history is ~0.66%. Previous MI ~4–6%. MI within 3–6 months >50% (depends on site of surgery).
  - Aggressive intervention with invasive monitoring and inotropes/vasodilators may decrease reinfarction rate substantially. Not yet proven and is resource intensive.
  - Heart failure: single most important risk factor.
  - Valvular lesions: e.g. aortic stenosis.
  - Hypertension: particularly if poorly controlled.
- **Perioperative factors (supply and demand factors)**
  - Hypertension: e.g. due to pain, hypercarbia, inadequate anaesthesia.
  - Prolonged tachycardia.
  - Hypotension: due to fluid loss and / or anaesthesia.
  - Excessive use of vasopressors/catecholamines.
  - Site of surgery: thoracic and upper abdominal operations are worse than others in this respect.
  - Hypothermia; hypoxia; hypercarbia and acidosis.

Marking points: There is potentially a lot of information to convey in this answer. The best approach, therefore, is to develop your answer from first principles using examples as appropriate.

—What is the role of the laryngeal mask in difficult intubation?

This is a question about a highly specific use for the laryngeal mask airway (LMA) which does not require a very long answer, but which aims to see if the candidate has a clear strategy under these circumstances.

Introduction

The LMA has in many ways revolutionised the management of the normal airway. Interest in the device has now extended to its use in resuscitation and for some time now an LMA has been found in most difficult intubation boxes. It has a role both in unexpected and in anticipated difficult intubation.

Unexpected difficult intubation.

- In cases in which intubation is not essential (fasted patient, elective surgery, IPPV with airways pressures 18–20 cmH$_2$0) surgery can proceed using the LMA.
- It can be used for airway rescue in the presence of applied cricoid pressure, and there are several case reports detailing success in failed obstetric intubation.
- The LMA can be used to guide a gum elastic bougie through the cords.
- It can be used to guide a size 6.0 endotracheal tube through the cords.
- It can also be used to guide a fibreoptic bronchoscope through the cords. This will have to have been loaded with a lubricated endotracheal tube (ETT), and the LMA kept in place.
- Leaving the LMA in place provides a means of maintaining the airway following extubation.

Anticipated difficult intubation

- In most patients in whom difficult intubation is certain (previous history, ankylosing spondylitis, anatomical deformity, etc.) the management of choice is awake fibreoptic intubation.
- The LMA can itself be inserted in an awake patient in whom the airway has been anaesthetised prior to its use as a guide to fibreoptic intubation, or as an aid to oral intubation.
- In patients in whom the degree of difficulty is less certain, any of the options discussed above can be employed.
- Other alternatives include the use of the intubating laryngeal mask.

> **Marking points:** Be careful not to stray from the boundaries of this very circumscribed question which seeks an orderly and logical approach to an important problem.

What problems does morbid obesity present to the anaesthetist?

This topic is a perennial favourite both in the written part of the exam and in the orals. There is potentially a lot to cover in the time available.

Introduction

Morbid obesity is defined usually by the body mass index (BMI) which is determined by the weight (kg) divided by the square of the height (m^2). A patient is morbidly obese when their BMI exceeds 35. The morbidly obese individual has only a 1 in 7 chance of reaching a normal life expectancy and their mortality for all forms of surgery is twice that of the non-obese population.

- Cardiovascular problems
    - Hypertension (50–60%, severe in 5–10%).
    - Increased blood volume and increased cardiac work.
    - Increased incidence of coronary artery disease and cardiomyopathy.
    - Increased risk (2×) of deep venous thrombosis and pulmonary embolus.
    - Less water per unit of body weight. Tolerate hypovolaemia badly. Tolerate changes of position badly.
- Respiratory problems
    - Difficult intubation.
    - Increased work of breathing due to mass effect of chest weight.
    - Spontaneous respiration restricted, diaphragmatic splinting.
    - Hypoventilation, reduced FRC (functional residual capacity), reduced lung volumes, pulmonary 'shunting', hypercapnia, hypoxia (perioperative), slow equilibration with inhaled anaesthetics.
    - Obstructive sleep apnoea (5%).
    - Extreme cases may manifest as the 'Pickwickian syndrome' – obesity, somnolence, polycythaemia, pulmonary hypertension and right heart failure.
- Gastrointestinal system problems
    - Prone to cholelithiasis, hiatus hernia, reflux and pulmonary aspiration.
- Endocrine problems
    - Increased likelihood of diabetes mellitus (5×), plasma insulin levels increase but binding to cell receptors decreases (insulin resistance).
- Metabolic problems
    - Is there an underlying cause, particularly hypothyroidism?
- Miscellaneous physical and technical problems
    - These patients are difficult to move, to lift and to nurse, venepuncture is difficult, estimation of drug dosage is problematic, non-invasive arterial pressure monitoring may be inaccurate, regional and local blocks are technically difficult, surgery is usually more prolonged.

Marking points: This is a large question and you will not have time to address all the potential problems in 15 minutes. You must, however, address those areas where safety is crucial: the risk of regurgitation and aspiration, respiratory problems and DVT prophylaxis.

Outline the methods for detecting awareness during general anaesthesia and give a brief account of their effectiveness

Few of these methods are available widely in clinical practice, but this is such an important area of anaesthetic practice that some knowledge of these research tools is expected.

Introduction

Unplanned awareness during general anaesthesia is a very serious complication of anaesthetic practice and much research effort has been devoted to the search for a practical and reliable method of detection. Most of those methods which do show promise are available only as research tools.

- In the spontaneously breathing patient who is not paralysed, awareness may be manifest by purposeful movement. Movement is a reliable indicator of light anaesthesia although a patient may have no recall.
- Frontalis (scalp) electromyogram (EMG): amplitude of the EMG decreases with increasing depth of anaesthesia, but this cannot be used in the paralysed patient.
- In the patient who is paralysed and ventilated: clinical signs of sympathetic overactivity – tachycardia, hypertension, diaphoresis and lachrymation. In the absence of other causes these may be reliable if present, but their absence does not exclude awareness.
- Isolated forearm technique (originally described by Tunstall in obstetric anaesthesia): effective (for first 20 minutes until ischaemic paralysis supervenes) but requires considerable cooperation by the patient and is not a practical technique for widespread use.
- Oesophageal contractility: amplitude and frequency of contractions of lower oesophageal smooth muscle reduce with increasing depth of anaesthesia. Limited value because of high rate of false positive/negative results. No longer commercially available.
- Sinus arrhythmia or R–R interval variation: useful, but depends on intact autonomic nervous system and healthy myocardial conducting system. Problems with for example beta-blockers, autonomic neuropathy, sepsis, conduction abnormalities.
- Fathom. Uses high resolution EEG plus an indication of the respiratory cycle. Is claimed to indicate the level of vagal efferent activity from the medulla oblongata.
- Evoked potentials: visual and auditory evoked potentials are effective but are technically demanding.
- EEG: effective but technically demanding and not practical for routine general anaesthesia.
- Cerebral function analysing monitor (CFAM): processed and simplified EEG, technically easier but has slow response time.
- Bispectral index: probably the most effective method currently available and works by comparing frequency harmonics in the frontal EEG. Rapid response and accurate. Not widely available.

> **Marking points:** Candidates will not fail because they do not mention all of the research methods, although the well-informed candidate will know of most of them. A candidate must emphasise both the importance and pitfalls of clinical monitoring.

What are the causes of awareness under general anaesthesia?

Insensibility, i.e a complete lack of awareness, is the raison d'etre of anaesthesia, and a patient who suffers unplanned awareness under anaesthesia has been failed by the specialty. Every anaesthetist, therefore, from the start of training, should know how to reduce to a minimum the risk of this happening.

Introduction

Anaesthesia exists to provide controlled insensibility. Anaesthetic awareness as a result of the failure so to do can range from vague recollection without pain to complete recall with severe pain, but the entire spectrum of awareness represents a major complication of anaesthetic practice. Its causes lie in equipment and its use; in pharmacology and its application and, very rarely, in the physiology of patients.

- **Equipment and apparatus.** Awareness may result from a failure of the apparatus to deliver adequate concentrations of anaesthetic agent. The anaesthetic machine must deliver an accurate fresh gas flow via an appropriate breathing system, using a vaporiser. Alternatively if total intravenous anaesthesia (TIVA) is being used an accurate syringe driver is required, together with a reliable system of infusion tubing. Awareness may result if there are failures in any part of these systems. These would include leaks, faulty or empty vaporisers, a misconnected or disconnected breathing system, inaccurate pumps and occluded infusion tubing.
- **Equipment and apparatus.** Awareness may result from a failure of the anaesthetist to use the equipment properly. Circle systems can present a particular difficulty.
- **Monitoring.** Failure to monitor the concentrations of inspired and expired volatile agent may result in inadequate anaesthetic agent being delivered. TIVA is more difficult to monitor in this regard.
- **Pharmacology.** Awareness, by definition, results from inadequate anaesthesia. The dose of induction agent may have been inadequate, as may be the alveolar concentration (it is important to remember that the minimum alveolar concentration (MAC) value that is quoted is only the MAC^{50}) or the computed blood concentration in target controlled infusion (TCI).
- **Pharmacology.** Awareness is not prevented by hyperventilation, by the use of nitrous oxide and oxygen alone, or by the use of opioids. Muscle relaxants drugs are not anaesthetics: anaesthesia must not be discontinued until their effects have been reversed.
- **Physiology.** Vanishingly rarely a patient may be 'resistant' to anaesthetic agents. Alcohol and other drugs of abuse are convenient scapegoats but the evidence is unconvincing. Similarly high anxiety is frequently cited as the reason why some patients may need higher than normal induction doses. Either way the anaesthetist should be alert to the clinical signs indicative of inadequate anaesthesia.
- **Physiology.** On occasion a patient may be so moribund (or so inadequately resuscitated) that adequate anaesthesia may be incompatible with maintaining cardiac function.
- **Anatomy.** During a difficult intubation the induction agent may wear off before the effects of the muscle relaxant.

Marking points: This is a core topic and most of the causes listed above would be expected.

What do you understand by the 'stress response' to surgery? Outline briefly the effects of anaesthesia on this response

The stress response to injury is a topic of perennial interest. Clinicians do not agree whether or not it is desirable to abolish it, but considerable research effort has been expended in studying the attenuating effects of general and regional anaesthesia.

Introduction

The 'stress response' is the term used to describe the widespread metabolic and hormonal changes which occur in response to trauma, including surgical trauma. It is a natural response whose net effect is to increase catabolism and release endogenous fuel stores.

Endocrine response

- **Autonomic nervous system: sympathoadrenal response**
  — Mediated via hypothalamus.
  — Increased medullary catecholamines.
  — Increased presynaptic norepinephrine (noradrenaline) release.
  — Predictable cardiovascular stimulation.
  — Modification of visceral function (renal and hepatic).
  — Renin–angiotensin system stimulates aldosterone release: Na^+ and H_2O retention.
- **Hypothalamic–pituitary–adrenal axis**
  — Hypothalamic releasing factors stimulate anterior pituitary.
  — There are increases in: ACTH (Adrenocorticotrophic hormone) (stimulates adrenal glucocorticoid release); somatotrophin (growth hormone: stimulates protein synthesis and inhibits breakdown, stimulates lipolysis, antagonises insulin) and prolactin (?Why - as it has little effect).
  — Other anterior pituitary hormones, including thyroid hormone, change little.
  — Posterior pituitary produces arginine vasopressin (antidiuretic).
- **Cortisol**
  — Release from adrenal cortex after stimulation by ACTH (may increase 4×).
  — Catabolic: protein breakdown, gluconeogenesis, inhibition of glucose uilisation, lipolysis.
  — Anti-inflammatory: inhibits leucocyte migration into damaged areas; inhibits synthesis of inflammatory mediators such as prostaglandins.
- **Insulin**
  — Main anabolic hormone: relative lack perioperatively; fails to match catabolic effects.
- **Inflammatory response**
  — Release of cytokines (interleukins, tumour necrosis factor and interferons) and development of 'acute phase response'.

Modification of the response by anaesthesia

- The net effect is catabolism (to provide endogenous fuel from carbohydrate, fat and protein) accompanied by sodium and water retention. In evolutionary terms this may have helped an animal to survive injury.
- Current thinking has it that the response is unnecessary in the context of modern anaesthesia and surgery: there is continued interest in attempting to ablate it.
- **Opioids**
  — Suppress hypothalamic and pituitary secretion. High dose opioids may attenuate the response substantially, but at the cost of profound sedation and respiratory depression.

- **Etomidate**
  - Inhibits the 11ß-hydroxylase step of steroid synthesis: cortisol and aldosterone production decreases. This drug is not used deliberately to attenuate the response.
- **Benzodiazepines**
  - Inhibit cortisol production (probably a central effect).
- **α_2-Agonists**
  - Reduce sympathoadrenal responses, indirectly decrease cortisol production.
- **Regional anaesthesia**
  - Source of much interest: extensive extradural block ablates the adrenocortical and glycaemic responses to surgery (difficult to achieve in upper GIT and thoracic surgery).
  - There is increasing acceptance of claim that targeted and sustained regional anaesthesia has beneficial effect on surgical outcome.

Marking points: There is a lot of potential detail in a topical question such as this, but much remains speculative and so the subject eludes focus. You will be able to give the impression of knowing sufficient about the topic if you have grasped the overall picture and can reproduce some of the key words.

Describe the diagnosis and management of local anaesthetic toxicity

The use of local anaesthetic drugs in regional anaesthesia and in peripheral nerve blocks is increasing as anaesthetists refine the management of postoperative pain. Fatal overdoses still occur and so the recognition and management of toxicity is an important safety issue.

Introduction

The interest in local anaesthetic drugs such as ropivacaine and levobupivacaine, which are claimed to be less toxic, demonstrates that dangerous overdose is of continued concern to anaesthetists. With one or two exceptions the features of toxicity are the same with all local anaesthetics, and can be related to their membrane-stabilising actions. They can be classified according to the systems involved, but because the effects occur simultaneously it is more logical to describe the clinical manifestations as blood levels increase.

Causes

- Local anaesthetic toxicity relates both to the absolute blood level and also to the rate of rise. It occurs after inadvertent intravascular injection, after premature release of the tourniquet in intravenous regional anaesthesia (IVRA), and after excessive doses have been used for infiltration.
- If the rate of rise is very rapid (e.g. after iv injection) then the first manifestations may be convulsions and / or cardiac arrest in ventricular fibrillation.

Clinical features

- Early symptoms: circumoral tingling and numbness, pallor, tinnitus. This is related to the rich blood supply and dense innervation of the face, mouth and tongue. It occurs at blood levels e.g. of lidocaine (lignocaine) of ~2–3 μg ml^{-1} and of bupivacaine of ~1.5–2.0 μg ml^{-1}.
- As levels increase: agitation, restlessness and anxiety. Twitching of limbs and excessive eye movements. Some patients may become drowsy (lidocaine has been used in status epilepticus). Unless the ECG is being monitored there are unlikely to be any cardiovascular signs or symptoms.
- At levels of ~12μg ml^{-1} (lidocaine) and 4.0 μg ml^{-1} (bupivacaine) patients will convulse. With lidocaine cardiac arrest is usually secondary to hypoxia following convulsions and coma, with decreased contractility and impaired conduction being contributory factors. Bupivacaine toxicity is associated with the sudden onset of refractory ventricular fibrillation, the drug binding avidly to myocardial Na$^+$ channels.

Management

There is no specific treatment for local anaesthetic toxicity: management is supportive.

- Airway; Breathing: Circulation: will need O$_2$, may require IPPV, small dose of anticonvulsant for fits (benzodiazepine or thiopental).
- Inotropes for circulatory failure, but beware arrhythmogenic potential of catecholamines.
- In cardiac arrest due to bupivacaine, bretylium is the anti-arrhythmic of choice: resuscitation will need to be prolonged.

Marking points: This is an important safety question and significant omissions would be marked severely.

Describe the complications associated with abdominal laparoscopy.

Laparoscopic surgery has evolved from relatively simple diagnostic and therapeutic gynaecological procedures to prolonged and complex intra-abdominal surgery. It is a common procedure of whose hazards all anaesthetists should be aware.

Introduction
The use of abdominal laparoscopy by general surgeons, by urologists and by gynaecologists is now commonplace. The procedure involves the blind insertion of at least two trocars, one to insufflate gas under pressure and the second to introduce the laparoscope. These contribute to a number of complications, the major ones of which are outlined below.

Trauma associated with the instruments
- **Puncture of a viscus.** At particular risk are a distended stomach (may be inflated if the patient has been ventilated vigorously prior to intubation) and bowel. The liver can be also be impaled.
- **Vascular trauma.** The great vessels, abdominal aorta and inferior vena cava can be damaged, as can mesenteric vessels. Bleeding is usually torrential requiring immediate laparotomy.

Problems associated with gas insufflation
- **Gas embolism.** May occur in about 1 in 2000 laparoscopies and is associated with high insufflation pressures (>~25 mmHg) or rarely, direct injection into a vessel. Will cause circulatory collapse. CO_2 is safer in this regard than the alternative gas N_2O which is less soluble and will remain within the circulation longer.
- **Impaired cardiac function.** At pressures of >20 mmHg preload and cardiac output decrease and SVR (systemic vascular resistance) rises. High and sustained insufflation pressures (>~30 mmHg) may cause compression of the vena cava with decreased venous return, CVP and cardiac index (by up to 50%).
- **Pneumoperitoneum will cause diaphragmatic splinting.** For this reason some anaesthetists believe it mandatory to use IPPV for prolonged procedures.
- **Vagally mediated bradycardia** from peritoneal distension.
- **CO_2 absorption** may cause rise in end-tidal CO_2 during long procedures. More a theoretical than an actual problem as absorption across the peritoneum is relatively slow.
- **Surgical emphysema and pneumothorax** have been reported after lengthy procedures.
- **Postoperative pain.** May be related to formation of H_2CO_3 in the peritoneal cavity. Referred shoulder pain is common.

Problems associated with position
- Patient may be head up (laparoscopic cholecystectomy) with risks of hypotension and cerebral hypoperfusion. Patient may be head down (gynaecological and surgical laparoscopy) with risks of cerebral oedema and retinal detachment (prolonged surgery).

Marking points: Laparoscopy is a common procedure whose main consequences and complications should be familiar.

What signs would lead you to suspect that a patient under general anaesthesia was developing malignant hyperthermia? Describe your immediate management.

Malignant hyperthermia (MH) is a rare clinical syndrome which is usually triggered by drugs used in the course of a general anaesthetic. Its mortality remains at ~10%, much less than the 70% of the early years, but still significant, particularly as the affected patients are often young and fit. The fall is due largely to earlier diagnosis and to rapid treatment with dantrolene, and it remains vital that anaesthetists have a high index of suspicion for early recognition of the condition.

Introduction

Malignant hyperthermia (MH) still carries a mortality of around 10%, and although it is uncommon, early recognition of the clinical features is vital. These clinical features reflect the fact that MH is a hypermetabolic state which results from decreased control of intracellular calcium.

Recognition

- Preoperatively: personal or family history (if positive, however, is likely to have been investigated).
- Musculoskeletal abnormalities: there is no evidence to support the claim that various myopathies (e.g. hernia and squint) and skeletal abnormalities (e.g. scoliosis) are associated with MH.
- At induction: masseter spasm following suxamethonium may be the first manifestation; there may also be generalised muscle rigidity (both usually subside after ~5 minutes).
- During early maintenance of anaesthesia: signs of hypermetabolic state:
    Tachycardia (+/− ventricular ectopic beats).
    Tachypnoea (if breathing spontaneously).
    Increasing $ETCO_2$ (and rapid exhaustion of soda lime).
    Biochemistry at this stage shows high P_aCO_2 and elevated K^+.
    May get brief hypertension, but sympathetic influence on BP is opposed by tissue mediated vasodilatation and BP may be unchanged.
- As anaesthesia continues:
    Rising patient temperature.
    Cyanosis.
    Biochemistry shows higher P_aCO_2, falling pH (lactic acid levels can increase 15–20×), rising K^+ and falling P_aO_2.
- Later signs:
    Continuing pyrexia (may reach 43°C).
    Coagulopathy.
    Hypoxia and hypercapnia.
    Myoglobinuria (rhabdomyolysis).
    Multiple ventincular premature beats (VBS).
    Generalised muscle rigidity (muscle ATP exhaustion).
    Acidosis: pH as low as 7.00.
    Hypotension; circulatory failure; cardiac arrest.

Management

- Discontinue all triggers (particularly the volatile agents) and obtain volatile-free breathing system if practicable.
- Hyperventilate with O_2 to prevent hyperpania.
- Dantrolene 1.0–2.0 mg kg^{-1} and repeated if necessary (up to 10 mg kg^{-1}). Early administration is crucial, but the drug is time consuming to prepare.
- Partially correct acidosis with iv $NaHCO_3$ 0.3 mmol kg^{-1}.

- Dextrose/Insulin to reduce hyperkalaemia (potent cause of arrhythmias).
- Active cooling: external with ice packs; internal with cold iv fluids, cold gastric lavage, cold peritoneal lavage.
- Admit to ITU.

Marking points: MH is a rare life-threatening disorder which is treatable, provided that diagnosis is swift and that management includes early administration of dantrolene and the use of supportive measures. Your answer must make this clear.

What is the pathophysiology of malignant hyperthermia? How does dantrolene affect the process? How would you investigate a patient in whom the diagnosis is suspected and who presents for non-urgent surgery?

Malignant hyperthermia (MH) is a rare syndrome which is usually triggered by drugs used in the course of a general anaesthetic. Its mortality remains at ~10%, much less than the 70% of earlier years, but still significant, particularly as the affected patients are often young and fit. The fall is due largely to earlier diagnosis and to rapid treatment with dantrolene, and it remains vital that anaesthetists have a high index of suspicion for early recognition of the condition.

Introduction

Malignant hyperthermia (MH) still carries a mortality of around 10%, and although it is uncommon, early recognition of the clinical features is vital. These clinical features reflect the fact that MH is a hypermetabolic state which results from decreased control of intracellular calcium.

Pathophysiology

- Following depolarisation Ca^{2+} is released from the sarcoplasmic reticulum (SR): the increased intracellular Ca^{2+} removes inhibition of the contractile elements by troponin and the muscle contracts. Reuptake is affected rapidly by intracellular Ca^{2+} pumps. Contraction and relaxation are energy-dependent processes (requiring ATP).
- MH is a disorder of Ca^{2+} control. In skeletal muscle cells exposure to triggering agents (such as suxamethonium and volatile anaesthetic agents) initiates abnormal release of Ca^{2+} from the SR.
- The site of this abnormality appears to be at the Ca^{2+} release channel of the SR, where (and this is a simplification of a complex process) the ryanodine receptor fails.
- The ryanodine receptor protein incorporates the Ca^{2+} release channel and spans the cytoplasmic gap between the sarcolemma of the T-tubule and the membrane of the SR.
- Increased intracellular Ca^{2+} has both direct and indirect stimulatory effects on metabolism.
  - Direct: increased glycolysis via phosphorylase activation.
  - Indirect: increased demand for ATP which governs contraction and relaxation.
  - Hyperstimulation of aerobic and anaerobic metabolism increases the production of CO_2, lactic acid and H^+ ions.

Dantrolene

- Prevents the release of Ca^{2+} from the terminal cisternae of the SR of striated muscle (vascular smooth muscle and cardiac muscle are less dependent on Ca^{2+} for contraction and are not affected). It does not affect Ca^{2+} reuptake.

Investigation preoperatively

- History and family history (MH is an autosomal dominant, but genetically heterogeneous).
- Resting CPK may be raised (in ~70% of susceptible individuals), although the test lacks sensitivity and specificity.
- Commonest protocol uses *in vitro* muscle contracture tests (IVCTs) in which living skeletal muscle is exposed separately to caffeine and to halothane. The combined IVCT is ~94% specific (false positive rate is ~6%) and 100% sensitive (false negative rate 0%).

- Patients fall into three groups: MHS (MH-susceptible), MHE (MH-equivocal) and MHN (MH-nonsusceptible).
- Newer techniques:
  - Ryanodine contracture test may prove to be 100% specific for MH.
  - Chlorocresol also affects Ca^{2+} release channel and shows equal promise.

Marking points: There are detailed monographs on MH which fail to make comprehensible the complex pathophysiology of MH. It is therefore not difficult to pass this question as long as you demonstrate a passing acquaintance with the overall hypothesis and appreciate that contracture testing is the gold standard. You should know how dantrolene is believed to work. The examiner may be as confused as you are about the genetic heterogeneity of the ryanodine receptor but will recognise quickly any deficits in your knowledge of the only drug which is of help in the management of MH.

What features would lead you to suspect that a patient undergoing surgery had suffered venous air embolism? With what procedures may this complication be associated?

Subclinical air embolism is common, but on occasion the anaesthetist is faced with cardiovascular collapse. This is an important critical incident which they should be able to diagnose, and part of the diagnosis is dependent on an awareness of procedures which place patients at higher risk. The question does not ask about arterial or paradoxical air embolism.

Introduction
The circulation can usually accommodate gas bubbles and subclinical air embolism is common. On occasion, however, gas embolism may be associated with circulatory collapse and so early diagnosis and treatment are essential.

Clinical features
The venous and pulmonary circulation can accommodate moderate volumes of gas. It is only with significant air embolism (volumes >2 ml kg^{-1}) that typical clinical features appear.
- Air enters the veins (this may be audible as a hissing sound) and via the right heart gains access to the pulmonary circulation:
  — Pulmonary vascular resistance increases and left atrial filling decreases.
  — LV filling may decrease and cardiac output and systolic BP may fall.
  — Ventricular ectopics are common.
  — 'Mill-wheel' continuous murmur is usually audible only with massive embolism.
  — If the air bubble is large it acts as an air lock and the circulation will fail.
- Arterial oxygenation and CO_2 elimination are affected. There is an acute drop in ETCO$_2$ and a rise in $P_a CO_2$.
- Gasping respiration (if breathing spontaneously), bronchoconstriction, pulmonary oedema.
- Further aids to diagnosis:
  — Marked increase in CVP if in place; aspiration may confirm presence of air.
  — Doppler ultrasound from right atrium: very sensitive (2× as good as capnography).
  — Transoesophageal echocardiography (better than praecordial Doppler).

Procedures implicated
Patients are at risk if:
- Surgery is performed in the sitting position in which the pressure in veins which are higher than the heart is subatmospheric. Examples include some neurosurgical procedures and some shoulder surgery in which the patient is in the 'deck chair' position.
- Surgery involving exposure of large areas of tissue, e.g. mastectomy.
- Intravascular cannulation (CVP, PA (Pulmonary artery) catheters, etc.) or decannulation is performed in vessels which are higher than the right heart.
- Gas is injected under pressure: examples include laparoscopy, uterine insufflation, gastrointestinal endoscopy, loss of resistance to air techniques, air embolus generated by the exothermic reaction of joint cement.
- The circulation is externalised, e.g. cardiopulmonary bypass.

Marking points: Prevention of this complication depends on understanding the mechanisms by which it can occur, and on identifying those procedures during which it is more likely to occur. Your answer must demonstrate both these facts.

Outline the diagnosis and management of massive venous air embolism.

This is a variation on the previous question, but which in this case also asks you to manage this life-threatening complication.

Introduction
Small air bubbles which gain access to the venous circulation are usually innocuous, but large intravenous volumes of gas may be associated with sudden cardiovascular collapse. Air embolism may be unexpected and a successful outcome will depend upon rapid diagnosis and immediate initiation of treatment.

Diagnosis is assisted by awareness of high risk procedures
- Air embolism can occur during any procedure in which:
  — Surgery is performed in the sitting position in which the pressure in veins which are higher than the heart is subatmospheric, e.g. posterior fossa craniotomy and shoulder surgery in the 'deck chair' position.
  — Surgery involving exposure of large areas of tissue, e.g. mastectomy, scalp reflection, head and neck surgery.
  — Intravascular cannulation (CVP, PA catheters, etc.) or decannulation is performed in vessels which are higher than the right heart.
  — Gas is injected under pressure: during laparoscopy, uterine insufflation, gastrointestinal endoscopy, loss of resistance to air techniques, air embolus generated by the exothermic reaction of joint cement.
  — The circulation is externalised, e.g. cardiopulmonary bypass.

Diagnosis
- Air enters the veins (this may be audible as a hissing sound) and via the right heart gains access to the pulmonary circulation:
  — Pulmonary vascular resistance increases and left atrial filling decreases.
  — LV filling may decrease and cardiac output and systolic BP may fall.
  — Ventricular ectopics.
  — 'Mill-wheel' continuous murmur only audible with massive embolism.
  — If the air bubble is large it acts as an air lock and the circulation will fail.
- Arterial oxygenation and CO_2 elimination are affected. ETCO$_2$ falls and P_aCO_2 rises.
- Gasping respiration (if breathing spontaneously), bronchoconstriction, pulmonary oedema.
- Marked increase in CVP if in place; aspiration may confirm presence of air.
- Doppler ultrasound from right atrium: very sensitive (2× as good as capnography) or transoesophageal echocardiography may confirm air bubbles and cardiac dysfunction.

Management
- Prevention of further air entry:
  — Inform surgeon of probable diagnosis.
  — Flood wound with NaCl 0.9%.
  — Compress wound site if feasible.
  — Discontinue N_2O (will increase functional impact of air bubbles).
  — Increase venous pressure by PEEP and/or fluid.
- Minimise possible cardiovascular impact:
  — Change position if possible: left decubitus.
  — Aspirate air from circulation: best site is SVC just above the right atrium (unlikely to have PA catheter in place).
- Cardiorespiratory support:
  — Maintain cardiac output: fluids and inotropes as indicated.

— 100% oxygen.
— IPPV with PEEP (may also attenuate pulmonary oedema).

Marking points: Air embolism is most dangerous when it is unexpected. Your answer must demonstrate that you both know about the predisposing circumstances and can treat it expeditiously should it occur. It is a test of your emergency skills.

Describe the anaesthetic arrangements involved in a gynaecology day-case list of 15 patients.

Textbooks do not usually include information on this type of subject. The question aims to assess whether you have a grasp of important skills of anaesthetic management and organisation.

Introduction
A large day-case surgery list is a logistic and anaesthetic challenge which depends on teamwork, communication and considerable organisation. When it goes well efficient day care is a rewarding part of anaesthetic practice, and with the increasing pressures to perform more and more surgery as day cases it is important that it should do so.

Preoperative selection
- Patients are unlikely to be seen by an anaesthetist prior to the day of surgery, hence the need for:
  — Detailed selection protocols for use by surgeons and clinic nurses.
  — Pre-admission medical and anaesthetic history questionnaire.

On the day of surgery
- Logistical arrangements
  — Staggered admission of patients to allow unhurried admission and preoperative anaesthetic assessment. May need planned breaks (could coincide with delays, e.g for instrument sterilisation) to allow this.
  — Adequate nursing staff: theatre, recovery and wards.
  — Adequate ancillary staff for patient transport.
  — Large list mandates careful and efficient checking procedures.
- Anaesthetic techniques
  — Should allow rapid awakening with minimal hangover.
  — Adequate analgesia and control of postoperative nausea and vomiting (PONV) both causes of overnight admission.
- Discharge
  — Ideally list should be arranged to allow staggered discharge by anaesthetist.
  — Discharge protocol (conscious level, accompanied, pain free, no nausea, etc.).
  — Written discharge instructions.

> **Marking points:** This question does not so much expect right or wrong answers as evidence that you understand both broader and specific anaesthetic problems associated with managing a long day-case list. Commonsense should allow you to pass this kind of question.

A patient requiring surgery claims to be allergic to latex. How would you confirm the diagnosis? Outline your perioperative management.

Latex is ubiquitous in the surgical environment and changes in production methods as well as increased exposure have led to an apparent increase on the number of individuals who are sensitive. It is an important cause of unexplained intraoperative collapse, and anaesthetists require both a high index of suspicion as well as a clear management plan for the treatment of a patient with this allergy.

Introduction

It is only in the last decade that latex has been identified as a cause of intraoperative anaphylaxis. With increasing awareness of the problem it has emerged that as many as 10% of healthcare professionals are latex sensitive, and because the substance is ubiquitous in the surgical and anaesthetic environment it can present very real problems.

Individuals at risk

- The patient may fall into one of the following groups:
  - Confirmed diagnosis of latex allergy by skin prick testing or radioallergosorbent (RAST) test.
  - History of atopy and multiple allergy. Cross-reactivity occurs with some foods, among them avocado, kiwi fruit and chestnuts.
  - History of sensitivity to latex (e.g. reaction to rubber gloves).
  - Repeated exposure to latex products: healthcare workers, patients undergoing repeated urinary catheterisations.
- There are two forms of allergy:
  - Type 1 IgE-mediated hypersensitivity (anaphylaxis possible).
  - Contact dermatitis: of less acute importance. If the history is inconclusive skin prick testing is specific and sensitive in indicating IgE latex antibody.

Perioperative management

- The key is the identification and thereafter avoidance of anything which may contain latex. Hospitals should have protocols which include lists of latex free equipment: this is a risk management issue of particular importance in emergency surgery. Latex is ubiquitous and is found in:
- Nursing equipment:
  - Trolley mattresses, pillows, TED stockings (lower leg ones are latex free).
- Anaesthetic equipment:
  - Bungs in drug vials (remove before making up into solution), some giving sets, blood pressure cuffs, face masks, nasopharyngeal airways, breathing systems, electrode pads.
- Surgical equipment:
  - Gloves, elastic bandages, urinary catheters, drains.
- The keys to safe management are to maintain a latex-free environment, to expect to find latex-containing products everywhere, and to maintain complete familiarity with the expeditious treatment of an acute anayphylactic reaction.

Marking points: This is an increasingly common problem, and failure to recognise and treat a reaction to latex will become difficult to defend. This is a basic safety question and you must demonstrate that you recognise the potential severity of the problem and also realise that latex is everywhere within the surgical and anaesthetic environment.

What are the causes of heat loss during general anaesthesia? What are the effects of hypothermia in the perioperative period?

This topic is of clinical importance, particularly in light of evidence that the maintenance of perioperative normothermia may reduce infection rates and decrease hospital stay. The question also incorporates some basic science.

Introduction
The importance of maintaining normal body temperature throughout the perioperative period has been reinforced by recent work which suggests that when this is achieved surgical infection rates and hospital stay are both decreased.

Mechanisms of heat loss
- **Radiation**
  — May account for 50% or more of heat loss. The body is a highly efficient radiator, transferring heat from a hot to cooler objects.
  — The process is accelerated during anaesthesia if the body is surrounded by cool objects and prevented from receiving radiant heat from the environment. May lose heat internally to cold infused fluids.
- **Convection**
  — May account for up to 30% of heat loss. Air in the layer close to the body is warmed by conduction, rises as its temperature increases and is carried away by convection currents.
  — Accelerated during anaesthesia if a large surface area is exposed to convection currents (particularly in laminar flow theatres).
- **Evaporation**
  — Accounts for ~20–25% of heat loss. As moisture on the body's surface evaporates it loses latent heat of vaporisation and the body cools. This is a highly developed mechanism for heat loss in health, but undesirable during surgery.
  — Accelerated during anaesthesia if there is a large moist surface area open to atmosphere (especially e.g. in major intra-abdominal surgery, intrathoracic work, reconstruction in plastic surgery, major orthopaedics).
- **Conduction**
  — Not a significant cause of heat loss during normal circumstances (~3–5%).
  — Accelerated during anaesthesia only if the patient is lying unprotected on an efficient heat conductor (e.g. metal).
- **Respiration**
  — Losses occur due to evaporation and the heating of inspired air (10%).
  — Should be minimised during anaesthesia by the use of heat and moisture exchangers or use of formal humidifiers.
- **Anaesthesia**
  — Alteration of central thermoregulation (hypothalamic).
  — Vasodilatation will increase heat loss.

Effects of hypothermia
Profound hypothermia with core temperatures of 28–30°C is unlikely to occur during anaesthesia unless it has been deliberately induced, but it is common to see patients whose temperatures have dropped by several degrees celsius. The effects of these temperature falls can be summarised as follows:
- **Cardiorespiratory systems**
  — Arrhythmias.
  — Decreased cardiac output.
  — Decreased oxygen delivery (shift to the left of oxygen-haemoglobin

dissociation curve: increased affinity, and vasoconstriction).
— Oxygen consumption increases during mild hypothermia (34°C).
— Oxygen consumption may increase by 500% during shivering on rewarming.
— Increase in blood viscosity.
— Mild acidosis.
● **Metabolic effects and effects on drugs**
— Metabolic rate decreases by ~6–7% for each 1°C fall in core temperature.
— Enzymatic reactions and all intermediate metabolism affected below 34°C.
— Drug actions are prolonged: particularly neuromuscular blocking agents.
● **Surgical outcome**
— There is recent convincing evidence that hypothermia compromises immune function and increases postoperative infection rates. Wound healing is adversely affected and hospital stay may be prolonged.

Marking points: The main mechanisms by which heat is lost will be required because an understanding of these allows a rational approach to prevention. Evidence suggests that the effects of hypothermia are significant and a broad overview of the effects of mild hypothermia will also be expected.

What hazards does a patient encounter when they are positioned in the lithotomy position for surgery? What additional hazards are introduced when the operating table is tilted head-down? Describe briefly how these hazards may be minimised.

Surgical malpositioning is an important cause of morbidity, and prevention of some of the problems requires both anatomical and physiological knowledge. Failure to take appropriate care to avoid morbidity leaves the anaesthetist vulnerable and this is an important area of practice.

Introduction

The anaesthetised patient is unable to protect themselves in any way from the effects of malpositioning, and it therefore behoves the anaesthetist to ensure that none of those structures which the awake patient would automatically protect are in any way at risk. The lithotomy position is particularly unnatural.

Lithotomy hazards

- **Lumbar spine**
  - In lithotomy rotation of the pelvis flattens the normal convexity of the lumbar spine and places increased strain on interlumbar and lumbosacral ligaments. This strain is reduced by the use of supporting pillows beneath the hips at the sides.
- **Appendages**
  - Fingers must be protected. If the arms lie flat by the sides the digits are vulnerable to being trapped by the hinged operating table.
  - They must not be in direct contact with the metal of the lithotomy poles with which they are commonly level.
  - This is prevented by supporting the arms in a neutral position away from the sides.
- **Nerves: several are vulnerable**
  - **Sciatic.** If thighs and legs are externally rotated, or if the knees are extended, the sciatic nerve may be stretched between its points of fixation (sciatic notch and neck of fibula).
  - **Femoral.** May follow prolonged lithotomy in flexion of thighs, abduction and external rotation of thighs. May kink the nerve at the inguinal ligament (Avoid both of these by minimising these excessive movements.)
  - **Common peroneal** (lateral popliteal). Classic lower limb nerve injury. May be stretched against the head of the fibula by flexion of hips and knees in lithotomy, or may be pressed against the supporting straps. Avoid by padding and by minimising stretch.
  - **Posterior tibial.** May be compressed against lithotomy stirrup which supports posterior part of the knee. Avoid such stirrups.
  - **Saphenous.** At risk of pressure against vertical poles. Ensure adequate padding.
- **Vessels**
  - Calf compression may result in venous thrombosis. Compartment syndrome after prolonged surgery has been reported.
- **Circulation and cardiac function**
  - Lithotomy has the effect of diverting blood that would have pooled in the lower limbs back to the core. Rarely, in a patient with precarious cardiac function this effective transfusion can precipitate ventricular failure and pulmonary oedema. More commonly this transfusion can mask the severity of blood loss by increasing venous return.

Hazards associated with head-down (Trendelenburg) position

- Circulation
  - — Head-down tilt exaggerates the circulatory effects already described.
- Respiration
  - — Pressure of viscera on diaphragm increases work of breathing.
  - — Gas exchange may deteriorate as closing volume exceeds FRC.
  - — These effects can be attenuated by IPPV.
- Central nervous system
  - — CSF pressure and cerebral venous pressure increase and so cerebral perfusion pressure decreases. Cerebral oedema (hydrostatic) has been described.
  - — Retinal detachment has also been described as a complication (Intraocular pressure (IOP) increases.)
  - — Shoulder retainers which prevent the patient moving backwards may cause pressure injury to the brachial plexus if the Trendelenburg is steep.

Marking points: The question seeks your understanding of the potential morbidity associated with a very common surgical position. Failure to cite the lesser complications will not lead to failure of the question, but if you do not identify the major problems and the means of avoiding them then you cannot pass.

What factors predispose a patient to aspirate gastric contents into the lungs during general anaesthesia? How can the risk be minimised? How should pulmonary aspiration be treated?

Pulmonary aspiration was implicated by Simpson in the first reported anaesthetic death in 1848 and 150 years later the topic is of enduring importance to anaesthetists. This question tests your knowledge about a core topic related to anaesthetic safety.

Introduction
Prevention of pulmonary aspiration of gastric contents is one of the central tenets of safe anaesthetic practice. The process requires passive regurgitation or active vomiting in the presence of depressed laryngeal reflexes and there are a large number of patients who potentially are at risk.

Predisposing factors
- Gastric volumes
  - May be high in the patient who is not fasted prior to surgery.
  - May be high in presence of outlet obstruction (pyloric stenosis or intestinal obstruction).
  - May be high in motility disorders (e.g. diabetic gastroparesis).
  - May be high if emptying is delayed by pain, trauma (acute gastric dilatation), labour (contentious), opioid analgesia, high-fat and high-solid content of a recent meal.
  - May be distended by air insufflated during manual bag and mask ventilation.
- Oesophageal sphincter and lower oesophagus
  - Usually remains tonically constricted.
  - Distal oesophagus is intra-abdominal and is constricted by 'pinchcock action' of diaphragmatic crura.
  - Many causes of sphincter incompetence: drugs (including general anaesthetic agents, anticholinergics, opioids); abdominal masses (e.g. gravid uterus); reflux disease (at both extremes of age); and also associated with hiatus hernia, achalasia, autonomic neuropathy, scleroderma, NG tube placement.
  - Tumours or strictures.
- Laryngeal incompetence
  - Anaesthesia (drug induced).
  - Tracheal intubation (mechanical effect which may impair competence for up to 8 hours).
  - Head injury and cerebrovascular accident.
  - Postictal (also in eclampsia with additional confounding features of pregnancy).
  - Coma (metabolic or drug-induced).
  - Trauma.
  - Hypothermia.
  - Bulbar problems: acute polyneuropathies (e.g. Guillain–Barré), motor neurone disease, muscular dystrophies.

Prevention

- Adequate fasting (at least 4 hours for solids; 2 hours for fluids). Longer if high fat.
- Antacid therapy as premedication: H$_2$ receptor antagonists (typically ranitidine); sodium citrate, proton pump inhibitors (typically omeprazole).
- Rapid sequence induction as standard anaesthetic technique in high risk subjects.

- High index of suspicion: pregnancy, obesity, drug abuse, hiatus hernia with symptoms.
- Emptying of stomach contents. Not currently popular and success is uncertain.
- Avoid general anaesthesia and sedation in favour of regional techniques.

Treatment

- Prompt recognition: clear airway, intubate and use tracheal suction before initiating IPPV.
- Oxygen.
- No evidence to support use of pulmonary lavage (acid damage occurs within 20 seconds).
- No evidence to support corticosteroids: suppress inflammatory defence reaction and may promote secondary bacterial infection.
- If no symptoms after ~2 hours respiratory problems are unlikely to supervene.
- Prophylactic antibiotics are not indicated.
- If earlier symptoms appear patient requires supportive therapy and observation. ARDS is possible; oxygenation meanwhile via CPAP (spontaneously ventilating), IPPV (if not), and if condition is deteriorating.

Marking points: It is clear that this is a core safety topic and you will be expected to give a good account of all three areas. It is recognised that you will not have time to include great detail.

What factors contribute to postoperative cognitive deficits in elderly surgical patients? How may these risks be minimised?

Confusion in the immediate postoperative period is common enough in the elderly patient almost to be regarded, wrongly, as routine. Thoughtful perioperative management may reduce the problem and it is this which the question seeks to test.

Introduction

Postoperative cognitive deficits (POCD) are those which relate to changes in personality, to difficulties with tasks requiring organisation of thought, to problems with social relationships and to short term memory lapses. Given the heterogeneity of the elderly surgical population it is clear that the problem is likely to be multifactorial. It may be oversimplistic to assume that it is all related to failures of cerebral oxygenation. The phenomenon occurs in about 25% of patients.

Preoperative factors

- Pre-existing mental infirmity
  — Alzheimer's disease, other dementias, mild confusional states. It is hard to influence these, although it should be recognised that a simple change of environment may result in total disorientation in time and space for some elderly patients.
- Pre-existing cerebrovascular and ischaemic heart disease
  — Co-morbidity is common. Preoperative management should aim to optimise the various conditions.

Perioperative factors

- Hypocapnia
  — Hyperventilation causes cerebral vasoconstriction and reduction in perfusion.
- Hypotension
  — Intuitive assumption would cite blood pressure falls as significant. This is not supported by any available evidence.
- Hypoxia
  — The role of hypoxia is believed to be indirect via neurotransmitter effects. Postoperative oxygen therapy may reduce risks of cardiac and thence cerebral effects, but is not directly influential on POCD per se.
- Drug effects
  — Effect of anaesthetic agents may be mediated via effect on memory processing.
  — Central anticholinergic syndrome.
- Metabolic disturbance
  — Postoperative hyponatraemia.
- Infection
  — Pyrexia and sepsis.

Specific procedures may be associated with increased POCD

- Cardiopulmonary bypass
  — Clear evidence that cognitive deficits occur in all age groups.
  — Prolonged extracorporeal perfusion is deleterious.
- Vascular surgery
  — Influence of aortic cross clamp times is significant.
  — Prolonged surgery and long clamp times deleterious.
- Surgery with embolism risk
  — Joint replacement surgery: air and fat embolus.

—   Carotid end-arterectomy.
● **Neurosurgery**
—   Direct interference with cerebral circulation.

> **Marking points:** This question is more complex than it appears because of the lack of evidence that obvious factors such as hypotension and hypoxia are central to the problem. This matters less than your demonstration that you would assess and manage the patient well enough to pre-empt some of the responsible factors.

What immunological consequences may follow homologous blood transfusion?

This is a very focused question which does not therefore require any discussion of potential infection risks or the problems of massive transfusion

Introduction

Amongst the many possible adverse consequences of homologous blood transfusion, immunomodulation was recognised many decades ago, and it actually enjoyed early favour in renal transplant surgery as a deliberate immunosuppressive therapy. Research has not confirmed the mechanisms by which transfusion achieves this, and there remains no consensus about the significance of its effects.

- **Mild allergic reactions.** Complicate ~1–3% of transfusions, are associated with presence of foreign protein in the blood and include:
  — Non-haemolytic febrile reactions.
  — Urticarial reactions accompanied by pruritus.
  — Alloimmunisation.
  — Hypersensitivity reactions including anapyhylaxis: transfusion of IgA to IgA-deficient patients who have formed anti-IgA.
- **Major haemolytic reactions:** rare (USA incidence of reactions 1 in 6000; fatal in 1 in 600 000).
  — May be immediate: usually ABO incompatibility.
  — Can be delayed: usually in recipients sensitised to RBC antigens following previous transfusion or pregnancy. Antibody level at transfusion is low, but an anamnestic response is triggered with increased levels and delayed haemolysis. The Rh and Kidd systems are involved rather than ABO.
  — Host attacks foreign RBCs via complement and antibody.
- **Delayed immunomodulation**
  — Early evidence following renal transplantation confirmed 20% increase in 1-year graft survival.
  — Significance waned with advent of effective immunosuppressants (ciclosporin A).
- **Current areas of interest**
  — **Postoperative infection rates:** blood transfusion as an independent variable may increase infection rates from single figures to 25%. (data not universally accepted).
  — **Tumour recurrence:** largest group of patients studied (mostly retrospective) are those with colorectal cancer. Studies are contradictory: no consensus whether tumour recurrence rates are increased by transfusion as an independent variable.
  — **Inflammatory bowel disease:** transfusion may reduce disease recurrence by 2–3× in patients with Crohn's disease (autoimmune aetiology).
  — Effects are more marked with repeated transfusion.
- **Mechanisms.** Unclear, theories include:
  — Clonal deletion: foreign MHC antigen deletes T cells with receptors for that MHC.
  — Tolerance: may be due to block on T-cell receptor site.
  — Active suppression: down-regulation of cellular immunity.

Marking points: This is a specialist area of current interest about which there is scientific speculation. You will gain by describing the postulated theories, although this is not expected. You will be required to demonstrate that you recognise these specific problems of transfusion.

Outline the effects of old age upon morbidity and mortality in anaesthesia

Anaesthesia for the elderly is of perennial relevance and as the population ages it will become even more so. This question should pose few problems but it is important to focus the many points down to those which command a high priority.

Introduction

Almost 15% of the population of the UK is aged over 65, and they are a group in whom surgery is more common, and in whom mortality is higher. In the CEPOD reports 75% of reported cases of mortality were aged over 70 years and the overall mortality rate was 10%. Old age is associated with significant co-morbidity which is superimposed upon the normal changes of ageing, both of which have important implications for anaesthesia.

- **Co-existing disease is common**
  - Ischaemic heart disease, hypertension, chronic airways disease, cerebrovascular disease, osteoarthritis, diabetes mellitus, dementia (20% if >80 years), Parkinson's disease, physical frailty, malnutrition, polypharmacy, sensory impairment (vision and hearing).
- **Central nervous system**
  - Progressive structural change with cerebral atrophy (brain weight decrease of >10%); decrease in neurotransmitter concentrations; decreased cerebral blood flow and oxygen consumption.
  - Maximum alveolar concentration (MAC) decreases with age (both GA and LA: ~5% per decade after age 40): receptor sensitivity (e.g. to benzodiazepines) may increase, protein binding (e.g. of opioids) may decrease.
  - Temperament: may be more stoical and phlegmatic with age.
- **Autonomic nervous system**
  - Functional decline: orthostatic hypotension (in 25% of >65 years) as baroreceptor function declines; decrease in neurotransmitter concentrations; decreased cerebral blood flow and oxygen consumption.
  - Temperature control is impaired: also have lower basal metabolic rate (BMR) and may have less subcutaneous fat (if frail and elderly).
- **Cardiovascular system**
  - Functional decline: cardiac output decreases (by 20% at age 60) with decreases in HR, SV and contractility.
  - Decreased sensitivity to inotropes (receptor numbers decrease).
- **Respiratory system**
  - Progressive decline with age: FRC = Closing volume at ~65 years (upright) but encroaches on FRC at age 44 if supine.
  - $(A - a)DO_2$ widens (increased V/Q mismatch).
  - Decreased sensitivity to hypoxia and hypercapnia.
  - Decreased lung compliance.
- **The airway**
  - Edentulous, osteoporotic mandible, poor facial tissue and oropharyngeal muscle tone, cervical spondylosis and osteoarthritis.
- **Gastrointestinal system**
  - Slower gastric emptying, parietal cell function impaired, hiatus hernia and reflux more common.
- **Renal system**
  - Renal blood flow decreases by 10% per decade and GFR (glomerular filtration rate) is decreased by 30–45% in the elderly; concentrating function impaired, fluid handling impaired, dehydration more likely.

- **Drug handling**
  - — Hepatic and renal function decrease; protein binding decreases; receptor sensitivity alters (increased for CNS depressants; decreased for inotropes, beta-adrenoceptor blockers).

Marking points: It would be hard not to pass this question (just) were you simply to take a systems approach and state that everything declined. Examiners will want to see some sense of priority with one or two quantitative examples to reassure them that you are not just guessing.

What are the risks associated with carotid endarterectomy? How may anaesthetic technique reduce these risks?

Carotid endarterectomy is a common vascular procedure which has attracted recent interest because of the increasing use of regional blockade. The conscious level of the awake patient is an excellent monitor of cerebral blood flow, the maintenance of which must underpin any anaesthetic technique.

Introduction

Transient ischaemic attacks (TIAs) have been described as 'fragments borrowed from the stroke that is to come' and this risk is relatively high: 1% of the population aged over 75 years will die from carotid atherosclerosis. A larger number will suffer non-fatal strokes. Carotid endarterectomy is a prophylactic procedure which aims to reduce this toll.

Risks of the procedure

- Mortality is in range of 5%.
- Patients have concomitant cerebrovascular and ischaemic heart disease: it is crucial to maintain cerebral perfusion pressure, particularly in the head-up position.
- Surgery requires cross-clamping: cerebral perfusion is dependent on collateral circulation.
- Surgery may dislodge plaque debris.
- Surgery may be complicated by perioperative bleeding (aspirin treatment is common).

Anaesthetic options: general anaesthesia

- Potential advantages
  - Airway control.
  - $P_a\text{CO}_2$ control.
  - Cerebral protective effect of barbiturates or deep volatile anaesthesia.
  - Use of hypothermia if required.
  - Easier for the surgeon.
- Potential disadvantages
  - CVS instability associated with maneouvres to secure the airway (intubation, etc.).
  - Maintenance of high normocapnia is not always easy to achieve during IPPV.
  - Deep volatile or barbiturate anaesthesia may compromise circulation and make neurological status more difficult to assess.

The anaesthetist, therefore, can attenuate the risks of the procedure by manipulating the circulation to try to ensure that cerebral perfusion pressure is maintained. There is, however, no reliable monitor of the adequacy of cerebral perfusion: hence the increasing popularity of regional anaesthesia for this operation. Techniques include cervical epidural anaesthesia, local infiltration, and local infiltration together with deep cervical plexus block. The latter is the most popular in the UK.

Anaesthetic options: regional anaesthesia

- Potential advantages
  - Changes in cerebral perfusion will be accompanied by rapid warning changes in patient cerebration: this is the most significant advantage.
  - Decreased requirement for shunting (which itself carries significant morbidity).
  - Lower cardiovascular morbidity.

- **Potential disadvantages**
  — Needs cooperative and motivated patient.
  — No airway control (important if cervical epidural used).
  — Hypothermia not an option.
  — Myocardial morbidity is unaltered.
  — Generic disadvantages of the local anaesthetic techniques used.
  — Problematic if conversion to GA is necessary.

The large randomised controlled clinical trial to determine whether general or regional anaesthesia is better for carotid endarterectomy has yet to be undertaken.

> **Marking points:** The answer must emphasise the importance of maintaining cerebral perfusion whatever the technique used. You must be aware that local and regional anaesthetic techniques are an important option, even though you may not have seen them employed.

What is the glucocorticoid response to surgery? Describe your approach to steroid replacement both in patients who are currently receiving corticosteroids and in those who have discontinued treatment.

The stress response to injury can be important in patients who are receiving corticosteroids. The traditional concern is related to the danger of precipitating an Addisonian crisis in patients whose hypothalamo–pituitary–adrenal axis is suppressed. There are those who believe the anxieties to be over-stated and certainly the use of potentially dangerous supraphysiological replacement regimens should be abandoned.

Introduction

Treatment with corticosteroids has the potential to cause adrenal suppression, and the exaggerated fear of precipitating an Addisonian crisis following surgery has resulted in the common use of supraphysiological replacement regimens. A logical approach to replacement rests on an appreciation of the normal response and that provoked by differing degrees of surgical trauma.

Steroid response to surgery

- **Autonomic nervous system: sympathoadrenal response**
  - Mediated via hypothalamus.
  - Increased medullary catecholamines.
  - Increased presynaptic norepinephrine (noradrenaline) release.
  - Modification of visceral function (renal and hepatic).
  - Renin–angiotensin system stimulates aldosterone release: Na^+ and H_2O retention.
- **Hypothalamo–pituitary–adrenal axis**
  - Hypothalamic releasing factors stimulate anterior pituitary.
  - Get increases in: ACTH via corticotropin-releasing hormone (CRH).
- **Cortisol**
  - ACTH stimulates adrenal glucocorticoid release (specific cell-surface receptor: G-protein activation, adenyl cyclase stimulation and increased intracellular cAMP).
  - Catabolic: protein breakdown, gluconeogenesis, inhibition of glucose utilisation, lipolysis.
  - Anti-inflammatory: inhibits leucocyte migration into damaged areas; inhibits synthesis of inflammatory mediators such as prostaglandins.
  - Normal response: maximal rise at 4–6 hours with peak cortisol usually subsiding within 24 hours but sustained for up to 72 hours in major (e.g. cardiac) surgery. Values may range from 800 (fourfold increase) to >1500 nmol L^{-1}.
  - Cortisol output: minor surgery (hernia) <50 mg in 24 hours; laparotomy or thoracotomy stimulates release of 75–100 mg.

Rationale underlying perioperative steroid replacement

Administration of steroids is assumed to result in suppression and atrophy of the hypothalamo–pituitary–adrenal (HPA) axis via feedback inhibition of hypothalamic and pituitary function. Replacement minimises risk of perioperative cardiovascular instability.

Supraphysiological doses of exogenous steroids, however, risk their numerous complications: excess catabolism, hyperglycaemia, immunosuppression, peptic ulceration, delayed wound healing, myopathy (can occur acutely), steroid psychosis (relates to sudden large increases in blood level), fluid retention and electrolyte disturbance.

Replacement regimens

- Ideally are based on laboratory evaluation of HPA axis (short synacthen or insulin tolerance tests if possible) and assessment of likely degree of surgical stress.
- Patients on prednisolone 10 mg daily (or equivalent) have a normal response to HPA testing and require no supplementation.
- Patients who have received this amount within 3 months from surgery should be assumed to have some degree of HPA suppression (test if possible).
- Patients on high dose immunosuppressant therapy must continue this perioperatively.
- If taking >10 mg daily and undergoing minor to moderate surgery:
  — Continue usual dose preoperatively.
  — Hydrocortisone 25 mg iv at induction.
  — Hydrocortisone 100 mg in first 24 hours (continuous infusion).
- If taking >10 mg daily and undergoing major surgery:
  — Continue usual dose preoperatively.
  — Hydrocortisone 25 mg iv at induction.
  — Hydrocortisone 100 mg per day for 48–72 hr (continuous infusion).

Marking points: Steroid replacement regimens are analogous to those used in the management of diabetes, although they are less common. In both situations the examiner wishes to see that you understand the rationale behind them and that you can prescribe a safe and sensible treatment plan.

What are the implications of anaesthetising a patient in the prone position?

Patients are placed in the prone position both for major procedures such as spinal surgery, but also for relatively more trivial operations such as pilonidal sinus excision or short saphenous vein varicose vein surgery. It is something that you will encounter, therefore, early in your anaesthetic career and you must be aware of the potential problems.

Introduction

A patient who is allowed to breathe spontaneously in the prone position has an FRC that is greater than if they were supine, and has less likelihood of aspirating gastric contents. Those are probably the only benefits to the patient apart from the important fact of optimising surgical access: otherwise the position confers nothing but disadvantage.

Respiratory effects

- FRC is greater than in the supine position (an advantage if breathing spontaneously), but the usual prone position may encourage the diaphragm to move cephalad.
- If the abdomen is not free from pressure breathing is compromised.

Airway

- Less likelihood of aspiration while actually in the prone position.
- Access to airway is restricted: should be secured using an armoured tube (although there are some anaesthetists who do use laryngeal mask airways in the prone position).

Circulation

- Anaesthetised patients do not tolerate changes in position well: applies particularly to the obese and to the hypovolaemic (should be fluid resuscitated first). Spinal surgery may also be associated with significant blood loss.
- Venous return may decrease due to pooling of blood in dependent cephalad half and legs.
- Abdominal compression may affect venous return via inferior vena cava: the shoulders and pelvis must be supported so that the abdomen is free.
- Intravenous lines may be dislodged during turning or may be inaccessible after turning: need secure fixation and use of extension tubes.

Musculoskeletal

- Damage can occur during turning (which must be done with adequate personnel using a log roll technique). The neck is particularly vulnerable.

Pressure effects

- Patients are at risk at a number of sites:
  — Eyes and globe: the retinal artery is an end-artery and thrombosis leading to blindness has been reported.
  — All tissues must be free from pressure on electrodes, monitoring wires or iv lines.
  — Hard pillows under the pelvis may compress the lateral cutaneous nerve of thigh.
  — The ulnar nerve is vulnerable at the elbow.
  — The brachial plexus is vulnerable to traction damage if the arms are too far abducted in the forward position with the forearms flexed. Arms should be close to patient's side, kept in pronation with hands either side of the head.

A patient presenting for total hip replacement tells you that he has a pacemaker. What further information do you require and how will this influence your anaesthetic management?

The traditional management of patients with pacemakers seemed to rely on the use of the theatre magnet which could never be found. Modern pacemakers have long since rendered this advice redundant and the subject is now of sufficient complexity and affected patients are common enough to make it a popular examination topic.

Introduction

Pacemaker technology is complex and detailed information will need to be obtained about the specific unit. It is also important to identify the underlying primary pathology.

Reasons for a permanent pacemaker

- Complete heart block.
- Sick sinus syndrome.
- Bifascicular and trifascicular block.
- Tachyarrhythmias.

Pacemaker details

- Is it temporary or permanent?
- They have a three-letter classification (more accurately it is a five-letter classification):
    - **Pacing.** Chamber that is paced: V – ventricle; A – atrium; D – dual.
    - **Sensing.** Chamber that is sensed: V – ventricle; A – Atrium; D – Dual; O – None.
    - **Responding.** Mode of response: T – Triggered (senses A +/– V depolarisation and paces stat); I – Inhibited (senses A +/– V depolarisation and aborts it); D – Dual (does both); O – Does neither.
    - **Programmability** and implanted **Defibrillator functions** make up 4th and 5th letters.
    - Commonest example is VVI: sensing and pacing in the ventricle, this is a ventricular demand pacemaker which is inhibited from pacing by R waves.
- Is it functioning? When was it sited? When was it last serviced?
- CXR: will show position and reveal its type via radio-opaque code.

Implications for anaesthesia

- **Suxamethonium**: fasciculations may be misinterpreted as cardiac impulse and inhibit pacemaker output (depending on type).
- **Surgical diathermy**
    - Cutting (~0.5 mHz) and coagulation (~1.5 mHz) provide interference that may be sensed as intrinsic activity.
    - Demand pacemakers default to a set rhythm in presence of constant interference.
    - External magnet (is a special pacemaker magnet) will bypass the sensing mode in a simple programmable demand unit.
    - Multiprogrammable units may be reprogrammed by diathermy, and this instability may be enhanced by an external magnet.
    - Can reprogramme these to asynchronous (fixed rate) mode.
    - A paced ventricle with neither sensing nor response modes (VOO) is unaffected.
    - Should use bipolar diathermy, minimal energies, short bursts.
    - Indifferent electrode should be sited distant from the pacemaker unit.

- **Defibrillation**
  - — If paddles are paced directly over the pacemaker the circuitry will be damaged.
  - — Otherwise defibrillation can be used if indicated.
- **Postoperatively**
  - — Unit will require checking to see if change in function has inadvertently occurred.

Marking points: Failing to remember all the nomenclature will not cost you the question, but you must demonstrate awareness of the main safety issues.

What factors would alert you to the fact that a patient might be difficult to intubate?

This is a core area of knowledge, and safe patient management mandates that every anaesthetist should be familiar with the main factors that may make tracheal intubation difficult. They also need the pragmatic understanding of the fact that there is no single nor any combination test that reliably will predict difficult intubation in more than about 75% of cases.

Introduction

Successful tracheal intubation requires the axial alignment of three planes – the oral, the pharyngeal, the laryngeal – and many factors can conspire to make this difficult, although in practice the incidence of difficult intubation is estimated only at ~1% and failed intubation at ~0.15%.

History
- Patient may be aware of previous dificulties. Records may confirm it or document view of glottis as graded by Cormack and Lehane (Grades 1 to 4).
- May have a condition associated with difficult intubation: rheumatoid arthritis, scleroderma, ankylosing spondylitis, acute trismus (Ludwig's angina), or congenital abnormality such as Klippel–Feil, Treacher–Collins or Goldenhar syndromes. There are many more.

Mouth opening and oral cavity (oral and pharyngeal plane)
- Should be at least 3 cm. Note that the effective opening may be reduced by prominent upper incisors. Actual opening is a function of the temporomandibular joint (TMJ) and may be affected acutely by pain or chronically by disease processes which affect the joint (rheumatoid arthritis, scleroderma, acromegaly, burns contractures).
- Macroglossia, high arched palate, prominent and over-riding upper incisors may increase difficulty.
- Jaw mobility: as demonstrated by ability to protrude lower incisors beyond upper incisors.
- Micrognathia, macrognathia.

Extension of the head at the atlanto-occipital joint (pharyngeal and laryngeal plane)
- Can be limited by conditions such as ankylosing spondylitis, arthritis, cervical spine surgery, cervical spine injury. It should be 35° in the normal individual.

Viewing of the larynx (laryngeal plane)
- Short, thick neck.
- High anterior larynx.

Problems at the laryngeal inlet
- Compression by external mass: goitre, haematoma (acutely).
- Supraglottic obstruction: infection, foreign body, trauma, tumour, angio-oedema.
- Subglottic obstruction; stenosis.

Predictive tests
- Mallampati test:
    – Class 1 to 4: as a simplification this relates size of base of tongue to oral cavity.
    – Many false positive results and 50% false negatives.
- Thryromental distance:
    – Indicator of head extension, position of larynx (whether high), size of

mandible.
- – Less than 7 cm is an indicator of potential difficulty.
- Hyoid-mandibular distance (in extension):
  - – Should be at least 3 cm (the laryngoscope displaces the tongue into this space).

None of these tests is either sensitive or specific enough to predict difficult intubation. Various combination scores have been suggested such as that proposed by Wilson:

- Wilson score:
- — Identifies and scores risk factors: obesity, head and neck mobility, mouth opening and jaw mobility, retrognathia and prominent incisor teeth. Predicts ~75% of difficult intubations with a false positive rate of ~12%.

Radiology

A number of X-ray markers have been associated with difficult intubation: their routine clinical use is not widespread:

- Gap between occiput and spinous process of C1.
- Gap between spinous processes of C1 and C2.
- Posterior and anterior depth of the mandible and their proportions.
- Atlanto-odontoid distance (>3 mm).
- Occipito–C1 gap.

> **Marking points:** This is a core topic, but there is unlikely to be enough time to include all the information in this answer. You should make clear that you understand the principles of why a patient may be difficult to intubate and give some examples to demonstrate that understanding. If you know about this subject do not waste time by detailing the Cormack and Lehane grading or the Mallampati classification.

A patient proves impossible to intubate. What factors determine the rate of haemoglobin desaturation? What can be done to maintain oxygenation in this situation?

This situation, although not particularly common (1 in ~750 intubations), is one which every anaesthetist must be able to manage safely and expeditiously. This question explores your understanding of the underlying principles and your practical management of a potentially difficult problem.

Introduction
Patients die from failure to oxygenate and not from failure to intubate, and although the clinical situation may be complicated by the need for rapid sequence induction because of a full stomach or gastrointestinal pathology, it should always be retrievable.

Basic principles
- The basal requirement for oxygen is ~250 ml min^{-1}.
- The functional residual capacity (FRC) in an adult is ~2000–2500 ml. Under normal circumstances, therefore, oxygen reserves will be exhausted in ~2 minutes.

Oxygen reserves
- Pre-oxygenation: either for 3–5 minutes or 3 vital capacity breaths will replace alveolar air with 100% oxygen. If nitrogen washout has been completed then 8–10 minutes may elapse before desaturation starts to take place.
- FRC is decreased or is exceeded by closing capacity in the following groups:
  — Children <6 years, adults >45 years, pregnancy, obesity.
- Pre-existing pulmonary disease causing shunt will reduce effectiveness of pre-oxygenation.
- Carboxyhaemoglobin: heavy smokers acutely may have 15% CoHb ($t_{1/2}$ is 4 hours in air): oxygen-carrying capacity is decreased.
- Haemoglobin concentration: in the presence of hypoxia the SpO$_2$ reading will be an underestimate (there is a linear relationship between the inaccuracy and decreasing Hb).

Desaturation rate also depends on oxygen consumption
- **Increased:** rise in metabolic rate, children, pregnancy, sepsis, pyrexia.
- **Decreased:** fall in metabolic rate: hypothermia, myxoedema, drugs.

Maintenance of oxygenation
- Patients die from failure to oxygenate, not failure to intubate: so management should include:
  — Bag and mask ventilation +/– airway adjuncts with O$_2$ 100% to restore oxygenation and elimination of CO$_2$ (can maintain cricoid pressure if this is a RSI (rapid sequence induction) but ease if it compromises ventilation: hypoxia is worse than aspiration).
  — Proceed to laryngeal mask airway: can be used as an aid to intubation (6.0 endotracheal tube (ETT); gum elastic bougie; replace ETT with larger size railroaded over the bougie).
  — If ventilation is also impossible a rapid decision to proceed to cricothyroidotomy will be necessary to ensure oxygenation.

Marking points: Your answer should demonstrate that you appreciate in which patients this situation is even more urgent and that you understand the fundamental priority of management.

What safety features should be incorporated into a patient controlled anaesthesia (PCA) system for adults and what is the purpose of each? Having sent a patient to the ward with PCA what instructions would you give to the nursing staff?

PCA is now widely used and should be familiar to every anaesthetist. This question on a core topic is directed overtly towards its safety aspects and is testing your appreciation of all the potential risks of a very common technique.

Introduction
Patient-controlled analgesia systems always comprise a large reservoir of opioids and some means of delivering a dose as the patient demands. It is clear, therefore, that there are several areas of potential hazard.

Administration of excessive dose
This should be prevented by:
- **Appropriate concentration:** in the PCA syringe, ideally it should be prepared by pharmacy.
- **Appropriate lock-out time** (usually 5 minutes). Electronic pumps are programmable; disposable sets rely on capillary refill to replenish the chamber. This physical process cannot be speeded up and so these arguably are inherently safer than electronic pumps which may malfunction.
- **Maximum hourly dose.** Of importance if a background infusion is added.
- **Alarms.** Microprocessor pumps should incorporate alarms which warn of excessive dose.
- **Anti-siphoning device.** A one-way valve should be incorporated into any system which is linked via a Y-connector to a fluid infusion giving set. Backflow otherwise can occur into the tubing of the fluid infusion which may then deliver a large bolus. As an alternative the PCA can be delivered via a separate dedicated line. The device should not be placed above the level of the patient.
- **Security.** Electronic pumps are robust and lockable so that the patient (or other party) can neither gain access to the syringe, which typically will contain 120 mg morphine, nor alter the programme. Disposable devices are much more vulnerable in this respect.

Safety instructions
These are to ensure that should the opioid be delivered in excessive dose or have excessive effect the patient will come to no harm.

- Sedation scoring and respiratory rate
  — Sedation is a more sensitive indicator of opioid overdose than respiratory rate.
  — Example: '0' = awake and responsive, '3' = unrousable to tactile stimulation.
  — Frequency: hourly for 4 hours, 2 hourly for 8 hours, 4 hourly thereafter.
  — Same for respiratory rate and other clinical indices.
  — This instruction varies between units: if in doubt err on the side of high frequency, because this is even safer and you cannot be faulted for that.
- Reversal of narcosis
  — Written prescription for naloxone. Nursing staff should be allowed to administer the drug according to a set protocol in the absence of immediate medical help.
- Equipment failure
  — Syringe volume should be checked against cumulative consumption on display.
  — Any discrepancy should result in discontinuation of PCA pending review.

- Medical help
  - 24 hour access to pain and / or emergency team for advice and assistance.

Other monitoring and instructions

- **Location:** nurse in open ward rather than in a side-room.
- **Pulse oximetry**
  - Often unhelpful. SpO_2 may be normal in presence of respiratory failure, but if hypoventilation is extreme then the patient will desaturate.
- **Pain scoring**
  - Frequency as above.
  - Example: '0' = no pain at rest or on movement, '3' = continuous pain at rest or severe pain on movement.
- **Postoperative nausea and vomiting**
  - Prescription for breakthrough anti-emetic and protocol for discontinuing PCA pending medical review.

Marking points: This is a question about basic safety and is not asking you to describe the advantages and disadvantages of PCA. Note that the instructions to nursing staff are not limited to the safety aspects. It should be very straightforward and so most of the points above must be covered. It is a core subject and will be marked accordingly.

You plan to anaesthetise a patient for total hip replacement under subarachnoid block with sedation. What do you understand by the term 'sedation' in this context, and what drugs and techniques are available?

'Sedation' is a term that is used to describe a spectrum which ranges from conscious minimal sedation to general anaesthesia by another name. Safe techniques of sedation can be difficult to achieve and this question seeks to explore your understanding of the options and their problems.

Introduction

Conscious sedation is a term intended to describe a state in which a drug or combination of drugs is used to cause a modest depression of conscious level without compromising airway, breathing or circulation. Such a sedated patient will remain cooperative, conscious and in contact with their surroundings. This state is not easy to achieve.

Sedation techniques

- **Local anaesthesia.** The key to successful sedation is successful local anaesthesia. It is potentially disastrous if the anaesthetist tries to overcome an indifferent local block by increasing the dose of sedative drugs.
- **Patient selection.** Patients need to be advised that they will not be unconscious during the procedure, but that they may be amnesic. This should be discussed, because amnesia is not popular with all patients and it is clearly inappropriate during, for example, caesarean section, where the use of an amnesic agent would result in the loss of an emotionally important event.
- **Monitoring.** Sedation may be used in patients who are too frail for general anaesthesia. All patients must be monitored as though they were undergoing full general anaesthesia.
- **Drugs.** These may be administered by any route: inhalational, orally, im, iv or even pr (very unusual in adults). In practice iv and inhalational methods are the most popular because they can be titrated against response.
- **Propofol.** Target-controlled infusion (TCI). This technique uses a microprocessor-controlled infusion pump that has been programmed to predict a target blood level, typically 1.0 to 4.0 μg ml^{-1}. Wide interindividual variation means that the pharmacokinetic model with which the pump is programmed may not prove accurate in a particular individual.
- **Inhalational agents.** These include nitrous oxide and low concentration volatile agents. These can be titrated against response. Nitrous oxide in concentrations up to 50% provides good adjunctive analgesia with modest sedation ('relative analgesia') but is emetic. Volatile agents can be effective but are unacceptable to many adults.
- **Benzodiazepines.** Typically midazolam. Is a good anxiolytic and is amnesic. Low dose administration (up to ~10 mg maximum) is often effective, but higher doses may result in disinhibition and a lack of cooperation which is followed by prolonged sedation after the surgical stimulus has ceased. Can be antagonised by flumazenil, but note that the elimination half-lives are not the same and patients may become re-sedated.
- **Ketamine** (low dose). Can be effective when given at ~ one tenth of normal dose (0.1 mg kg^{-1}) although sympathomimetic and psychotomimetic effects may still be problematic.
- **Opioids:** short-acting drugs such as alfentanil and remifentanil. Opioids are not primarily sedatives. Are probably best given as very low dose adjuncts to other sedative agents to counter physical discomfort being experienced by the patient.
- **Others:** chloral hydrate, clomethiazole, chlorpromazine and other

phenothiazines, butyrophenones droperidol and haloperidol. Some of these drugs are major neuroleptic agents with alarming side effect profiles and should be used with great care.

Marking points: There is some commonsense in this question which aims to test whether you have a safe and practical approach to sedoanalgesia. The emphasis should be on safety.

Outline the causes and the physiological effects of hypercapnia. A patient has a $P_a\text{co}_2$ of 12 kPa. How does this affect oxygenation?

This is a question about the applied physiology of a gas whose expired concentration is measured during almost every anaesthetic. It tests your understanding of the clinical effects based on basic science knowledge.

Introduction

The normal partial pressure of carbon dioxide in arterial blood is between 4.5 and 6.0 kPa depending on the reference laboratory, and so hypercapnia may be defined as a $P_a\text{co}_2$ of greater than 6.0 kPa. It may further be classified into 'moderate' (6.0–9.0 kPa) and 'severe' (>9.0 kPa) hypercapnia with clinical features which vary accordingly. The main causes are listed below.

Hypoventilation
- **Mechanical:** obstruction, splinting of diaphragm.
- **Pharmacological:** opioid drugs, residual neuromuscular blockade.

Increased ventilation of dead space
- Apparatus: catheter mounts, endotracheal tubes (ETTs), breathing system filters, masks.
- Pulmonary hypertension: impairs perfusion of well-ventilated upper zones.
- Tachypnoea: lower tidal volumes mean higher proportion of anatomical dead space, and may not ventilate less compliant areas of lung which need larger volumes to expand them.
- PEEP: may increase ventilation in upper zone while decreasing perfusion by reducing venous return.

Inspired CO_2
- Rebreathing due to inappropriate fresh gas flows.
- Failure of CO_2 absorption.

Increase in CO_2 production (normal is ~200 ml min^{-1})
- Malignant hyperpyrexia.
- Pyrexia: rise to 40°C increases CO_2 output by ~25%.
- Overactivity of thyroid.
- Muscle activity (and shivering).
- High carbohydrate intake (especially in ITU feeding).

Physiological consequences: mediated via the sympathetic nervous system

Cardiovascular
- Sympathetic response causes tachycardia (bounding pulse), peripheral vasodilatation, may see hypertension with widened pulse pressure (increased cardiac output with decreased SVR).
- Relationship between $P_a\text{co}_2$ and cardiac output is direct between ~2.5 and 10.5 kPa.
- Direct effect is depressant: negative inotropic effect is masked by sympathetic response until level of ~9.0 kPa is reached.

Respiratory
- Depends if the hypercarbia has a primary respiratory cause. If not, e.g. as in malignant hyperthermia, then see signs of stimulation, tachypnoea.
- The CO_2 response curve is linear, with minute ventilation increasing in proportion to the rise in $P\text{co}_2$.

Central nervous system
- May get CO_2 narcosis in a non-habituated individual at ~12.0 kPa.
- Cerebral blood flow increases linearly by ~7.5 ml 100 g min^{-1} for each 1 kPa rise from baseline to maximal at ~10.5 kPa. At this level no further vasodilatation is possible.

Effect on oxygenation
- Hypoventilation due to CO_2 narcosis may lead to desaturation (unless respiratory failure is masked by high concentration supplemental oxygen).
- Decrease in pH shifts OHDC (Oxygen-haemoglobin dissociation curve) to the right with decrease in O_2 affinity and increased delivery.
- Alveolar gas equation quantifies by how much alveolar oxygen is decreased by increased alveolar CO_2.
- $P_AO_2 = P_IO_2 \, (F_IO_2 \times \text{Atm. Pressure} - \text{SVP of water}) - P_ACO_2 / RQ$.
- In this example, assuming normal barometric pressure at sea level an RQ of 0.8, and a patient breathing room air, a P_ACO_2 of 12 reduces P_AO_2 to ~5 kPa. If the patient's P_ACO_2 were 5 kPa their P_AO_2 would be ~13.5 kPa. Hypercarbia can affect oxygenation very significantly.

Marking points: This is a core topic and you will be expected to demonstrate understanding of the basic principles. The effect of hypercapnia on oxygenation is important.

What are appropriate criteria for the selection of adult patients for day-case surgery under general anaesthesia?

Within recent memory procedures that formerly involved prolonged hospital stays (such as cataract surgery) are now performed as day cases. Anaesthesia has contributed significantly to this development and it is an important area of clinical practice about which you should be well informed.

Introduction

The current political and economic objective is to ensure that within less than 10 years 60% of all surgery will be carried out on a day-case basis. While this may have many social and domestic benefits for patients, the key to its safety and success lies in adequate patient selection processes. The important criteria are both physical and social.

General well-being and previous history

- In general fit, well and mobile. Able to climb one flight of stairs without dyspnoea. Chronological age is no bar: biological age is important.
- Should not be obese (BMI > 30). Evidence suggests that risk of adverse respiratory events is increased by up to four times in this group.
- No significant previous problems with anaesthesia and surgery.

Surgery

- Advent of drugs and techniques such as TIVA with propofol, sevoflurane and desflurane removes a time limit. Body cavity surgery or that in which blood loss is a potential problem should be avoided.

Cardiovascular exclusions

- Hypertension (BP > 180/110 mmHg) although there is currently some concern that isolated systolic hypertension is as significant as diastolic hypertension.
- Angina pectoris if poorly controlled or worsening.
- Cardiac failure or myocardial infarction within 6 months.
- Peripheral vascular disease or cardiac valvular disease with symptoms.

Respiratory exclusions

- Significant chest disease including asthma. An adequate history is vital: exercise tolerance > 250 m (walking on flat); recent in-patient admission (<3 months); disease that requires corticosteroids.

Central nervous system exclusions

- Transient ischaemic attack or cerebrovascular event within previous 6 months.
- Epilepsy. If control is poor or >3 fits in the past year. (This is rather arbitrary.) In patients in whom control is good the issue is debatable: the propofol data sheet warns that if administered to a patient with epilepsy 'there may be a risk of convulsion', but etomidate may provide an adequate, albeit less satisfactory alternative induction agent.
- Any severe disorder: e.g. multiple sclerosis, myasthenia, dystrophies.

Metabolic and endocrine

- Diabetes mellitus. Insulin (IDDM) or non-insulin dependent if poorly controlled. IDDM can be accommodated provided surgery is early and time allowed to return to oral intake. May depend on the individual likelihood of postoperative nausea and vomiting (PONV).

Other systems

- Significant renal and hepatic disease.

- Alcohol or drug abuse.
- Significant psychiatric disease.

Medication which should usually preclude day-case surgery
- Monoamine oxidase inhibitors.
- Anticoagulants.
- Corticosteroids.
- Antiarrhythmic agents.

Social criteria
- Accompanying responsible adult and adult supervision (not care) overnight.
- Distance: within 60 minutes travelling time.
- Adequate domestic circumstances: telephone, heating, sanitation, etc.

Marking points: It is very easy to list a huge number of pathological conditions which simple clinical judgement confirms to be completely unsuitable for day-case surgery. This question seeks your assessment of the more difficult areas such as hypertension, obesity and stable disease. There is no single correct answer to this question. Most hospitals have day-case protocols which can form a basis for your answer, but your own commonsense and clinical judgement are also important.

An 8-year-old child presents for extraction of four deciduous molar teeth in the dental chair. Describe the anaesthetic management and identify the problems that may be encountered.

Statistically, chair dental anaesthesia is very safe with a mortality of less than 1 in 250 000, but it is a politically charged and topical issue. You may be unfamiliar with the technique itself, but you should be aware of the broad safety issues that are involved.

Introduction
Anaesthesia in the dental chair exemplifies the challenge of the shared airway during an anaesthetic that is usually very brief. Although it is transient the standards of anaesthetic care must match those in any other area of practice.

Preoperative assessment
- Imperative: as in any other form of anaesthesia. Standard medical history (likely to be brief in a population that is fit and well), including anaesthetic history and family anaesthetic history. Common problems: asthma (in ~15% of children) and recent upper respiratory tract infection (coryza).
- Why does the child require general anesthesia? Four quadrant surgery usually requires GA, and sedation techniques, apart from the use of nitrous oxide in relative analgesia (RA), are inappropriate. Some 8 year olds cope well with local anaesthesia and so request for GA may indicate possible difficulties with cooperation.

Anaesthetic technique
- **Induction.** If given the choice ~50% of children will opt either for inhalation or intravenous induction. Empowering the child in this way may make them less apprehensive and more likely to cooperate.
- **Persuasion.** The child cannot be forced to undergo anaesthesia and dental extraction. Restraint should not be used: technically it is an illegal assault (Children's Act) which may ensure that a child becomes permanently phobic about dental treatment.
- **If inhalational:** N_2O/O_2 and sevoflurane volatile induction and maintenance of anaesthesia (VIMA). Whether or not venous access should then be obtained is a moot point. Some anaesthetists argue with justification that the cannulation is likely to take as long as the extractions. If the anaesthetist is cannulating then to whom should be delegated the control of the airway? 'Cannulation is not necessary until it is necessary' (because of an adverse event).
- **If intravenous: propofol.** It is a poor drug for dental anaesthesia in children (large volume, viscous, painful on injection, associated with myoclonus at the end of induction, prolonged emergence from anaesthesia because of the relative overdose that is required), but there is now no acceptable alternative. Methohexitone is no longer available.
- **Monitoring:** SpO_2 and ECG are mandatory (electrodes on the forearms give an adequate signal and the child does not need to be disrobed.) The transient nature of the procedure means that only a single, largely uninterpretable, blood pressure reading would be obtained intraoperatively. Capnography and gas analysis are inaccurate and unhelpful (unless a laryngeal mask airway is used).
- **The airway.** Nasal mask vs LMA. The LMA requires deeper and longer anaesthesia. This procedure (four teeth) takes an experienced extractor about 60 seconds and deep anaesthesia of this nature is neither necessary nor desirable. In skilled and experienced anaesthetic hands airway maintenance does not pose problems.

- **Position.** Contentious. Studies have demonstrated that anaesthesia in the semi-sitting position is not associated with hypotension and cerebral hypoperfusion. Airway problems are greater in the supine position, and dental forceps for lower extractions are designed for use in the upright position. (The matter polarises opinion and you should be able to justify your choice.)

Potential problems

- **Airway.** May be obstructed by the pack (relatively common), by debris (rare), by bleeding (rare) by laryngospasm (rare). Vomiting is very uncommon. Aspiration has not been reported.
- **Breathing.** May be rendered transiently apnoeic by induction agent (rare).
- **Circulation**
  - Cardiac arrythmias. Problematical with halothane (should not now be used) but much less so with sevoflurane. Hypoxia and hypercarbia are potential precipitants if surgery is prolonged, and airway management is suboptimal.
  - Hypovolaemia. Potentially a problem with young children fasted in hot weather for excessive periods.

Marking points: Chair dental anaesthesia is a topic that polarises anaesthetic opinion. You will fare best if you follow the party line (iv access, full monitoring, supine position) in a written answer, although in the oral you might get more opportunity for rational discussion of the issues.

What are the physiological changes that occur when a patient undergoes electroconvulsive therapy (ECT)? What are the potential complications and in which patients is ECT contraindicated?

Anaesthesia for ECT is transient, it often takes place in isolated sites and is undertaken in a group of patients who are sometimes viewed as peripheral to the mainstream acute hospital population. This means that it may not be taken as seriously as it should. The physiological effects may be transient, but they are extreme, and are consequences of which anaesthetists should be aware.

Introduction

Electroconvulsive therapy is an empirical, and controversial treatment, whose use is confined largely to patients with refractory psychiatric disorders, mainly psychotic depression but also catatonia, mania and schizophrenia. An electric shock (pulsatile square wave discharge of ~35 J) is delivered to one or both cerebral hemispheres to induce a grand mal convulsion.

- **Grand mal fit.** A short latent phase is followed by a tonic phase of general contracture of skeletal muscle which lasts ~15 seconds. This is succeeded by a clonic phase which lasts 30–60 seconds. The central electrical seizure (as demonstrated by EEG) outlasts the peripheral myoclonus.
- **Autonomic effects: parasympathetic.** The discharge is short lived, but is associated with typical parasympathetic effects. At their worst these include bradycardia and vagal inhibition leading to asystole.
- **Autonomic effects: sympathetic.** As the clonic phase of the seizure begins there is a mass sympathetic response which peaks at ~ 2 minutes. Plasma epinephrine (adrenaline) and norepinephrine (noradrenaline) levels at 1 minute exceed baseline by 15 and 3 times respectively. Predictable effects include tachyarrhythmias and hypertension, with increased tissue and in particular myocardial and cerebral oxygen consumption.
- **Cerebral effects.** The cortical discharge is accompanied by a large increase in cerebral blood flow (5–7×) and $CMRO_2$ (Cerebral metabolic rate for oxygen) (4×). Intracranial pressure rises accordingly.
- **Musculoskeletal effects.** The grand mal convulsion is accompanied by violent contractions of all skeletal muscle which have been associated with vertebral fractures and other skeletal damage.

Complications: associated with anaesthesia

- There are the generic complications associated with any of the induction agents in use (methohexitone was the agent of choice, but is no longer available) and problems with suxamethonium, which is given to attenuate the force of the muscle contraction on the skeletal system.
- Bag, valve, mask ventilation in a paralysed patient without intubation does not itself represent a problem, although ECT does increase intragastric pressure. The action of suxamethonium may outlast that of the induction agent, but awareness is negated by the postictal state.

Complications: associated with the (modified) convulsion

- These are predictable in light of the autonomic and other effects described above:
  — Cardiac arrhythmias and hypertension.
  — Raised ICP (and intraocular pressure).
  — Skeletal and tissue damage (e.g. to tongue).

Contraindications: also predictable in light of the effects described

- Recent cerebrovascular or myocardial event (within 3 months).

- Hiatus hernia (can perform rapid sequence induction but will need higher dose of suxamethonium).
- CNS mass lesion or raised ICP.
- Glaucoma.
- Severe ischaemic heart disease.
- Osteoporotic bone disease (risk of fractures is higher).

Marking points: This question has been phrased deliberately to concentrate on the physiological changes associated with ECT rather than the anaesthetic implications of the procedure. If you are struggling with the facts then it may help to return to first principles by considering the physiological consequences of a grand mal fit. Complications and contraindications are relatively non-specific and so a commonsense approach may just get you a '2'.

List the factors which may cause atrial fibrillation. How would you recognise the onset of this rhythm during anaesthesia and how would you treat it?

Atrial fibrillation (AF) is one of the commonest arrhythmias and both acute and chronic forms have anaesthetic implications. Sudden onset AF is a rhythm that you will be expected to recognise and treat.

Introduction
Many conditions are associated with AF, but the most common are ischaemic and hypertensive cardiac disease. Sudden onset AF may be a feature of sepsis, it may be an indicator of other serious disease but in some individuals it may be idiopathic. Immediate management depends upon whether the rhythm causes haemodynamic instability.

Causes of atrial fibrillation
— Ischaemic heart disease.
— Hypertensive cardiac disease.
— Acute sepsis.
— Cardiomyopathies.
— Congenital heart disease.
— Thyrotoxicosis.
— Chronic airways disease – COPD.
— Mitral valve disease.
— Alcohol excess.
— Accessory conducting pathways.
— Idiopathic.
— Perioperative cardiac surgery.

Recognition intraoperatively
- ECG is the only definitive method of diagnosis, which is confirmed if there is complete disorganisation of atrial activity, an absence of the 'p' waves of atrial contraction, the presence of fine fibrillatory 'f' waves, and an 'irregularly irregular' ventricular rate due to variable conduction. Atrial rate is 350–500 and ventricular rate 60–170 beats per minute.
- Adenosine 3 mg stat can aid diagnosis if the rate is very rapid (inhibits adenyl cyclase, decreases cAMP and slows AV conduction).
- Atrial fibrillation can occur in conjunction with an AV accessory pathway (e.g. Wolff–Parkinson–White), i.e. get AF with pre-excitation. Lead II alone will not reveal this abnormality.
- Other monitors may support diagnosis indirectly:
  — SpO_2 waveform will identify the irregular ventricular rate.
  — $ETCO_2$ may drop if the sudden onset is associated with marked fall in cardiac output. The loss of the atrial component to ventricular filling can be significant.
  — NIBP (non-invasive blood pressure) may not produce an adequate reading in the presence of markedly irregular pulse.

Treatment
- If CVS is stable, control of ventricular response rate by agents that slow AV conduction:
  — Beta-adrenoceptor blocker: e.g. esmolol 1 mg kg^{-1}.
  — Ca^{2+} channel blocker: e.g. verapamil 5–10 mg.
  — Class III (delay repolarisation): ibutilide 1 mg by slow (10 minutes) infusion (new agent which is effective but which is associated with delayed torsade

de pointes).

— An AV nodal blocker should be given before a Type 1 arrhythmic (block fast Na^+ channels). If the atrial rate is slowed it may allow 1 : 1 AV conduction with a paradoxical increase in rate; hence should achieve AV block beforehand.

— Digoxin takes between 1 and 3 hours to exert its effect and is of minimal benefit acutely.

- If CVS is unstable and there is haemodynamic compromise:
  — Synchronised DC cardioversion: start at ~100 J.
- If there is AF with pre-excitation:
  — If stable: procainamide 50 mg min^{-1} to total of 10 mg kg^{-1}.
  — If unstable: synchronised DC cardioversion.

Marking points: AF is common and although it is unusual to have to treat the arrhythmia acutely in theatre it is sometimes necessary. This is a critical event which you must be able to manage safely. If you do not then you will fail the question.

What are the indications for induced hypotension? What drugs may be used to achieve it? What are the problems with the technique and how can they be minimised?

The old adage, which bears repeating, is that induced hypotension must never be used to make the difficult easy, but the impossible possible. It is not a technique that should be undertaken lightly and you should be aware of the potential problems with the drugs that you suggest. This is a question about the safety of applied pharmacology.

Introduction
Bleeding from the surgical field does not occur solely because the systemic blood pressure is high: equally it may reflect a hyperdynamic circulation or venous congestion. Interest in hypotensive anaesthesia comes and goes, and concerns about blood transfusion have renewed interest in the technique, although many still believe that it is justified for only a very limited number of specialised procedures such as choroidal tumour resection in the eye.

Indications
- Traditionally, hypotensive anaesthesia was used to produce a dry operating field in middle ear, spinal, maxillofacial, urological, plastic and vascular surgery, as well as in the clipping of intracranial aneurysms.
- Many of these indications no longer apply: intracranial surgeons, for instance, prefer to maintain cerebral perfusion pressure, and overall blood loss is unchanged for many procedures, prompting concerns that the patient may be put unnecessarily at risk for operative convenience.
- The final stance adopted by some anaesthetists is that hypotensive anaesthesia should be avoided except in those few situations in which surgical success would be impossible without transient periods of profound hypotension, such as is needed for the excision of choroidal tumours.

Drugs used to induce hypotension: singly or in combination

Beta-adrenoceptor blockers
— Influence on BP is probably due to decreased cardiac output via decreased heart rate, plus some inhibition of the renin–angiotensin system.
— Esmolol. Relatively selective β_1 antagonist. Ultra short-acting with a $t_{1/2}$ of ~9 minutes.
— Labetalol. Both an α and β antagonist (ratio is 1 : 7), so get decreased SVR without reflex tachycardia. Elimination $t_{1/2}$: 4–6 hours.

Ganglion blockers
— Antagonists at nicotinic receptors at autonomic ganglia (sympathetic and parasympathetic) but no effect at nicotinic receptors of neuromuscular junction.
— Trimetaphan is the most commonly used (20–50 μg kg^{-1} min^{-1}).
— Direct vasodilator effect in peripheral vessels.
— Causes histamine release and reflex tachycardia is common.

Direct vasodilators
- **Nitroglycerin (glyceryl trinitrate (GTN))**
— Mediates hypotensive action via nitric oxide: NO activates guanylate cyclase which increases cyclic GMP within cells, which in turn decreases available intracellular Ca^{2+}.
— Causes venous more than arteriolar vasodilatation, hence decreases venous return and preload. Decreased myocardial oxygen demand due to decrease

in wall tension.
— Rapid onset (1–2 minutes) and offset (3–5 minutes) allows good control of BP: no rebound hypertension on discontinuing infusion. Rate: 0.1–4.0 μg kg min^{-1}.
— Increases ICP.
• **Sodium nitroprusside (SNP)**
— Mediates hypotensive action via NO as with GTN.
— Arterial and venous dilatation: hypotension and reflex tachycardia.
— Rapid onset (1–2 minutes) and offset (3–5 minutes) allows good control of BP: but may see rebound hypertension when infusion is stopped. Rate: 1.5 μg kg min^{-1}.
— Complex metabolism leads to production of free CN$^-$ which is potentially very toxic (irreversible binding of cytochrome oxidase) at levels of >8 μg ml^{-1}. Total dose should not exceed 1.5 mg kg^{-1}.
— Giving set must be protected from light.
• **Hydralazine**
— Hypotension via direct vasodilatation plus weak α antagonist action.
— Mediated via increase in cyclic GMP and decrease in available intracellular Ca^{2+}.
— Arteriolar tone affected > venous.
— Reflex tachycardia is common.

Alpha-adrenoceptor blockers
• **Phentolamine**
— Non-selective α antagonist ($\alpha_1 : \alpha_2$ is 3 : 1) with weak ß sympathomimetic action.
— Influence on BP is via block of α_1 vasoconstriction with decrease in peripheral resistance plus mild ß sympathomimetic vasodilatation.
— α_2 blockade increases norepinephrine (noradrenaline) release.
— Rapid onset (1–2 minutes), duration up to ~15–20 minutes.

Sympathetic block as part of regional anaesthesia with local anaesthetics
— May cause hypotension and decrease systemic pressure while increasing flow.

Potential problems
• Can be avoided only with scrupulous technique and monitoring.
• Should include direct intra-arterial blood pressure monitoring.
• Rate of fall is important: Precipitate falls in blood pressure can be associated with catastrophic drops in perfusion of essential areas, such as the retinal circulation.
• **Central nervous system**
— Damage may result from impaired cerebral perfusion.
— Hypoperfusion may be exacerbated by head-up position and hypocapnia, also by pre-morbid disease: e.g. hypertension shifts autoregulation curve to the right (normal range 60–130 MAP (mean arterial pressure)) although drug-induced hypotension moves it to the left.
— In the anaesthetised patient cerebral function can be monitored by the CFAM (cerebral function analysing monitor) and more sensitively by somatosensory evoked potentials. Any technique used to induce hypotension must be capable of rapid reversal should these monitors show evidence of critical hypoperfusion.
• **Myocardium**
— Hypotension may reduce O_2 consumption and so may be less potentially damaging, but in presence of marked hypotension patients are very susceptible to blood volume changes.

— Reflex tachycardia may decrease coronary flow (decreased diastolic filling time).
— Patients with coronary artery disease with a fixed stenosis are at risk because perfusion is purely pressure dependent.
— Monitoring is by ECG: crude. Ideal method measures coronary sinus lactate and oxygen content (research tool only).

- **Kidneys**
  — Hypotension will reduce RBF (renal blood flow) and GFR. Acute renal failure following induced hypotension is unlikely except in the presence of pre-existing impairment of renal function.
  — No evidence that use of mannitol or diuretics to maintain urine output is beneficial.

Marking points: This is a safety question and so it is better for you to show limited enthusiasm for induced hypotension, which many anaesthetists believe to have a very restricted role. Knowledge of the drug actions will be expected, as will an account of the end organs which are vulnerable. As always, if you damage the patient you will do badly in the question.

What criteria are appropriate for the discharge of patients who have undergone day-case surgery? Why might overnight admission be necessary?

The current political and economic objective is to ensure that within less than 10 years 60% of all surgery will be carried out on a day-case basis, which means that increasing numbers of higher risk patients will undergo day surgery, which itself is likely to include procedures of greater complexity, such as laparoscopic cholecystectomy. Strict selection and discharge criteria are essential for the safe delivery of this service.

Introduction

Day-case surgery currently is expanding in terms of numbers of patients, is treating more patients with intercurrent disease and of greater age, and is undertaking surgery of increasing complexity. Such a service can only be delivered safely if meticulous attention is paid to selection and discharge criteria.

Discharge criteria

- May partly depend on inclusion criteria for day-case surgery, in which some units will treat elderly and ASA III patients.
- Such patients must have disease that is stable and well controlled; must be undergoing surgery of only limited complexity; and must have a higher level of post-anaesthetic and postoperative care and supervision at home.
- **From recovery**
  - Full movement of all limbs (unless involved in the surgery).
  - Adequate respiration with good cough.
  - Circulation stable.
  - Awake and orientated.
  - Pain must be under control.
  - SpO_2 maintained on room air.
- **From the day unit**
  - Must be able to ambulate (with some assistance if necessary).
  - No new cardiovascular or respiratory symptoms.
  - Must be free from nausea and vomiting and should have been able to take fluids.
  - If regional (e.g. caudal analgesia) has been used motor function must be restored.
  - Bladder function must have returned; urine passed.
  - Sensorium must be clear: patient should be alert and well orientated.
  - Pain must be under control and likely to remain so by the use of oral analgesics.

Social criteria

- Accompanying responsible adult and adult supervision overnight.
- Distance: within 60 minutes travelling time.
- Adequate domestic circumstances: telephone, heating, stairs, sanitation.

Reasons for overnight admission

- Failure to satisfy any of the criteria above.
- Surgical complications (such as bleeding).
- Cardiovascular or respiratory instability.
- Postoperative nausea and vomiting. Worse in females with other contributory factors including type of surgery (gynaecological), unrelieved pain, dehydration.
- Pain.

Marking points: This is a straightforward question which you should be able to pass with a minimum of common sense. Social circumstances are important as well as the control of postoperative nausea and vomiting (PONV) and pain, which are the two main reasons for admission.

What place does preoperative medication (premedication) have in current adult anaesthetic practice?

What is now referred to as 'preoperative assessment' is an anaesthetic activity that used more commonly to be known as 'seeing the pre-meds': a term which reflected the fact that almost all adults were given premedication, usually comprising an opioid mixture such as papaveretum and hyoscine. That practice largely has stopped, but there is now more interest in preoperative medication in a wider sense. This question is assessing whether or not you have developed that wider view, which is taking anaesthesia into the area of perioperative care.

Introduction

The use of premedication in adults has developed from the traditional administration of an opioid/anti-emetic/sedative mixture into the use of a much wider range of perioperative medication which aims to optimise the patient's outcome. Indications and examples are outlined as follows.

None

- There are many patients for whom the preoperative anaesthetic visit alone provides adequate mental preparation, and who require no further medication.

Continuation of preoperative therapy

- Most treatment should be continued. Examples of those drugs which should be stopped incude MAO (monoamine oxidase) inhibitors and warfarin (depending on the INR and the surgical procedure).

Anxiolysis

- Anxiety is common, and one of the benzodiazepines such temazepam, diazepam or lorazepam can be prescribed. Patients may have unrealistic expectations of their effects and it is wise to explain that such drugs may have only minimal effect. Some patients moreover may be very perturbed by the accompanying amnesia, which is particularly marked with lorazepam.
- Some anaesthetists believe it more effective to treat the symptoms of anxiety by prescribing beta-adrenoceptor blockers. The practice is not widespread.

Sedation

- This is linked to anxiolysis. Optimal sedation, in which the patient is calm, relaxed and rousable, is not easy to achieve, not least because of the wide interindividual variability in response to oral sedatives. Ward and theatre pressures mean that parenteral preparations may not be given at the appropriate time.
- Examples of drugs used include the benzodiazepines and hyoscine plus opioid mixtures (much less popular than hitherto, but nonetheless effective).

Analgesia and neuroleptanalgesia

- Preoperative analgesia is essential if a patient is in pain prior to emergency surgery.
- NSAIDs are examples of drugs which can be used preoperatively to allow blood levels to peak at around the time of maximal tissue trauma.
- Pre-emptive analgesia prior to major surgery by using central neuraxial anaesthesia is used by some anaesthetists, but is as yet unproven.
- Neuroleptanalgesia in which drugs such as droperidol are used is probably best avoided. Droperidol is a good anti-emetic and sedative agent which may, however, precipitate a 'locked-in' depersonalisation syndrome in which patients appear outwardly relaxed while inwardly feeling intensely agitated.

Control of secretions

- Considered essential prior to procedures such as bronchoscopy or awake fibreoptic intubation.

Control of gastric pH and volumes

- Patients who are considered to be at high risk of gastric reflux and pulmonary aspiration of gastric contents (emergency surgery, particularly for the acute abdomen, pregnancy, morbid obesity, diabetic gastroparesis, hiatus hernia) should receive combination premedication to:
  - Empty the stomach: using e.g. prokinetic drugs such as metoclopramide or domperidone (oral or suppository preparation only). Cisapride has been withdrawn.
  - Neutralise the stomach contents with non-particulate agent: e.g. 0.3 molar sodium citrate.
  - Decrease gastric acid production: proton pump inhibitors such as omeprazole or H_2- receptor antagonists, e.g. ranitidine.

Modification of the sympathetic response

- Some clinicians use preoperative drugs such as beta-adrenoceptor blockers or α_2 agonists to modify the pressor responses to laryngoscopy in patients with hypertension or coronary artery disease. This is less common than using agents at the time of induction.
- Recent interest has centred on the use of the beta-adrenoceptor blocker atenolol as a means of reducing silent myocardial ischaemia as well as adverse cardiovascular events in the perioperative period.

> **Marking points:** This question requires that you think wider than the traditional concept of premedication. Once you do so then this answer becomes very straightforward. Anaesthetists have often held very individual attitudes towards premedication, and there are no 'right' answers. Have confidence in your own clinical practice and tell the examiner what you do and why: if it is sensible you will pass.

An adult patient is known to be very difficult to intubate. Describe a technique of awake fibreoptic intubation. What supplemental nerve blocks may be needed?

The aim of fibreoptic intubation is to secure the airway while causing the patient the minimum of distress. The aim of this question is to demonstrate your knowledge of at least one technique that is effective and safe. There are various ways of achieving this: the specimen answer below describes some of the options and also covers the generic points that will apply to whichever variation you choose. The question invites you to focus on one technique, so describe the one with which you are most familiar.

Introduction
The development of fine-bore fibreoptic bronchoscopes with high quality optics has meant that the technique of fibreoptic intubation has largely superseded those various techniques, such as retrograde intubation, with which anaesthetists used to manage the difficult airway.

Equipment requirements
- Appropriate equipment includes:
    - Fibreoptic endoscope (and defogging material).
    - Topical local anaesthetics.
    - Local anaesthetic drugs for infiltration.
    - Range of oral and nasal endotracheal tubes (ETTs).
    - Range of airway adjuncts, including laryngeal mask airways (LMAs) and a cricothyrotomy device.
    - Presence of a surgeon capable of creating a surgical airway if needed.
    - Appropriate sedative drug.

Preparation
- Patient preparation includes:
    - Preoperative drying agent: atropine 0.6 mg, glycopyrrolate 0.2 mg or hysocine 0.4 mg (amnesic and sedating).
    - Anxiolytic premedication if indicated.
    - Sedation if indicated: with caution, as the patient must not be rendered apnoeic.
    - Supplemental oxygen.
    - Standard minimal monitoring.
    - Nebulised lidocaine (lignocaine): effectively anaesthetises the entire upper airway.

Intubation
- Decide on the nasal or oral route.
    - **Nasal:** must anaesthetise nasal mucosa and nares with a local anaesthetic plus vasoconstrictor to minimise risk of bleeding. Typically cocaine (maximum dose 1.5 mg kg^{-1}).
    - Nasal route is technically easier because of the more direct route to the glottis.
    - **Oral:** tongue and posterior pharynx must be anaesthetised e.g. with lidocaine 10% metered pump delivering 10 mg with each spray (beware overdose) or lidocaine 4%.

'Spray as you go' technique
- Lidocaine 4% (usually) is introduced into the airway under direct vision via an injector channel in the fibreoptic endoscope.

Supplemental nerve blocks
- Glossopharyngeal
  - — Provides sensory innervation to the oral pharynx, supraglottic area, base of tongue and vallecula. Can be blocked by submucosal infiltration behind the tonsillar pillars.
- Superior laryngeal (branch of the vagus)
  - — Sensory innervation to vocal cords above the larynx and the epiglottis.
  - — Can be blocked by bilateral injections performed either by walking off the greater cornu of the hyoid to penetrate the thyrohyoid membrane, or by walking off the superior alae of the thyroid cartilage.
- Recurrent laryngeal (branch of the vagus)
  - — Sensory innervation below the vocal cords including the trachea.
  - — Usually blocked via a transtracheal injection that is made through the cricothyroid membrane (using e.g. lidocaine 4%×4 ml) during inspiration. (Cough distributes the solution more widely.)

Technique
- Intubating technique
  - — Load the appropriate sized nasal or oral ETT onto the lubricated endoscope and then gently direct the tip via the preferred route.
  - — Identification of the structures at each level is essential. Disorientation should prompt withdrawal of the endoscope until a familiar landmark is identified.
  - — Structures viewed include the inferior turbinate bones, the soft and hard palate, the epiglottis and the laryngeal inlet.
  - — Once through the larynx and into the trachea (confirmed by the view of tracheal rings and carina) the ETT can be advanced and secured after confirmation of placement by clinical signs and especially by $ETCO_2$. Railroading the tube in the awake patient can be difficult. If the carina is touched by the end of the endoscope or tube the patient may cough it out of the airway.
  - — Anaesthesia can be initiated by whichever means appropriate (inhalational or intravenous).

Marking points: You cannot pass this question simply by stating that you would just 'spray as you go', even if that is the technique currently favoured by many anaesthetists. Your description must also include the preparation of patient and equipment. The question about supplemental nerve blocks is to test your knowledge of the applied anatomy of the area. Innervation of the laryngeal region is core anaesthetic anatomy.

What factors may lead to inadvertent intra-arterial injection of a drug? How would you recognise it? Describe your management of such an event.

Intra-arterial injection is a rare and serious mishap whose consequences may be grave. Anaesthetists must be able to recognise accidental injection and to manage the effects, particularly if highly damaging agents such as thiopental or phenytoin are injected.

Introduction

Iatrogenic intra-arterial injection can occur in the context of general anaesthesia or in the intensive care unit. This is a very serious mishap whose potentially grave consequences will depend on the substance that is injected. Much more common is intra-arterial injection by drug abusers in whom the damaging substances may be difficult to identify but which can cause catastrophic ischaemic damage.

Anaesthesia

Inadvertent intra-arterial injection usually involves induction agents and can occur at several sites, most commonly in the antecubital fossa.

- **Antecubital fossa**
  - In ~10% of patients the brachial artery divides above the elbow and the ulnar artery may then run superficial to the bicipital aponeurosis (the grâce à dieu fascia) which protects the artery at the elbow. In these subjects the artery lies immediately deep to the median cubital vein and is unprotected.
- **Wrist**
  - In some subjects a superficial branch of the radial artery leaves the volar surface of the arm to cross the radial side of the wrist where it can be mistaken for a vein.
- **Foot**
  - Small arteries may be mistaken for veins in patients in whom venous access is difficult.

Intensive care

- Accidental injection occurs when an intra-arterial catheter is mistaken for a venous cannula. Drugs that have been so injected include phenytoin, benzodiazepines and antibiotics.

Accident and emergency

- Individuals (usually drug abusers) may present following inadvertent intra-arterial injection. The substances are frequently impure non-parenteral agents (such as benzodiazepines which are presented in gelatine capsules) which increase the risk of superadded infection to compound the arterial damage that they can cause.

Recognition of intra-arterial injection

- Pain (in the awake patient) distal to the injection site, typically the hand. May be very severe.
- May see ischaemic colour changes in the distal limb. Pale, mottled, cyanosed. Due to arterial spasm. Thrombosis may follow.
- Later signs: secondary to ischaemia and thrombosis as above, trophic skin change, ulceration, oedema. Gangrene may supervene in the worst cases.

Management

Will depend on the substance injected and on the clinical features as above. Thiopental, for example, causes substantial damage. At body pH thiopental precipitates into crystals which occlude small arterial vessels, provoke intense vasospasm mediated via local norepinephrine (noradrenaline) release, and may lead to complete arterial thrombosis which may not manifest for some days. Propofol, by contrast, seems relatively innocuous. It is, however, worth treating any such mishap initially as for the worst case scenario, because clinical experience of intra-arterial injection of many drugs is limited.

- Leave needle or cannula in place (very important).
- Inject heparin 500–1000 units to reduce thrombosis risk.
- Inject warm NaCl 0.9% to dilute substance.
- Inject antispasmodic: traditional advice is to infuse papaverine 40–80 mg. Other suggestions have included prostacyclin at rate of 1 μg min^{-1}, tolazoline (noradrenaline antagonist) and phenoxybenzamine. Sound though the recommendation may be, these drugs may well not be immediately available, and this advice may be impractical.
- Dexamethasone 8 mg stat may reduce arterial oedema.
- Sympathetic block: stellate ganglion (SGB) or brachial plexus. Stellate ganglion block is probably quicker to perform but will not provide the analgesia afforded by a brachial plexus block. Optimal management is probably immediate SGB followed by axillary (or femoral) catheter placement to allow continuous analgesia and vasodilatation.
- Maintenance anticoagulation is recommended for up to 14 days. Hyperbaric oxygen has also been suggested as a means of minimising final ischaemic damage.

Marking points: Clinical experience of this event is not extensive, but it will aid your credibility if you do convey a pragmatic and realistic clinical approach to the problem rather than simply repeating a list of often impractical recommendations. When did you last see an ampoule of papaverine? You must demonstrate that you can recognise the mishap when it occurs.

Describe the complications of tracheal intubation.

This is essential knowledge for anaesthetists and so this question should present no problems apart from the requirement to describe the complications in some order of priority.

Introduction

Tracheal intubation is perceived, at least by non-anaesthetists, as the core anaesthetic skill. It is certainly a routine procedure in anaesthetic practice, but it does also carry with it the potential to cause untold harm.

A tracheal tube bypasses every natural protective reflex of the airway by means of neuromuscular paralysis or profound anaesthesia. There are potential problems, therefore, with the tube itself, with the mechanics of its insertion, and with the drugs that are required to allow its placement.

Complications associated with the tube

- Oesophageal intubation. Should this go unrecognised the patient will proceed to hypoxic cardiac arrest and death, or suffer disastrous neurological damage. This is the most catastrophic complication of anaesthesia, not least because it is avoidable. Patients die because of a failure to oxygenate, not intubate.
- Disconnection. A secondary complication, but as important as tube misplacement. Unrecognised disconnection will have the same disastrous consequences.
- Endobronchial placement. Hypoxia will ensue if not corrected.
- Obstruction. Herniation of cuff, kinking of tube, obstruction within tube.
- Airway stimulation. Laryngospasm, bronchoconstriction.
- Trauma
  - Tears in mucosa of oesophagus, larynx, trachea: cause mediastinal emphysema.
  - Airway perforation.
  - Arytenoid cartilage dislocation.
  - Nasal tubes may dissect posteriorly and pass down the posterior pharyngeal wall: bacteraemia occurs in ~5% of patients after nasal intubation.
  - Cribriform plate perforation has been reported.
  - Sore throat and hoarseness are common.
- Pressure effects: due to the tube. The shape of a standard ETT may exert substantial pressure on the arytenoid cartilages, the posterior part of the vocal cords and the posterior tracheal wall. The tube is fixed externally (usually) and so movement of the tube occurs with each breath, and with any head movement.
- Pressure effects: due to the cuff. Less of a problem with low pressure, high volume cuffs, but these provide a less secure seal against airway contaminants. May be over-inflated if lung compliance is low (high airways pressure and leak back past the cuff). May cause nerve injury due to pressure on branches of the recurrent laryngeal nerve.
- Physiological trespass. An ETT is a conduit which bypasses normal airway reflexes and protective mechanisms. These include normal humidification. Dry and cool gases increase evaporative loss of heat and moisture. The ETT is also a potential conduit for debris, and a site for ignition during laser surgery.
- Effects of long term intubation (ITU). Trauma and pressure effects may lead to trauma, ulceration, healing with fibrotic scar tissue (causes stenosis), granulomas or with formation of webs over the injured areas. Erosion into the airway may occur. Vocal cord damage with paresis/paralysis, recurrent laryngeal nerve injury. Damage is commonest at the posterior laryngeal wall.

Complications associated with the mechanics of insertion (laryngoscopy and adjuncts)

- Pressor response. Laryngoscopy and intubation provoke intense sympathetic stimulation with tachycardia, possible tachyarrhythmias and hypertension. Important in patients with ischaemic heart disease, hypertension, hypertension of pregnancy.
- Neck extension. Traditional warnings have been given about patients with atlanto-axial instability (rheumatoid arthritis, Down syndrome, etc.) although current thinking suggests that the risk of spinal cord damage is overstated.
- Trauma. Lips, teeth, oropharynx and larynx. Introducers, stillettes and bougies may contribute to trauma and may also perforate the airway.
- Barotrauma. Intubation facilitates the delivery of high pressures directly to the airway.

Drugs

- The bypass of the potent normal airway protective reflexes requires neuromuscular blockade or profound anaesthesia.
- There is a large range of potential complications associated with neuromuscular blocking agents, particularly suxamethonium (anaphylaxis, autonomic effects, myalgia, apnoea), and with deep inhalational anaesthesia in individuals with cardiorespiratory disease.

Marking points: You will not have time to detail every recorded complication. It does not matter how you classify your answer but you must include those complications that are associated with the most serious outcomes.

Describe the anaesthetic management of a patient undergoing elective thyroid surgery.

Assessment of the patient for thyroid surgery involves some perioperative medicine and an airway that might prove problematical throughout the operative period. It is therefore a topic of obvious interest to anaesthetists.

Introduction

Anaesthesia for thyroid surgery can be challenging, particularly if it is complicated by endocrine instability or a large goitre which compromises the airway.

Preoperative assessment

- Is there evidence of deranged thyroid function?
- **Hyperthyroidism**
  — Thyrotoxicosis is a hypermetabolic state.
  — Cardiac output increases: tachycardia, tachyarrhythmias (atrial fibrillation) and signs of decompensation (left ventricular hypertrophy, failure).
  — Impairment of adrenal function and increased drug metabolism.
  — Patients should be euthyroid before surgery.
- **Hypothyroidism**
  — Myxoedema is a hypometabolic state with more serious implications.
  — Myocardial dysfunction is common and may be severe.
  — Respiratory depression with increased sensitivity to depressant drugs.
  — Anaemia and decreased blood volume.
  — CNS depression: at worst – myxoedema coma.
  — Hypoglycaemia, hyponatraemia and adrenal inadequacy.
  — Patients must be euthyroid before surgery.

Is there evidence of airway compromise?

- Symptoms of respiratory obstruction (positional, associated with exertion, etc.).
- Associated symptoms: dysphagia.
- Signs: goitre, impairment of neck mobility, etc. (standard airway assessment).
- Investigations:
  — CXR : evidence of tracheal compression and deviation.
  — Thoracic inlet views (lateral): show A–P tracheal abnormalities.
  — CT scan: for retrosternal thyroid swelling.
  — MR imaging: gives excellent views of the soft tissues in all planes.

Intraoperative considerations

- **Airway management**
  — Tracheal intubation (technique will depend on airway assessment, but may be fibreoptic) with an appropriate tube, e.g. armoured or pre-formed north-facing is commonly used because it secures the potentially vulnerable airway. The laryngeal mask airway is also favoured by some anaesthetists because it allows much better assessment of vocal cord function.
- **Patient positioning**
  — Head is extended and draped. Customary precautions should be taken (secure connections, padding of areas) for the patient whose airway is isolated from the anaesthetist. Exophthalmic eyes will require special protection.
- **Surgical problems**
  — Carotid sinus stimulation may affect baroreceptors and cause arterial pressure instability.
  — Blood loss may be significant, particularly from a large vascular goitre.
  — Pneumothorax: uncommon.

- **Injuries to the laryngeal nerves**
  - — Recurrent laryngeal nerve: supplies the muscles which control the laryngeal inlet.
  - — If both nerves are damaged then both cords oppose or overlap in the midline. This leads to inspiratory stridor and potentially to total obstruction.
  - — Partial paralysis affects the abductors more than the adductors, with unilateral injury the corresponding vocal cord is paralysed. Results in hoarseness.
  - — If one or both nerves are transected the vocal cord(s) adopt the cadaveric position in which they are partially abducted and through which airflow is less compromised. Phonation, however, may be reduced to a whisper.
  - — External branch of the superior laryngeal nerve: supplies the cricothyroid muscle which tenses the vocal cords. Damage causes hoarseness. If unilateral this will be temporary (the other cricothyroid will compensate); if bilateral it will be permanent.

Postoperative considerations
- **Airway obstruction**
  - — Haematoma formation.
  - — Laryngeal oedema.
  - — Tracheomalacia caused by pressure of chronic goitre.
- **Tetany**
  - — Inadvertent parathyroid resection causes hypocalcaemia and tetany.
  - — May also be accompanied by laryngospasm.
  - — Uncommon complication.

Marking points: The important factors that you should cover are the assessment of endocrine status, the assessment of the airway and the prediction of important potential postoperative problems.

A 45-year-old woman with type 1 diabetes mellitus which is controlled by insulin requires total abdominal hysterectomy. Describe the anaesthetic management.

Diabetes mellitus affects up to 4% of individuals in industrialised countries and it is curious, therefore, that there is no consensus about optimal perioperative management. This question assesses your appreciation of the associated medical problems and requires you to suggest a credible and safe regimen for glycaemic control.

Introduction

Diabetes mellitus is a heterogeneous group of endocrine disorders in which the common feature is a relative or absolute absence of insulin. The resulting disorder of glucose metabolism affects all body systems, the most important of which from the anaesthetist's point of view are the cardiovascular, renal and autonomic complications that may ensue.

Associated complications

- **Coronary and cerebrovascular disease**
  - — Incidence is 4–5× that of the non-diabetic population.
  - — Hypertension in ~40% of those with poor control.
  - — 'Silent ischaemia' may occur in the presence of other risk factors.
  - — Peripheral and cerebrovascular disease are common.
- **Renal dysfunction**
  - — Diabetic nephropathy is the main cause of end-stage renal failure, and affects >30% of all patients with type 1 disease.
  - — Intraoperatively renal function must not be worsened by hypovolaemic hypoperfusion or the use of prostaglandin inhibitors such as NSAIDs.
- **Autonomic neuropathy**
  - — Affects up to 40% of type 1 diabetics.
  - — Causes gastroparesis (implications for pulmonary aspiration).
  - — May cause cardiac and respiratory instability.
- **Musculoskeletal**
  - — High glucose levels causes glycosylation of collagen in cervical joints ('stiff joint syndrome') which may predispose to difficult intubation.
- **Infection**
  - — Occult infection is said to be present in 17% of diabetics: worsens glycaemic control.
- **Glycaemic control**
  - — Patient is the best guide to their normal glycaemic status.
  - — Glycosylated Hb (HbAc$_1$) indicates recent (1–2 months) control. Level of >8% suggests probable microvascular complications.

Anaesthetic management

- Anaesthetic technique need not be modified except in some relatively minor aspects:
  - — Use of epidural analgesia (if acceptable) is likely to shorten resumption of oral intake (earlier ambulation, less postoperative nausea and vomiting (PONV) compared with PCA).
  - — Beware influence of autonomic neuropathy and increased infection risks.
  - — Avoidance of NSAIDs as adjuncts in 'balanced analgesia'.
  - — Avoidance of Hartmann's solution (lactate is gluconeogenic).

Glycaemic control

- **Stress response.** Surgery induces the 'stress response' with the secretion of catabolic hormones (epiephrine (adrenaline), cortisol, glucagon, growth hormone, etc. and promotion of glycogenolysis, gluconeogenesis, proteolysis and lipolysis).

These hormones are counter-regulatory in that they oppose the actions of insulin.

- **Goals of therapy.** These should be to:
  — Achieve normoglycaemia (not mild hyperglycaemia) and to avoid protein catabolism.
  — Avoid electrolyte disturbance and ketoacidosis.
  — Avoid significant glycosuria and osmotic diuresis with dehydration and electrolyte loss.
- **Diabetic regimens:** various options exist but there is no consensus as to that which is best.
- **Glucose-potassium-insulin (GKI)**
  — Inherent safety of simultaneous infusion of insulin with glucose. Typical is the 'Alberti' regimen in which a GKI mixture of glucose 5% or 10% plus KCl 10 mmol is infused at 100 ml hr^{-1} with the contents adjusted according to blood glucose.
  — If glucose is: <5 mmol l^{-1} add 10 units (Actrapid); 5–12 mmol l^{-1} add 16 units; >13 mmol l^{-1} add 20 units.
  — This regimen is safe and simple, but has the disadvantages of excessive fluid loading and the need for frequent infusion changes if glucose concentration is unstable.
- **Variable rate infusion of insulin**
  — Separate intravenous infusion of insulin alone.
  — Start rate at 1 unit h^{-1} and increase as indicated (requirements vary widely).
  — Simultaneous infusion of glucose at rate of ~5 g for every 2 units of insulin infused.
  — Requires high level of supervision but offers better glucose control.
- **Subcutaneous insulin and sliding scale**
  — Not recommended. Absorption is variable and a sliding scale is destined to fail because it is essentially retrospective. A fixed dose is given according to a blood glucose reading which is historical. Likely to be very inaccurate.

Marking points: You should give an overview of the important coexisting problems and provide a safe and credible insulin regimen for glycaemic control. The question does not ask you to discuss the different options, but it is worth justifying briefly the technique that you use.

What is the anaesthetist's contribution to safe intraocular surgery under general anaesthesia?

The trend in intraocular surgery is away from general and towards day-case local anaesthesia, but there remains a core group which includes patients who are unable to lie flat (COPD or heart disease) or to lie still (Parkinson's tremor) who require general anaesthesia. This question asesses your ability to identify the criteria for safe intraocular surgery.

Introduction

Intraocular surgery is performed increasingly on patients using local anaesthesia, but in the dwindling group of patients who present for ophthalmic surgery under general anaesthesia for mainly medical reasons, it is even more important to satisfy the criteria for safe intraocular surgery.

Operative conditions

- **Position**
  - The eye should be akinetic and fixed in neutral gaze. Traction sutures necessitated by divergence may distort subtly the anatomy of the anterior eye.
- **Analgesia**
  - Ophthalmic surgery is not systemically disturbing. The cornea, conjunctiva and iris, however, are acutely sensitive. Profound analgesia of this local area is necessary to prevent reflex responses (and movement if the patient is not paralysed).
- **Absence of bleeding**
  - Local bleeding may complicate intraocular surgery, although it rarely contributes to an adverse outcome. It will be minimised if the anaesthetist can present the surgeon with a still, quiet operative field. Tachycardia and hypertension militate against that ambition. Care should be taken if anticholinergic drugs are given to obtund the oculo-cardiac reflex lest a hyperdynamic circulation results.
- **Smooth induction and eduction of anaesthesia**
  - Coughing, straining, partial airway obstruction, laryngospasm, vomiting, etc. are all factors which raise intraocular pressure and should be avoided.
- **Intraocular pressure (IOP)**
  - In vitreo-retinal intraocular work the surgeon controls IOP manometrically through a sealed infusion port in the pars plana, and so anaesthetic factors are less relevant. The exception is the situation in which a gas, typically sulphur hexafluoride (SF_6), replaces the vitreous. Nitrous oxide will increase the pressure in the gas bubble and should be discontinued before it is injected.
  - In other intraocular work IOP is important. Normal pressure is 10–22 mmHg and its prime determinants are:
  Choroidal blood flow and volume (influenced by P_aCO_2, venous drainage, hypoxia).
  Formation and drainage of aqueous humour (impaired in glaucoma and also influenced by venous pressure).
  External pressure on globe by contraction of extraocular muscles and of the orbicularis oculi muscle (or by local anaesthetic solution).
  - Coughing, straining, vomiting, etc. will increase the IOP by 40 mmHg or more.
  - Implications: if IOP is already high in glaucoma, further rises can precipitate acute crisis. If IOP is high and the globe is penetrated, expulsive haemorrhage may result. Once the eye is open IOP becomes atmospheric

and sudden pressure increases may cause vitreous loss or prolapse of the iris and the lens.

Implications for anaesthetic technique (summary)

- Avoid airway obstruction, coughing, Valsalva maneouvre, vomiting.
- Avoid venous obstruction and ensure good drainage (slight head-up tilt if surgically feasible).
- Avoid hypoxaemia.
- Avoid hypercarbia.
- Avoid suxamethonium (transient IOP rise due to extraocular muscle fasciculation).
- Acetazolamide and mannitol to reduce aqueous and vitreous humour volumes (if needed).
- Maintain quiet, still eye and a tranquil circulation.

Marking points: You need to know the main determinants of IOP pressure because from that you can work out the rest of this answer. Textbooks continue to emphasise the importance of a low P_aco_2, although many anaesthetists favour the use of the laryngeal mask airway and spontaneous ventilation in which the $ETCO_2$ can rise significantly. Surgeons do not generally complain, either because they are used to operating with a higher IOP caused by intraorbital local anaesthetic, or because it is the tranquil circulation that is responsible for good operating conditions. If you are confident enough in your own practice to cite these factors rather than following the traditional line then do so.

Anaesthesia and medical disease

A patient who has undergone heart transplantation requires non-cardiac surgery. What problems may this present for the anaesthetist?

Heart transplantation is well established and it is increasingly common for patients to present for non-cardiac surgery. The difficulties that such patients present are in fact quite modest, but it is important for anaesthetists to appreciate the physiological implications.

Introduction
Long-term survival after cardiac transplantation is continuing to improve and it is increasingly frequent for patients to present for non-cardiac surgery. Anaesthetic problems are related to the natural history of the transplanted heart, to its altered physiology and to the effects of the necessary immunosuppressive drug regimens.

Natural history of the transplanted heart
- **Heart transplantation is a treatment for end-stage cardiac disease**
  - In some patients, for example those with hyperlipidaemias, the underlying diathesis persists and may continue to affect coronary artery patency.
  - Graft atherosclerosis may also be accelerated by the chronic rejection process and so patients must be assumed to have coronary artery disease.
  - Transplanted hearts are denervated and so patients do not usually suffer from warning signs of angina pectoris (some believe that residual reinnervation can eventually occur).

Physiological changes
  - The donor heart is usually anastomosed to a residual atrium which retains its innervation, and whose activity may be discernible as a p wave on the ECG. The heart otherwise is denervated and lacks efferent and afferent components of parasympathetic and sympathetic nervous systems.
- **Sympathetic effects**
  - Although there is no neuronal supply the transplanted heart responds normally to circulating catecholamines. Sympathetically mediated tachycardia will take some minutes to develop and the effects of exogenous

inotropes and vasopressors will also be delayed.
— The Starling mechanism ensures that the cardiac response to stress is maintained. As left ventricular end-diastolic volume (LVEDV) increases so do cardiac contractility and cardiac ouput. This mechanism is very dependent on venous return and it is crucial to avoid hypovolaemia. The heart does not respond rapidly to changes in SVR.

- **Parasympathetic effects**
  — Vagal effects are absent.
  — Muscarinic bradycardias due to drugs such as anticholinesterases are absent.
  — The heart does not respond to atropine or to other vagolytics: a desired increase in rate will require directly acting agents (e.g. isoprenaline) or pacing.

Drug regimens

- Patients take long-term immunosuppressive drugs, typically:
  — Cyclosporin (check renal and hepatic function).
  — Corticosteroids (wide range of effects from diabetes to osteoporosis).
  — Azathioprine (check haematology).

Marking points: Problems with patients with transplanted hearts can be overstated, but they do follow from a logical consideration of the pathophysiological changes that are involved. Given that such patients do present for surgery outside specialist centres a broad overview of the subject will be expected.

What are the anaesthetic implications of dystrophia myotonica?

Dystrophia myotonica is one of the commonest muscular dystrophies (~1 in 20 000) and it involves a wide range of systems. It has wide-ranging implications for anaesthesia about which clinicians should be aware.

Introduction

Dystrophia myotonica is one of the commonest muscular dystrophies. It is inherited as an autosomal dominant disorder and has an incidence of about 1 in 20 000. It is a multisystem disease which is slowly progressive and usually presents between the second and fourth decades of life. The systems and the anaesthetic implications are outlined as follows:

- **Skeletal muscle**
    - Myotonia describes persistent contraction after voluntary use or stimulation.
    - The site of the myotonia is the muscle fibre itself: there are probably several gene defects but at least one causes abnormalities of Na^+ conductance in the cell.
    - Depolarising muscle relaxants lead to sustained contracture.
    - Response to non-depolarising relaxants is very unpredictable.
- **Smooth muscle**
    - Abnormalities lead to bulbar muscle weakness (dysphagia and aspiration), to reduced oesophageal motility and delayed gastric emptying.
- **Cardiac muscle**
    - Involvement leads to conduction defects and arrhythmias, and cardiomyopathy (In some patients cardiac function improves with exercise.)
- **Respiratory problems**
    - May be chronic hypoventilation and respiratory muscle weakness. There is fatigue of intercostals trying to overcome myotonic contraction of abdominal respiratory muscles.
    - Pulmonary aspiration due to bulbar weakness.
    - Primary CNS effects leading to somnolence.
    - Sensitive to respiratory depressant effects of all hypnotics, sedatives and narcotics.
- **Associated endocrine disorders**
    - Include dysfunction of thyroid and adrenal glands, and gonads. Associated diabetes mellitus is due to insulin resistance and reduced number of insulin receptors.

Anaesthetic implications

- Preoperative assessment of cardiorespiratory status is essential.
- Induction: reduce dose of hypnotic; avoid depolarising muscle relaxants; antacids to reduce problem if aspiration occurs; airway must be secured rapidly.
- Maintenance: keep warm (cold may act as myotonic trigger): expect unpredictable response to muscle relaxants (may not work at all); expect opioids to have marked respiratory depressant effect. Use regional/local anaesthesia wherever feasible.
- End of surgery: avoid anticholinesterase drugs (myotonic trigger); have low threshold for postoperative care, nurse in intensive care or at the very least a high dependency unit.

Marking points: The condition is rare but important, and has a number of significant anaesthetic implications. You must be able to demonstrate that you could anaesthetise such an individual safely.

What are the anaesthetic considerations in a patient with autonomic neuropathy?

Autonomic neuropathy may be associated with other conditions such as diabetes and alcoholism, or may be a rare primary condition such as the Shy–Drager syndrome or familial dysautonomia. This question is not testing your grasp of rarities but is exploring your basic knowledge about the importance of the autonomic nervous system in anaesthesia.

Introduction

The functions of the autonomic nervous system in maintaining homeostasis are never more obvious than when they are absent due to congenital or acquired autonomic neuropathy. Predisposing causes may further complicate the picture, but the consequences of autonomic failure are essentially the same.

Predisposing causes

- Diabetes mellitus, chronic alcoholism, nutritional deficiencies, Guillain–Barré syndrome, Parkinson's disease and AIDS are among conditions which may lead to autonomic neuropathy.
- Anaesthetic management will be influenced accordingly.

Diagnosis

- Family history (congenital) and medical history as above may suggest diagnosis.
- Signs and symptoms include:
    — Orthostatic hypotension (no reflex pressor response to maintain CVS stability).
    — Labile blood pressure.
    — Flushing.
    — Erratic temperature control (night sweats).
    — Episodic diarrhoea; nocturnal diuresis and sodium loss (loss of diurnal rhythms).
    — Loss of response to hypoglycaemia.
    — Abnormal response to Valsalva manoeuvre.
    — Absence of sinus arrhythmia.

Anaesthetic considerations

- Hypotension on induction: sudden cardiac arrest has been described – full monitoring is mandatory – diabetics and other groups may have silent cardiac ischaemia.
- May be more sensitive to analgesics (? pain perception altered).
- Gastroparesis (antacids and airway protection).
- Care with fluid management: tolerate hypovolaemia badly.
- Ventilation: are prone to atelectasis and may need IPPV.
- Positioning: loss of reflexes mandates care – changes of posture tolerated poorly.
- Response to cautious administration of vasoactive drugs (e.g. atropine and vasopressors) is similar to normal patients.
- Temperature control: continuous monitoring required.

Marking points: The main purpose of this question is to determine whether you know the diagnostic features of autonomic neuropathy, whatever the cause, and are able to adapt your anaesthetic technique safely to accommodate the likely consequences.

Describe your management of a patient who requires surgical removal of a phaeochromocytoma.

This is an uncommon but important condition which is challenging anaesthetically, and which requires the rational use of applied pharmacology. This alone has made phaeochromocytoma a popular examination topic. 'Management' includes preoperative medical management.

Introduction
Phaeochromocytoma is a rare tumour of chromaffin cells which in over 90% of cases arises from the adrenal medulla. The tumours secrete norepinephrine (noradrenaline), epinephrine (adrenaline) or dopamine into the circulation, and the presenting features reflect which of these catecholamines predominates. Norepinephrine-secreting tumours commonly present with severe and refractory hypertension, while epinephrine- and dopamine-secreting tumours may lead to paroxysmal tachycardias and episodic attacks of high anxiety and features of sympathetic hyperactivity. Individual tumours secrete catecholamines in different proportions and the clinical features vary accordingly.

Preoperative management
- **Assess end-organ hypertensive damage:** particularly myocardium and kidneys.
- **Pharmacological control:** hypertension and arrythymias and to restore normovolaemia.
  - Alpha-adrenoceptor antagonists (alpha-blockers): traditionally phenoxybenzamine which binds irreversibly to receptors. Its actions may therefore persist well into the postoperative period. It is non-selective and by blocking presynaptic alpha$_2$-receptors removes the feedback inhibition to norepinephrine release. Central effects may cause sedation. An alternative is doxazosin (selective alpha$_1$-blocker) in once daily dose.
  - Beta-adrenoceptor antagonists (beta-blockers) to control tachycardia (epinephrine/dopamine tumours and also after phenoxybenzamine). Common choice is labetalol (alpha- and beta-blocker).
  - Magnesium sulphate (reduces catecholamine release) has also been advocated in place of adrenoceptor blockade.

Anaesthetic management
- Discontinue adrenoceptor antagonists ~12 hours preoperatively: the aim is to produce CVS stability (until tumour is handled).
- Monitoring: direct intra-arterial and central venous pressure is essential in addition to standard monitoring.
- Induction of anaesthesia after volaemic status is confirmed adequate.
- Analgesia: regional – thoracic epidural (very effective) or high dose opioid (may partly depend on surgical approach: open or laparoscopic).
- CVS control during tumour manipulation: may get norepinephrine surge with marked pressor response, or epinephrine/dopamine response with tachycardia/tachyarrhythmias. Treat with e.g. the alpha-blocker phentolamine and/or a beta-blocker, e.g labetalol or short-acting esmolol.

Postoperative management
- Main postoperative problem: persistent hypotension.
  - Persistent effect of phenoxybenzamine (refractory to alpha-agonists and which may require excessive fluid administration).
  - Suppression by tumour activity of contralateral adrenal output, plus receptor down-regulation.
  - May need inotrope infusion, e.g. norepinephrine as appropriate to maintain BP.

- Invasive monitoring must continue postoperatively and patients should be nursed in a high dependency or intensive care unit.

Marking points: Important safety points are preoperative treatment and intravascular resuscitation, invasive monitoring, management during tumour handling and targeted postoperative care. The condition is rare, but the question is common and predictable.

A patient who is HIV seropositive is scheduled for laparotomy. What factors determine the risks of transmission to anaesthetic staff? How may this risk be minimised?

Infectious diseases, particularly conditions such as hepatitis B and C, tuberculosis and HIV, pose significant and increasing risks to healthcare workers. This question tests both your appreciation of the particular risk associated with HIV, as well as the safety of your approach.

Introduction

HIV / AIDS is one of a number of infectious diseases, among them hepatitis B and C, and tuberculosis, which pose increasing risks to healthcare workers. Risks in the UK are much less than say in sub-Saharan Africa or in New York City, but it is important to appreciate that theatre staff are a group at increased risk.

- **Infective agent.** The virus responsible for HIV / AIDS appears to be present in all bodily fluids of infected subjects, and has been isolated from, amongst others, blood, semen, saliva, CSF, tears, urine and amniotic fluid.
- **Infectivity.** Compared with hepatitis B a substantial viral inoculum is required before acute seroconversion will occur. The two main routes of infection are by needlestick injury or by splashing of fluids on mucous membrane or broken skin.
- **Risks.** Increased with increasing prevalence in the surgical population that is being served.
- **Risk of needlestick injury.** This can occur due to carelessness, to failure properly to dispose of contaminated sharps, and to engage in potential hazardous procedures such as resheathing needles after use. The worst type of needlestick injury would appear to be a deep subcutaneous or intramuscular stab. A hollow needle is likely to bear a larger inoculum than a solid one. A single stab carries a 0.3% chance of transmission.
- **Risk of splashing by contaminated fluids.** All fluids potentially are contaminated and an individual is at risk if broken skin is exposed or if mucous membranes are unprotected. The risk of transmission is much lower than after needlestick and is estimated at 0.09%.
- **Universal precautions.** These risks can be minimised by the use of universal precautions which, some argue, should be employed routinely for all cases. Such was the recommendation in 1987 by the Centre of Disease Control (CDC) in Atlanta, USA. The precautions of particular relevance to the anaesthetist include:
  — Use of gloves. A needlestick through a single layer of glove is associated with a 10–100-fold decrease in inoculation risk.
  — Use of masks and visors to protect mucous membranes.
  — Safe and immediate disposable of all sharps.
  — No recapping of needles.
  — Use of sealed suction bottles with immediate disposal of all bodily fluids.
- **Postexposure prophylaxis**
  — Should begin within 1–2 hours after exposure, although can still be initiated 1–2 weeks after the incident.
  — Typical regimen includes three antiretroviral agents. Toxicity and non-compliance may be problems.

Marking points: Anaesthetists should know about this for their own protection. For the purpose of this answer do not focus too greatly on universal precautions: some of the information specific to HIV will be required.

A 20-year-old patient requires open reduction and fixation of a forearm fracture sustained 12 hours previously. He has sickle cell disease. Describe the anaesthetic management.

This is a straightforward scenario which tests the safe perioperative management of an important condition.

Introduction

Sickle cell disease is a disorder of abnormal haemoglobin synthesis which involves a single amino acid substitution on the beta chain of haemoglobin, with the production of Haemoglobin S (HbS). Individuals who are homozygous for S beta-globin chains have sickle cell disease. The abnormal HbS is believed to protect erythrocytes from invasion by the malaria parasite, but this potential survival advantage is offset by the fact that red cells 'sickle' into distorted shapes when exposed to oxygen tensions of less than 5.3 kPa (40 mmHg). This has clear implications for anaesthetic management.

Preoperative management

- **End-organ effects of repeated sickling: history, examination and investigations**
  — Cardiovascular: left ventricular hypertrophy and cardiomegaly are common by age 20.
  — Respiratory: pulmonary infarction and atelectasis.
  — Central nervous system: vaso-occlusion and thrombosis cause neurological deficits.
  — Renal: medullary infarction, loss of concentrating ability.
  — Reticulo-endothelial system: autoinfarction of the spleen and hyposplenism.
  — Haematology: FBC will show anaemia, typically 6–8 g dl⁻¹.
- **History, examination and investigations**
  — Exclusion of other injury.
  — Assess volaemic status (may be dehydrated if fasted for emergency surgery).
- **Preoperative transfusion**
  — Consult haematologist to discuss case.
  — Transfusion: exchange (to achieve HbS <40%) or top-up (Hb 10–12 g dl⁻¹) is contentious. Evidence suggests it should be reserved for thoracotomy, laparotomy (and adenotonsillectomy) and not used for peripheral surgery.

Perioperative management

Details of technique are less important than the fundamental principles:

- **Ensure oxygenation** (above 5.3 kPa in all parts of the circulation)
  — Humidified oxygen throughout and into the postoperative period.
- **Avoid hypothermia** (contributes to sickling)
  — Vigorous warming throughout and into the postoperative period.
- **Avoid low flow or stasis in circulation**
  — Adequate hydration (warm fluid) throughout and into the postoperative period.
  — Avoid arterial tourniquets.
  — Position to avoid stasis in limbs or dependent parts of circulation.
- **Avoid acidosis**
  — Hypercarbia may contribute.
- **Ensure adequate analgesia**
  — Unrelieved pain has undesirable cardiorespiratory sequelae (oxygen consumption and catecholamine release).

Anaesthetic options

- **General anaesthesia**
  — Must incorporate principles above, but various options are acceptable.

- **Local anaesthesia**
  - Must incorporate principles above, so intravenous regional anaesthesia is not an option.
  - Brachial plexus block will provide good analgesia (could continue postoperatively with axillary catheter) and vasodilatation. Axillary block may need supplementation if the musculocutaneous nerve is spared.
- **Antibiotic treatment**
  - Hyposplenism is associated with increased infection risk.

Marking points: This is an important safety question and the underlying principles of management must be covered. If your perioperative management contains any omission or commission that would risk precipitation of a sickling crisis then you will fail the question.

A 38-year-old woman requires total abdominal hysterectomy. She has multiple sclerosis. How does this influence your anaesthetic management?

Multiple sclerosis (MS) is the most common demyelinating disease and is more prevalent in northern latitudes. The anaesthetic implications are relatively modest but with a relapsing neurological disorder there is always concern about the use of regional nerve blocks, and this is a condition with which you should be familiar.

Introduction

Multiple sclerosis (MS) is a demyelinating disorder which is characterised by unpredictable episodes of remission and exacerbation of symptoms. Demyelination does not occur in specific areas and so patients exhibit a wide spectrum of neurological deficit.

Preoperative assessment

- **Disability.** Assessment of degree of disability and pattern of symptoms: cardiovascular and respiratory problems per se are not usually a feature of the disease.
- **Drug therapy.** There is no specific treatment, but patients may be on a variety of therapies which may include ACTH or corticosteroids, immunosuppressives, interferon or cannabinoids (for pain).
- **Investigations.** No specific investigations are indicated.
- **Relapses.** These can be provoked by surgical and other trauma, emotional stress, infection, pregnancy (not probable in this case) and increases in body temperature (as little as 0.5°C) which can block conduction in impaired neurones.
- **Prognosis.** The unpredictable nature of MS and these factors above mandate careful discussion with the patient about the likely influence of anaesthesia and surgery on the natural history of their disease. This is especially important if peripheral nerve or central neuraxial block is contemplated.

Perioperative management

- General anaesthetic agents for induction and maintenance do not exacerbate the disease.
- Patients with severe disease associated with muscle atrophy may have a hyperkalemic response to suxamethonium.
- Non-depolarising muscle relaxants can be used without problems.
- Anticholinergic drugs should be avoided on the theoretical grounds that they may cause pyrexia.
- There must be scrupulous attention to temperature control.
- Any prodromal symptoms / signs of infection should be treated aggressively.
- Regional anaesthesia is contentious. Some authorities believe that the loss of myelin in the spinal cord renders it more vulnerable to histotoxic change due to local anaesthetics, although there are several clinical studies which suggest that the incidence of relapse is no more common after spinal anaesthesia. Peripheral nerve blocks and extradural blocks theoretically present less of a potential risk. Intrathecal opioids do not exacerbate symptoms. The issue should be discussed in full with the patient.
- It is sensible to conduct a postoperative neurological review to document any changes in symptoms.

> **Marking points:** MS is common and the important management points in this answer are the avoidance of even mild hyperthermia, the avoidance of suxamethonium in the presence of muscle wasting and the necessity for full preoperative discussion with the patient.

A 75-year-old man with chronic obstructive airways disease requires a transurethral resection of the prostate. Outline the advantages and disadvantages of subarachnoid anaesthesia for this patient.

This question does not require a general generic discussion of the advantages and disadvantages of spinal anaesthesia. You should focus your answer round the fact that the patient has chronic obstructive pulmonary disease. Both the surgical condition and the medical disease are common.

Introduction
Transurethral urology lends itself well to regional anaesthesia, but despite this not all urological surgeons share the anaesthetists' enthusiasm and if given a choice prefer general anaesthesia. Coexisting pulmonary disease makes the arguments in favour of subarachnoid or extradural analgesia more persuasive, although there remain some disadvantages.

- **In the patient with COPD: main advantages lie in avoidance of general anaesthesia**
  — Full control of the airway and breathing.
  — No airway instrumentation with the attendant risk of provoking bronchoconstriction.
  — No risk of barotrauma (pneumothorax) with IPPV.
  — No respiratory depression.
  — No difficulty in resumption of adequate spontaneous ventilation.
  — Lower risk of postoperative chest infection.
- **Advantages specific for TURP**
  — Earlier and easier detection of the TURP syndrome.
- **Generic advantages of the technique**
  — Possible lower risk of venous embolism.
  — Good postoperative analgesia (although pain after TURP is not usually severe).
- **In the patient with COPD the disadvantages of spinal anaesthesia include:**
  — Respiratory compromise if the block spreads to involve the intercostal muscles.
  — Patients with COPD may find it difficult to lie flat.
  — Persistent coughing will interfere with surgery.
- **Generic disadvantages of the technique:**
  — Hypotension (in an elderly age group).
  — Unsuitable for the restless or uncooperative patient.
  — Some suggestion that there is increased fibrinolysis under subarachnoid block (SAB).
  — Risk of postdural puncture headache (small).

Marking points: It helps if the candidate gives some impression of having managed these conditions. You will not pass this question unless you focus on the coexisting pulmonary disease.

A 25-year-old intravenous drug abuser requires surgery for a compound tibial fracture. What problems may this present for the anaesthetist?

Substance abuse is very common, and some drug addicts can present a major anaesthetic challenge. Many do not, but the anaesthetist should be aware of the broad range of problems which may be encountered.

Introduction

Drug abuse is endemic, and although many individuals who take drugs may pass through relatively unnoticed there are some who present significant anaesthetic challenges.

Substances used

- A very wide range: opioids, cocaine, amphetamines (including methylene-dioxymethamphetamine, 'Ecstasy'), cannabis, benzodiazepines, solvents.
- Accurate (and truthful) history is usually hard to obtain.

Patient's affect

- Some drugs of abuse are associated with paranoia, but the subject, who may be stressed by withdrawal, may also be hostile, manipulative and uncooperative.

General health

- **Nutrition.** Frequently poor nutritional state, with anaemia and hepatic dysfunction.
- **Coexisting infection.** May have coexisting HIV, hepatitis B or C (and at risk of TB).
- **Contamination.** Injection of contaminated substances is associated with bacteraemias, myocarditis, endocarditis (tricuspid valve endocarditis has been described).
- **Poor oral hygiene.** Teeth may be at increased risk during airway maneouvres.
- **Venous access.** May be impossible due to widespread venous thrombosis (may have to resort to central veins).
- **Resistance.** May be resistant to CNS depressants (tolerance at cellular level).
- **Withdrawal.** Associated with acute autonomic hyperactivity. Management depends on specific drug history. This is not the time to withhold opioids if that is the class of drug to which the patient is addicted.
- **Anaesthesia in this case.** Options are as for any ORIF (open reduction and internal fixation):
  — GA plus opioid; GA plus peripheral nerve blockade.
  — GA plus extradural (may avoid postoperative problems with opioids).
  — Extradural or subarachnoid block alone (patient may not be phlegmatic enough to cooperate with these) or with target-controlled infusion for sedation.
- Intraoperative management
  — Titrate anaesthesia against response.
  — Patient should be assumed to be high risk and managed accordingly (protection of staff).
- Postoperative management
  — Withdrawal problems.
  — Analgesia: if patient rejects regional anaesthesia options, they may need higher dose opioids than usual. PCA may need to be reprogrammed. Security of the device is important.
  — It is usually simpler to permit an addict what they require to stay comfortable in the perioperative period. Drug rehabilitation can be considered thereafter.

Marking points: Many of these details are non-specific. Management of these individuals requires both an understanding of the main problems and an approach that is pragmatic and shows commonsense.

What features are important in the anaesthetic management of a patient with myasthenia gravis?

Myasthenia gravis is a rare disorder but is a popular examination topic because of its particular relevance for anaesthetists. There are few groups of patients whose main medication is a class of drug used predominantly in anaesthesia.

Introduction

Myasthenia gravis is an autoimmune disease of the neuromucular junction, in which IgG antibodies to the acetyl choline receptor reduce the number of functional receptors. Patients complain of muscular weakness which worsens with activity, and it is of particular anaesthetic relevance if respiratory or bulbar muscles are affected.

Associated disorders

- May influence management and should be excluded:
  - Autoimmune disorders: thyroid disease, collagen vascular diseases, diabetes mellitus, rheumatoid arthritis.
  - Myasthenic syndrome: associated with malignancy (Eaton–Lambert syndrome), classically carcinoma of the lung, the fatigue improves with exercise.

Anaesthetic considerations

- **Bulbar involvement**
  - Weakness will increase risk of pulmonary aspiration: may need rapid sequence induction. Myasthenia is said to make patients resistant to suxamethonium: a dose of 2 mg kg^{-1} reliably provides conditions for intubation as good as 1 mg kg^{-1} in those who are unaffected.
- **Respiratory weakness**
  - Decreases capacity to clear secretions.
  - Preoperative pulmonary function testing and physiotherapy is required.
  - Up to 30% may require postoperative ventilatory support (American data): some predictive factors include advanced generalised disease and steroid therapy; others are chronic respiratory disease; disease duration >6 years; VC <2.9 L; high dose preoperative anticholinesterase. Surgical procedure is clearly a crucial influence here.
- **Preoperative therapy**
  - Anticholinesterases: usually pyridostigmine (longer duration of action).
  - Steroids and other immunosuppressants are sometimes used.
  - Plasmapheresis occasionally used in the very weak patient prior to surgical treatment by thymectomy.

Perioperative management

- **Regional or local anaesthesia wherever possible.**
- **Anticholinesterase treatment.** Can continue oral anticholinesterase in which case patient may then need neuromuscular blocker, or omit and rely on propofol/opioid, or inhalational technique for tracheal intubation and subsequent relaxation.
- **Neuromuscular blockers**
  - Patients are very sensitive to their effects: should start at 10% of normal dose and expect very variable and unpredictable recovery.
  - Monitoring of neuromuscular function is essential.

Postoperative care

- HDU or ITU, not necessarily for IPPV but for good analgesia, physiotherapy and early intervention if necessary.
- Beware myasthenic or cholinergic crisis:

— Cholinergic crisis results from excessive anticholinesterase, manifest by excessive muscarinic activity (salivation, bronchorrhoea, diarrhoea, miosis, in addition to weakness).
— Myasthenic crisis due to relative underdose of anticholinesterase (may be provoked by infection, surgical stress): there are few muscarinic manifestations and pupils show mydriasis.

Marking points: Myasthenia gravis is rare but its management embodies some crucial safety points: preoperative assessment of respiratory/bulbar symptoms, care with neuromuscular blockers, postoperative specialist nursing, and the differentiation between myasthenic and cholinergic crises. You will be expected to comment on these.

A patient with hepatic porphyria requires general anaesthesia. Why may this be significant?

Porphyrias are not common in the UK, but the particular problems that some anaesthetic agents pose makes them of anaesthetic and examination interest. The biochemical details of haem biosynthesis are complex and details will not be required. There is also uncertainty about the precise relation between the enzymatic defects and the symptoms which makes a definitive answer more difficult. You will, however, be expected to know something about the scientific basis of the disorder, and in particular the dangers associated with certain anaesthetic drugs.

Introduction

The hepatic porphyrias are a heterogeneous group of disorders of porphyrin metabolism that are inherited as autosomal dominant conditions. There are acquired forms that are associated with liver disease and blood dyscrasias, but their manifestations are solely cutaneous. The symptoms of inherited porphyrias are variable but can be precipitated by exposure to various drugs, including some anaesthetic agents. These acute porphyrias include acute intermittent, variegate and hereditary coproporphyria.

Metabolic disorder

- Porphyrins are substances comprising four pyrrole rings which are essential for haem biosynthesis. Haem is a porphyrin–iron complex which can be synthesised in the mitochondria of all mammalian cells, and which is incorporated into haemoglobin and a large number of enzymes. These include the cytochromes, catalases and peroxidases.
- The initial biosynthetic steps include the formation of δ-amino-levulinic acid (ALA) which is catalysed by ALA synthetase (ALA-S). Beyond this step a number of porphyrin precursors of haem are synthesised. ALA-S is the rate-limiting enzyme in a unidirectional process.
- In hepatic porphyrias there are enzyme defects that affect different parts of the biosynthetic pathway distal to the formation of ALA. This appears to result in an inappropriate increase in ALA-S activity with the accumulation of haem precursors proximal to the enzyme block. (The block is only partial: haem biosynthesis is essential for life.)

Symptoms

- Acute attacks are associated with symptoms whose aetiology is unclear:
  - Neurological derangement: confusion, frank psychosis, coma, epilepsy, neuropathies (may be due to a defect in neural haem synthesis).
  - Cardiovascular instability: autonomic dysfunction, tachycardia, hypertension.
  - Respiratory system: may get weakness of respiratory muscles.
  - Gastrointestinal system: severe abdominal pain, nausea and vomiting.

Anaesthetic implications

- Acute attacks may be precipitated by dehydration (beware prolonged preoperative fasting), by infection, by hormonal changes (pregnancy and menstruation) and by some drugs.
- Drugs that are dangerous are those which induce the production of ALA synthetase and the formation of excess porphyrin haem precursors.
- The list of inducers is extremely long. Most patients have their own information leaflets which can be very useful, although it is easier for a pharmaceutical company to counsel caution than to state that a drug is definitely safe. Anaesthetic examples include:
  - Induction agents: barbiturates must be avoided. Propofol is safe.

— Inhalational agents: may induce ALA-S *in vitro*, but sevoflurane and desflurane are considered to be safe.
— Muscle relaxants: atracurium is safe (aminosteroids are probably safe, despite the fact that steroid hormones can be porphyrinogenic) alcuronium should not be used .
— Analgesics: most appear to be safe, pentazocine and clonidine are dubious.
— Local anaesthetics: avoid lidocaine (lignocaine) and its parent compound mepivacaine.
— Benzodiazepines: temazepam is safe.
— Anticholinesterases: safe.

Marking points: This is a complex disorder about which there is some uncertainty, which extends to the porphyrinogenicity of many drugs. You should at least be aware of the central importance of the enzyme ALA-S and of the salient features of a porphyric crisis should anaesthesia precipitate it.

A patient presenting for elective surgery is found to be anaemic. What are the implications for anaesthetic management?

Anaemia is common, and it used to be equally common for a haemoglobin concentration of less than 10 g dl^{-1} to trigger reflex cancellation of elective surgery and a request for transfusion. This question seeks a more considered approach to the problem.

Introduction
Anaemia may be a sign of serious intercurrent disease, and if it is severe, may decrease oxygen delivery to the tissues. At the very least oxygen delivery will be maintained only at the expense of increased cardiac output. The significance of anaemia, therefore, will depend on the age and physical status of the patient, as well as on the proposed surgery.

Causes
- Anaemia may be caused by mortal disease (e.g. malignancy) or simple dietary inadequacy. There are many possible causes which (ideally) should be identified:
  — Renal disease (urea and creatinine will be elevated).
  — Haematopoietic disease (blood picture and blood film).
  — Dietary inadequacy (decreased MCV).
  — Chronic blood loss, e.g. from uterine fibroids, from bladder pathology, because of NSAIDs (normochromic microcytic anaemia), malignancy, etc.
  — Dilutional because of increased plasma volume (pregnancy, athletes).

Management
- **Severity of the anaemia**
  — May be significant if patient has systemic or cardiac disease.
  — Symptoms may be associated with attempts to compensate: palpitations, headaches, dyspnoea, chest pain.
  — May be important if surgery involves significant blood loss.
- **Should the patient be transfused?**
  — O$_2$ delivery depends upon cardiac output (CO) and oxygen content (Hb × SpO$_2$% × 1.34).
  — At [Hb] <9 g dl^{-1} tissue oxygenation can be maintained only by increasing cardiac output, which provides the rationale for transfusion.
  — At [Hb] of 6 g dl^{-1} in the ASA grade I healthy patient (can compensate by increasing CO, but surgical blood loss may cause decompensation).
  — At [Hb] of 8 g dl^{-1} in the ASA grade II patient with controlled systemic disease (less reserve for increasing CO and greater requirement for O$_2$ delivery).
  — At [Hb] of 10 g dl^{-1} in the patient with symptomatic heart disease (increasing CO may cause unacceptable increase in myocardial O$_2$ demand).
  — There is no evidence to show that in non-cardiac disease preoperative normalisation of Hb concentration decreases morbidity or mortality. In ischaemic heart disease there is a relation between haematocrit <29% and further myocardial ischaemic episodes in the perioperative period.
  — Overtransfusion is undesirable: at a haematocrit of 45%, for example, cerebral blood flow falls.
  — Timing? At least 24 hours prior to surgery to allow restoration of 2,3 DPG (although clinical experience suggests that this may be more theoretical than real: patients who receive what are in effect exchange transfusions after massive haemorrhage maintain oxygen saturation).

Operative management of the anaemic patient

- Goals are to maximise oxygen delivery to tissues, minimise oxygen consumption and minimise blood loss.
  - Regional anaesthesia where appropriate.
  - Adequate F_iO_2 to maintain $SpO_2\%$ in the high 90s.
  - Careful positioning to reduce venous pressure.
  - Scrupulous surgical technique.
  - Hypotensive anaesthesia (some dispute its value).
  - Haemodilution so that net volume of blood lost is reduced.
  - Drugs may be useful: desmopressin (increases Factor VIII), tranexamic acid (inhibits plasminogen activation and fibrinolysis), ethamsylate (reduces capillary bleeding), aprotinin (inhibits the fibrinolysis).

Marking points: This question is less concerned about the many underlying causes of anaemia than about the recognition of its influence on oxygen flux, and the patients in whom this may be significant. The examiner wishes to see a reasoned science-based approach to management rather than a protocol-driven account based on arbitrary figures.

Anaesthesia and medical disease

How would you assess a patient with chronic obstructive pulmonary disease (COPD) who presents for laparotomy? What are the major perioperative risks and how may they be reduced?

A patient with severe COPD can present significant anaesthetic challenges, the main one being how to ensure that they may be kept off a ventilator and out of an intensive care unit. COPD is a spectrum of disease and the question is assessing your knowledge of the condition and your judgement in its management.

Introduction

The cardinal feature of chronic obstructive pulmonary disease is increased airways resistance to flow (hence the alternative title of chronic obstructive airways disease). COPD is characterised by a disease spectrum that ranges from chronic bronchitis which limits activity only mildly, to severe and incapacitating emphysema.

Preoperative assessment: history

- Exercise tolerance (stair climbing is a more reliable indicator than walking on the flat).
- Dyspnoea (on severe, moderate or minimal exertion, or at rest).
- Sputum and cough: chronic, or is there evidence of acute intercurrent infection?
- Medication: steroids, bronchodilators, domiciliary oxygen.
- Hospital and especially ITU admissions for exacerbations.
- Smoking history.

Preoperative assessment: signs

- Body habitus: are they barrel-chested, plethoric, asthenic?
- Dyspnoea: are they able to talk in sentences at rest?
- Respiratory pattern: is there 'fish mouth' breathing, use of accessory muscles?
- Auscultation: are there wheezes, crackles, adventitious sounds?
- Right heart failure: is there peripheral oedema, jugular venous distension, hepatomegaly?

Preoperative assessment: investigations

May just confirm the clinical impression gained from history and examination, but may help quantify the problem and assist in prediction of outcome.

- **CXR:** may show emphysematous bullae, hyperinflation, patchy atelectasis, fibrosis.
- **ECG:** may show right heart strain, low voltage.
- **FBC:** polycythaemia, leucocytosis.
- **Arterial blood gases on air:** evaluation of baseline preoperative status and confirmation of CO_2 retention if suspected.
- **Pulmonary function tests:** spirometry typically shows decreased FEV_1 and decreased $FEV_1 : FVC$ (forced vital capacity) ratio. A large number of variables can be defined. Flow–volume loops may be of more use in characterising airway obstruction. An $FEV_1 : FVC$ ratio of <50% is associated with increased morbidity and mortality after all forms of body cavity surgery.
- **Predictors:** $FEV_1 < 1$ L, $P_a CO_2 > 7$ kPa, $FEV_1 : FVC$ ratio <50% all predict requirement for postoperative ventilatory support (particularly after upper abdominal or thoracic surgery).

Perioperative risks: anaesthesia and surgery

Anaesthesia

- **Pulmonary function.** Exerts a generally deleterious effect.
  - Decrease in FRC (33%), VC (up to 50%), pulmonary compliance etc. follow all forms of general anaesthesia.
  - Atelectasis, hypoxaemia, hypoventilation are common.
- **Barotrauma**
  - Associated with IPPV and airways resistance.
  - Use of N_2O in presence of bullae or emphysematous blebs.
- **Airways reactivity**
  - Associated with intubation, airway manipulation.
  - May be provoked by histamine releasing anaesthetic agents (avoid).

Surgery

- Body cavity surgery is associated with significant morbidity:
  - Thoracic and upper abdominal > lower abdominal.
  - Prolonged surgery in supine position.
  - Diaphragmatic excursion is impaired, restricted respiratory expansion due to pain.

Risk reduction

The key to risk reduction is the optimisation of the patient's perioperative condition:

- **Smoking.** Cessation is difficult in patients with a lifelong habit, but reduction in postoperative respiratory morbidity will result if it can be achieved 2 months prior to surgery.
- **Pharmacology.** Optimise the regimen, particularly if there is a reversible component. Appropriate antibiotic treatment of any intercurrent chest infection.
- **Physiotherapy.** Pre-emptive and with use of techniques such as incentive spirometry.
- **Analgesia.** Good postoperative analgesia (i.e. by epidural) will reduce respiratory complications incident upon diaphragmatic splinting and basal atalectasis due to inhibition of deep breathing by pain.
- **Regional anaesthesia.** Use wherever feasible, but must beware anaesthetising the intercostal muscles with high neuraxial blocks, or using techniques which impair phrenic nerve function (interscalene block).
- **Ambulation.** Encourage early mobilisation.

Marking points: Clinical experience and judgement is as important as the respiratory numbers in deciding whether or not these patients are going to require postoperative intensive care. You need to emphasise those clinical features as well as outlining an anaesthetic strategy that will minimise that risk. Good preoperative preparation and optimal postoperative analgesia are crucial to that aim.

A surgical patient smokes 20–30 cigarettes a day and requires a general anaesthetic. Does this have any significance?

Cigarette smoking is common and it has diverse pathophysiological effects, both chronic and acute. It also excites an evangelical zeal in some clinicians which may impede objective appraisal of the evidence. This is a standard and predictable question which expects you to demonstrate knowledge of the applied physiology and pharmacology of smoking as well as an awareness that the risk–benefit analysis of preoperative cessation may be less simple than it seems.

Introduction
Cigarette smoking is common and it can have marked effects, both chronic and acute. Some of these may be of more theoretical than actual significance, but others may clinically be very important, particularly in the context of major surgery.

Chronic effects
- **Respiratory**
  - Heavy consumption causes chronic obstructive pulmonary disease (chronic bronchitis, asthmatic bronchitis and emphysema).
  - Emphysema is the most severe condition. In susceptible individuals (not all smokers are affected as badly) destruction of alveolar membranes follows an imbalance which favours destructive proteases mainly derived from neutrophils, overprotective circulating antiproteases, the most important of which is alpha$_1$-antitrypsin. Cigarette smoking increases the ratio of proteases to antiproteases.
  - Significant airflow resistance and hyperreactivity is demonstrated with much lower consumption (10 per day).
  - Pulmonary complications after major procedures are increased 6× in smokers and 20× in those with chronic lung disease (but these figures are based on very old data).
- **Cardiovascular**
  - Smoking is a risk factor for coronary artery disease (risk of sudden death over age 45 doubles in smokers of >20 per day). Cessation halves the risk in 1 year.
  - Nicotine is a sympathetic stimulant: increases HR, vascular resistance and myocardial oxygen consumption.
  - Interference with wound healing (vascular compromise).
- **Central nervous system**
  - Smoking (specifically nicotine) is powerfully addictive.
  - Increases risk of rupture of intracranial aneurysms.

Acute effects
- **Oxygen delivery**
  - An individual who is smoking may have a carboxyhaemoglobin (COHb) of up to 15% with consequent impairment of O_2 delivery to tissues.
  - COHb $t_{1/2}$ in air is ~4 hours, in 100% ~1 hour. Is also dependent on minute ventilation. If this is decreased (e.g. overnight) then COHb elimination will be delayed.
- **Cardiovascular affects**
  - Increased cardiac work secondary to impaired O_2 delivery.
  - Stimulation by nicotine: stimulates sympathetic postganglionic neurones; increases heart rate and causes peripheral vasoconstriction.

Should smokers be encouraged to stop preoperatively?

Major benefits are not seen until after 8 weeks following cessation. The risk–benefit analysis for smokers who have abstained for a shorter period is more complex.

- Within 12–24 hours of cessation: CO and nicotine levels return to normal. Decrease in COHb shifts the dissociation curve to the right and increases O_2 availability.
- Within 2–3 days upper airway ciliary function improves, but this is accompanied by an increase in sputum production (smokers have significantly lower mucus transport velocities).
- Within 2 weeks sputum volume declines to normal.
- Cessation precipitates increase in airways reactivity: laryngospasm and bronchoconstriction.
- Is associated with decrease in arterial, but an increase in venous thrombosis.
- After 8 weeks there is a decrease in postoperative respiratory morbidity (PORM) (by 66% in one series of coronary artery bypass graft (CABG) patients, although smokers who stopped more recently than 8 weeks had an increase in PORM from 33% to 57%).
- Abstinence is likely to provoke anxiety and withdrawal symptoms due to the potent and complex addiction.

Marking points: You may well be in the position of having to discuss smoking with patients preoperatively and it is important that your advice is well informed. This answer will be marked according to that criterion.

A patient in chronic renal failure requires a laparotomy. What are the anaesthetic implications?

Chronic renal impairment is a spectrum of disease which ranges from modest elevations in urea and creatinine to end-stage renal failure requiring full haemodialysis. This question expects you to produce an overview of the influence of impaired renal function on anaesthesia, and of anaesthesia on impaired renal function, with particular emphasis on the key safety points.

Introduction

At best chronic renal failure is manifest as moderate elevations in urea and creatinine, at worst it requires full haemodialysis. The pre-existing disease has implications for anaesthetic technique, which in turn will influence renal function. Both aspects need to be considered.

Implications of chronic renal failure for anaesthesia

- **Precipitant?** Is there an associated underlying cause? The commonest is diabetes mellitus.
- **Severity?** How great is the renal impairment? Mortality in end-stage disease is high: 4% overall and 20% after emergency surgery (sepsis, arrhythmias, cardiac failure).
- **Cardiovascular problems.** Chronic hypertension and cardiac insufficiency. Very labile BP and HR during anaesthesia, arrhythmias and hypertensive surges are common. Uraemic pericarditis or pericardial effusions may be present in severe disease.
- **Metabolic problems.** Hyperkalaemia. Impaired handling of other electrolytes.
- **Renal problems.** Decreased ability to compensate for fluid loads and fluid shifts. Unable to deal with acid–base perturbation. Impaired drug excretion.
- **Haematological problems.** Uraemia depresses erythropoiesis. Chronic anaemia is common with haemoglobin concentrations of 6–8 g dl^{-1} not unusual. Uraemic platelet dysfunction increases bleeding.
- **Immunological problems.** Infection risk increased due to immunosuppression.
- **CNS.** Uraemia depresses neurological function. Effect of hypnotic and sedative drugs may be enhanced: caution is required with doses. Neuropathies may be present.
- **Anaesthetic techniques:**
  - Preoperatively the patient should be euvolaemic. Recent dialysis normalises electrolytes and acid–base status at the expense of dehydration. Rehydrate cautiously. Careful fluid management thereafter.
  - K$^+$ may be elevated. Must avoid further rises so suxamethonium is contraindicated (unless recently dialysed).
  - May need DDAVP, cryoprecipitate and platelets to minimise excessive surgical bleeding.
  - Caution with opioids: metabolite of pethidine is convulsive (nor-pethidine). Metabolite of morphine is itself a potent opioid and is renally excreted (morphine-6-glucuronide).

Influence of anaesthesia on renal function

- General anaesthesia always leads to a (normally reversible) depression of renal function as measured by urine output, glomerular filtration rate (GFR), renal blood flow (RBF) and electrolyte excretion. Anaesthesia accelerates chronic renal impairment, albeit slightly.
- Central neuraxial and regional anaesthetic blocks have less effect.
- Surgical stress response: renin–angiotensin system stimulates aldosterone release with Na$^+$ and H$_2$O retention, and posterior pituitary produces arginine vasopressin (antidiuretic).

- Myocardial depression due to anaesthesia is associated with increase in renal vascular resistance: GFR and RBF decrease.
- Any decrease in systemic vascular resistance decreases GFR and RBF.
- Normovolaemia and cardiovascular stability minimise disturbance.
- Drug effects: fluoride-containing volatile inhalational agents are potentially, but not actually, nephrotoxic (even methoxyflurane required 7 MAC hours to cause damage); sevoflurane is 3.5% metabolised and is probably safe; desflurane ideal in this regard (minimal metabolism).
- Induction agents and opioids depress GFR and RBF.
- NSAIDs must be avoided: prostaglandin inhibition compromises intrinsic renal vasodilatation.
- Muscle relaxants: atracurium is ideal, vecuronium is 15% renally excreted.
- IPPV: may decrease urine volume and Na^+ excretion, stimulate ADH release and activate renin–angiotensin–aldosterone system.

Marking points: Chronic renal failure is a spectrum of disease and so you have to treat this (big) question with some generalisations. You must demonstrate safe management and so should mention cardiac, haematological, metabolic and volaemic status as well as the danger of drugs such as suxamethonium.

Outline the anaesthetic implications of managing patients with thyroid disease who require non-thyroid surgery.

Thyroid disease is common and so anaesthetists may frequently encounter patients who require non-thyroid surgery, who may or may not have the medical complications associated with hyperthyroidism and myxoedema. This question assesses your grasp of the range of challenges that thyroid disease may present.

Introduction

Thyroid disease is common, even in iodine-sufficient areas, and both deficiency and excess of thyroid activity present as multisystem disorders which have important anaesthetic implications.

Myxoedema

- Hypothyroidism (may present with non-specific clinical features which mimic those of other conditions) has a prevalence of ~20 per 1000 (5 overt, 15 subclinical).
- Severe untreated or undertreated disease may be characterised by:
  — Myocardial depression (bradycardia, decreased contractility, hypotension) due to depression of intracellular myocardial metabolism and deposition of protein and mucopolysaccharides within the myocardium.
  — Baroreceptor reflexes are impaired (hypotension).
  — Haematological changes: anaemia, decreased blood volume.
  — Respiratory depression (hypoventilation). Ventilatory responses to hypoxia and hypercarbia are blunted.
  — Metabolic disturbance: hypoglycaemia, hyponatraemia, adrenal insufficiency with impairment of the hypothalmo–pituitary–adrenal axis, decreased response to stress.
  — Drug handling: hepatic and renal clearance is decreased.
  — CNS changes: dulling of sensorium and ultimately, myxoedema coma.
- Anaesthetic implications
  — Unstable and labile CVS.
  — Extreme sensitivity to drugs that affect the CNS: includes most anaesthetic agents.
  — Increased probability of severe respiratory depression.
  — Precipitation of myxoedema coma by hypothermia, trauma (including surgical), infection and respiratory depressants.
- Anaesthetic management
  — **Elective surgery in severe disease**. Patients should be euthyroid: it may take up to 4 months before the cardiac and other effects are reversed, and surgery should be deferred.
  — **Elective surgery in mild disease**. Increased risk is disputed. Can probably proceed with cautious use of drugs, regional anaesthesia where possible, ambient temperature control, corticosteroid supplementation.
  — **Emergency surgery.** there is no choice but to proceed after instituting cautious replacement therapy (intravenous T_3 and T_4 by slow infusion) to avoid precipitating critical coronary ischaemia.
  — Extreme sensitivity to drugs that affect the CNS: i.e. to most anaesthetic agents.
  — Increased probability of severe respiratory depression.

Hyperthyroidism

- Hyperthyroidism is commoner than myxoedema, affecting 2% of women and 0.2% of men.
- Is a hypermetabolic state: the main anaesthetic implications are cardiac.
- Increased cardiac output and tachycardia: may have tachyarrhythmias (atrial fibrillation) and signs of decompensation (left ventricular hypertrophy, failure).
- May have impairment of adrenal function.
- Increased metabolism of drugs (may appear 'resistant' to anaesthetic agents and require higher doses: e.g. propofol has increased clearance and volume of distribution).
- 'Thyroid storm' is much written of and rarely seen: is an acute manifestation of thyrotoxic hypermetabolism with tachycardia and hyperpyrexia. May occur after surgery (6–24 hours).
- Anaesthetic management
  - **Elective surgery.** Patients should be euthyroid: it may take up to 2 months before antithyroid agents (carbimazole, propylthiouracil) are fully effective.
  - **Emergency surgery.** Acutely the effects of thyroid excess can be attenuated by the use of beta-adrenoceptor blockers. Fluid replacement must cover increased losses. Maintain normothermia. Corticosteroid supplementation may be needed.

Marking points: Both are multisystem diseases and you should be aware of their important cardiorespiratory implications. Particular safety issues are the sensitivity of myxoedematous patients to depressant drugs and the requirement that patients should be rendered euthyroid prior to surgery. You should outline a strategy for emergency surgery.

Describe the assessment of a patient with arterial hypertension. Why is it important that it should be treated preoperatively?

Hypertension is common and affects as many as 25% of the population. It is treated with a wide range of drugs, some of which have anaesthetic implications, and if it goes untreated is associated with substantial morbidity. You should demonstrate an understanding of why these patients may have perioperative problems.

Introduction

Blood pressure is a continuum and so the definition of what constitutes hypertension is debated, but whatever criteria are used it is clear that it is a common problem that may affect as many as 25% of the adult population and which has significant implications for anaesthesia.

Preoperative assessment

- **Identification and definition.** The nature of the hypertension should be identified. It has been traditional to ascribe hypertensive morbidity to diastolic hypertension caused by increased systemic vascular resistance. It is now believed that isolated systolic hypertension, which reflects an arteriosclerotic circulation, is a better marker for cardiac risk in the 50+ age group. Pulse pressure is a better predictor of adverse cardiac events. The wider the pressure (which means that the diastolic BP may be low) the greater the risk. An SBP (systolic blood pressure) of >160 mmHg represents hypertension. So-called 'white coat' (i.e. anxiety-induced hypertension) is part of the same phenomenon and is not benign. Degree of control should be assessed in the light of any drug therapy.
- **Aetiology.** Is commonly idiopathic (>90%) or associated with inelastic circulation as above. May be associated with other conditions such as renal and endocrine disease, obesity and alcoholism.
- **End-organ damage.** Symptoms, signs and investigations may reveal evidence of chronic damage to target organs.
  — Cardiac. Myocardial ischaemia, left ventricular hypertrophy or strain.
  — Renal. Urea and electrolytes, urinalysis.
  — Retinopathy. Fundoscopy.
  — CNS. Evidence of CVA (Cerebrovascular accident) associated with hypertension.
- **Pharmacology.** Hypertensive patients can be treated with a wide range of drugs and combinations of drugs:
  — Diuretics (e.g. bendrofluazide) May cause electrolyte derangement.
  — Beta-adrenoceptor blockers (e.g. atenolol). May interfere with capacity of patient to compensate for sympathetic block or for hypovolaemia.
  — ACE inhibitors (e.g. enalapril). If continued up until the time of surgery may be associated with severe intraoperative hypotension.
  — Angiotensin II receptor antagonists (e.g. losartan). Similar to ACE inhibitors but do not inhibit breakdown of bradykinin and other kinins.
  — Ca^{2+} channel blockers (e.g. nifedipine). In theory may potentiate neuromuscular blockers (particularly verapamil), little obvious effect in clinical practice.
  — K^+ channel activators (e.g. nicorandil). Insufficient clinical experience to date.

Importance of preoperative control

- **End-organ damage.** 50% of untreated hypertensives proceed to irreversible end-organ damage: cardiac and renal failure, hypertensive retinopathy, cerebrovascular events.

- **Blood pressure lability.** Of particular importance at times of intense sympathetic stimulation: laryngoscopy, intubation, extubation; surgical stimulus, postoperative pain.
- **Drug effects.** Untreated hypertensive patients may have exaggerated responses to vasoactive drugs, both pressors and vasodilators.
- **Autoregulation.** The autoregulation curve for cerebral blood flow shifts to the right, which increases the risk of critical hypoperfusion if the mean arterial pressure falls. It is likely that this phenomenon also occurs in other vascular beds.
- **Volaemic status.** The untreated hypertensive with a constricted peripheral vasculature is effectively hypovolaemic with depleted intravascular volume. In addition a non-compliant hypertrophied left ventricle may have diastolic dysfunction in which left ventricular end-diastolic volume (LVEDV) is decreased. These patients depend even more on adequate preload for cardiac performance. They tolerate actual or effective fluid shifts poorly and demonstrate marked haemodynamic fluctuations.
- Overall there is evidence from several studies that untreated hypertension is strongly associated with increased perioperative cardiac morbidity. It seems probable that other organs may also be at ischaemic risk.

Marking points: Accurate assessment of patients who may be at risk of haemodynamic instability because of hypertensive disease is basic to safe anaesthetic practice. You will be expected to be aware of all the main points in this answer.

A patient has a history of chronic alcohol abuse. What are the anaesthetic implications?

Considering that 15% of the population are said to be alcoholics and that 10% or more of hospital admissions are related to alcohol abuse, it is curious that anaesthetists do not encounter more frequent difficulties with such patients. Alcohol is a potent toxin that affects all systems, but it seems that only at the extreme end of the spectrum are all the theoretical problems manifest. The subject has both basic science as well as clinical interest, and the focus of this question is on both.

Introduction

Alcohol is a social facilitator that is also a powerful toxin that can exert major pathological effects on every system in the body. Although some 15% of the adult population are said to be alcoholics it appears that it is only at the extreme end of the spectrum of disease that anaesthetic problems are overt. It is probable, however, that morbidity can be avoided by management that is based on the predictable systemic derangements.

Cardiovascular

- Acute alcohol ingestion impairs LV function and causes peripheral vasodilatation. Chronic abuse can lead to a global cardiomyopathy with both LV and RV dysfunction, pulmonary hypertension and arrhythmias. CVS problems are the main cause of death in long-term alcoholics. Thiamine deficiency can lead to high output cardiac failure. Anaesthetic techniques should encompass these possibilites.

Central nervous system

- Acute disinhibition is well recognised and chronic ingestion may cause profound neuropsychiatric abnormalities. Some are linked to nutritional deficiency. Neuropathy and myopathy may be evident.

Gastrointestinal

- Gastric hyperacidity, gastroparesis and reflux oesophageal disease are common, with obvious implications for anaesthetic practice. Portal hypertension secondary to cirrhotic liver disease causes oesophageal varices. Bleeding from ruptured varices can be torrential and may occur following instrumentation of the oesophagus (endoscopy or even by a rigid NG tube).

Haematological

- Anaemia. Nutritional deficiency and/or chronic gastrointestinal blood loss.

Hepatic

- The liver has huge functional reserve and can continue to metabolise most drugs even in the presence of widespread pathological change. Protein metabolism is decreased, so levels of coagulation factors may be diminished (prolonged PT) as is albumin (decreased protein binding of drugs). Plasma cholinesterase levels are decreased in liver disease and so the actions of suxamethonium and mivacurium may be prolonged.

Effects of anaesthetic agents

- The alcohol abuser who is not acutely intoxicated is commonly resistant to the sedative effects of anaesthetic drugs. This is not due to enzyme induction, but appears to be a phenomenon of non-specific cellular tolerance.

Immune system

- Excessive alcohol consumption is immunosuppressive.

Respiratory system

- Has effects analogous to smoking (which habit it frequently accompanies): ciliary dysfunction, leucocyte inhibition, surfactant depletion. Postoperative chest infections are more common.

Metabolic

- **Hypoglycaemia.** Subjects who have recently ingested large volumes of alcohol are at risk of profound hypoglycaemia. The metabolism of alcohol to acetaldehyde is catalysed by alcohol dehydrogenase in a reaction which produces NADH from NAD^+. This effectively depletes NAD^+ which is important co-factor in the gluconeogenetic conversion of lactate to pyruvate.

Withdrawal syndrome

- Peak onset is ~12–36 hours following abstention from alcohol, and so can occur commonly in the first postoperative day. Severe withdrawal may manifest as delirium tremens (mortality may approach 10%), autonomic hyperactivity with cardiovascular instability, agitation, diaphoresis, abdominal cramping and diarrhoea. Convulsions may supervene. It is clear that the differential diagnosis between withdrawal and other postoperative problems that may present similar symptoms is important in this context. The withdrawal syndrome may last for several days: can be treated with benzodiazepines (commonly lorazepam) or with alcohol infusion itself.

Marking points: Every body system needs evaluation in the chronic alcohol abuser who presents for surgery: the important safety points that you should cover are the possibility of hypoglycaemia and the probability of a postoperative alcohol withdrawal syndrome.

Medicine and intensive care

Describe the diagnosis and management of Guillain–Barré syndrome.

Guillain–Barré Syndrome (Landry–Guillain–Barré syndrome) is one of the most common neurological disorders which requires intensive care. Anaesthetists need to be familiar not only with the ITU management of a complex disorder, but also with the clinical features which make ITU admission and IPPV more likely.

Introduction
Guillain–Barré syndrome is an acute demyelinating polyneuropathy of uncertain aetiology. It is believed to have an immunological basis as it frequently follows viral and other infections. Its presentation is variable, although motor weakness is more pronounced than sensory loss.

History
- Recent viraemia or bacterial infection, e.g. campylobacter, also immunisations and surgery.
- Ascending motor weakness is typical, onset over days (can be rapid).
- Sensory symptoms and paraesthesia, also pain in >50% and hyperpathia.
- Differential diagnosis: other causes of acute polyneuropathy/polyneuritis: poisons, drugs, organophosphates, heavy metals, alcohol, malignancy, inflammatory processes, transverse myelitis, poliomyelitis, Lyme disease, AIDS, myasthenia gravis.

Examination
- Motor impairment, loss of deep tendon reflexes, sensory changes.
- Signs of autonomic instability: postural hypotension, sweating, tachycardia, hypertension.

Investigations
- Lumbar puncture: increase in CSF proteins, white count unchanged.
- Serology: may have antibodies, e.g. to Ebstein–Barr virus, mycoplasma, campylobacter.
- Nerve conduction: reduced at various sites.

Management
- **Specific treatment with immunoglobulin or plasmapheresis.** No difference in

efficacy although iv immunoglobulin much simpler. Corticosteroids are of no benefit.

- **Supportive intensive therapy.** Criteria for intubation/ventilation include:
  — Bulbar involvement; inability to cough, swallow, protect airway.
  — Exhaustion of respiratory muscles: clinical assessment, FVC of <1 L or <15 ml kg^{-1}.
  — Blood gas evidence of respiratory failure; cyanosis (very late sign).
  — Autonomic instability.
- **General ITU management:**
  — Tracheal intubation (beware suxamethonium with denervated muscle).
  — DVT prophylaxis.
  — Analgesia, sedation, physiotherapy.
  — Early tracheostomy if rapid weaning unlikely.

Prognosis

- Mortality quoted at 5–10%; severe morbidity 10%; some but not all recover fully.
- Poor prognostic features:
  — Age >40 years.
  — Rapid onset of symptoms/signs.
  — Requirement for IPPV.
  — Markedly impaired conduction in peripheral motor nerves (<40 m s^{-1}; normal is >70).

Marking points: This is a relatively common ITU problem and the answer should demonstrate definite criteria for ITU admission and IPPV, the value of immunoglobulin and the potential dangers of suxamethonium.

Outline your management of a patient with status asthmaticus whom you are asked to see in the A&E department.

Anaesthetists become involved in these cases usually after initial management by others and at a stage when ventilation is required. Knowledge of management is obviously important, both because it informs treatment should a patient require intensive care, and because of the many situations in which an anaesthetist may have to confront severe bronchoconstriction.

Introduction

Status asthmaticus can be defined as the acute deterioration of asthma, with increasing dyspnoea and exhaustion to the point of collapse, which has not responded to the usual therapies. This is a medical emergency whose severity may go unrecognised until very late. Early diagnosis and assessment is vital.

Assessment

- **Clinical history** (from relatives if indicated): pre-morbid state, previous hospital admissions, precipitants, medication, duration of exacerbation.
- **Clinical examination**
  — Any causative or associated condition that needs immediate treatment: pneumothorax (spontaneous pneumothorax well recognised in asthmatics), acute bacterial infection.
  — State of exhaustion and conscious level. Can the patient talk? How much? Breathing characteristics: rate and pattern. Use of accessory muscles. Tracheal tug, intercostal recession. Pulsus paradoxus (exaggeration of normal phenomenon) is often quoted as a sign but has been shown to be unreliable and of limited value in assessment. Oxygen saturation? – very bad sign if it is lower than 98–99% on supplemental oxygen.
- **Investigations.** Peak expiratory flow rate (PEFR): serial measurements may be useful. Main laboratory test to guide management is arterial blood gas analysis. Acute asthma is associated with a normal P_aO_2 and a low P_aCO_2. A high normal P_aCO_2 is ominous and by the time that CO_2 retention or decreasing response to oxygen therapy occurs the patient is very likely to require ventilation. CXR and sputum sample if appropriate or practicable.

Management

- **Airway and breathing.** Humidified oxygen, nebulised beta$_2$-agonists; intravenous corticosteroids; antibiotics if indicated. Intravenous bronchodilators may be needed: salbutamol, aminophylline (check if patient has been taking theophyllines – this is a potentially dangerous agent).
- **Circulation.** Traditional teaching stated that these patients are dehydrated and required intravenous resuscitation. Severe asthma is associated with an increase in ADH secretion and some clinicians restrict fluids to two-thirds of maintenance requirements.
- **Further drugs.** If there is no response to first line drugs: nebulised or intravenous epinephrine (adrenaline); ketamine; volatile anaesthetics (traditionally halothane, but all volatiles are bronchodilators); magnesium sulphate.
- **Intensive care management.** If IPPV is required: cautious induction of anaesthesia.
  — Check hydration status.
  — Rapid sequence induction.
  — Volume cycled ventilator (if pressure cycled may be unable to ventilate).
  — Minimise airways pressures: slow rate, long expiratory time.
  — Allow permissive hypercapnia. Over-ventilation may drop cardiac output significantly.

— May need full muscle relaxation to assist ventilation.
— Will need adequate sedation throughout period during which ventilation is needed.

Marking points: Principles of management are important, but much less so than the ability to recognise when an asthmatic is seriously ill or deteriorating. You must make your criteria for ITU admission very clear.

What are the indications for tracheostomy in adults?

This is a straightforward question because the technique of percutaneous tracheostomy has made this an anaesthetic procedure. Beware concentrating too much on intensive care: there are other relevant indications with which you should be familiar.

Introduction
Tracheostomy can be an emergency life-saving procedure or one that is semi-elective. In every case it involves bypassing the upper airway and securing an airway directly into the trachea.

Indications
- **Airway obstruction (complete)**
  — Burns, trauma, angioedema, infection (Ludwig's angina, epiglottitis), supraglottic tumour.
- **Airway protection (from aspiration)**
  — Neurological disease, bulbar palsies, motor neurone disease, acute demyelinating disease (Guillain–Barré syndrome).
- **Airway protection (from excessive secretions, sputum retention)**
  — Typically ITU patients with respiratory muscle weakness or in any debilitated patient in whom the strength of coughing is severely impaired (mini-tracheostomy commonly).
- **Airway protection (during surgery)**
  — Semi-elective tracheostomy may precede major surgery on the head and neck.
  — Permanent tracheostomy is necessary after laryngectomy.
- **Weaning from ventilation in ITU**
  — Long-stay ITU patients can be difficult to wean from ventilators. The reasons are multifactorial and there is no consensus as to optimal timing.
  — Tracheostomy reduces the work of breathing (removes dead space by 30–50%) and allows ready clearance of sputum and secretions.

Marking points: Do not give details of a percutaneous technique or complications. The question has essentially asked for a list which having constructed logically you can arrange in order of priority.

Classify each type of heart block and describe the appropriate treatment in the perioperative period.

Ischaemic heart disease is very common and is a major cause of conduction abnormalities. Anaesthetic agents, in addition, may contribute to conduction deficits and so some knowledge of heart block is necessary for safe anaesthetic practice.

Introduction

Heart block describes the condition in which the wave of electrical excitation is delayed or blocked at the junctional tissues of the AV node and the Bundle of His. It can be permanent or appear as a temporary phenomenon.

Sick sinus syndrome (variety of disorders including sinoatrial block)

- Disorders of the SA (Sino-atrial) node represent dysfunctions of excitation rather than conduction and can be excluded from this classification.

1st degree AV block

- Impulses are slowed, but all are conducted.
- Characterised by delayed AV conduction: manifest on the ECG by a P–R interval >0.2 s.
- Treatment is rarely necessary. Atropine can be given, as can isoprenaline by infusion.

2nd degree (or partial) AV block

- Impulses are slowed and not all are conducted. Is divided into two forms.
- **Möbitz Type 1 or Wenkebach block**
    - P–R interval shows progressive lengthening until the propagation of an atrial impulse is completely blocked (progressive fatigue of AV node and recovery during dropped beat).
    - Treatment not often necessary: includes atropine and isoprenaline. Pacing very rarely.
- **Möbitz Type 2**
    - P–R interval is either normal or prolonged but is fixed except when there is an intermittent failure of AV conduction and beats are dropped, either in irregular ratios or in a 2 : 1, 3 : 1 or 4 : 1 pattern.
    - It may proceed without warning to complete heart block. Atropine and isoprenaline infusion can be used as temporary measures pending (mandatory) pacing.

3rd degree (or complete) AV block

- None of the impulses are conducted, and there is complete dissociation of atria and ventricles.
- Isoprenaline infusion may be necessary to raise the pulse to ~60 b.p.m. as temporary measure until pacing can be established. Typical treatment regimen: isoprenaline 2 mg (2 ampoules) in glucose 5% or NaCl 0.9% (4 μg ml^{-1}). Infuse at rate up to 10 μg min^{-1}.

Bundle branch and fascicular blocks

- Are ECG abnormalities associated with blocks of conduction in either the left or right main branch bundles or in the anterior or posterior fascicles of the left bundle branch.
- Left anterior or left posterior hemiblock plus right bundle branch is bifascicular block which can proceed to complete heart block. Perioperative temporary pacing is indicated.

Pacemakers

- Patients may present with pacemakers already in place. Need checking preoperatively.

Postoperatively

- Cardiological advice is likely to be needed.

Marking points: Fine detail of complex arrhythmias are not required. What you must demonstrate is that you can recognse potentially dangerous conduction deficits and can treat them appropriately. A bradycardia which compromises cerebral and cardiac perfusion needs urgent treatment and you must be able to describe an appropriate treatment regimen.

What are the causes of muscle weakness in the intensive care patient?

This is an important phenomenon because of its influence on weaning patients from ventilators and because some of the causes are treatable.

Introduction

The longer a patient remains in intensive care the more remote may become the original reason for admission and the more immediate the generic problems which are associated with prolonged multi-organ dysfunction. Weaning patients from supportive ventilation is one of these problems to which muscle weakness makes a significant contribution.

Potentially treatable causes

- Nutritional deficiency
  — Prolonged catabolism with loss of muscle mass.
- Electrolyte abnormality
  — Hypokalaemia, hyper- and hypo-magnesaemia, hypophosphataemia.
- Myasthenia gravis or myasthenic syndrome
- Infection or postinfective polyneuropathy
  — Guillain–Barré syndrome (under-diagnosed in this context). May respond to immunoglobulin treatment (or plasmapheresis).
  — Poliomyelitis (unlikely).

Non-treatable causes

- Polyneuropathy of critical illness
  — Seen in sepsis and multi-organ failure, burns and trauma: very significant cause.
  — Axonal degeneration of motor and sensory nerves.
- Disuse atrophy (prolonged assisted ventilation)
- Prolonged (>5 day) use of neuromuscular blocking drugs
  — Occurs both with aminosteroids and non-steroid relaxants.
  — Tetraparesis may last several months.
  — Appears to be a myopathic process in presence of normal neuromuscular transmission, analogous to steroid myopathy.
  — Asthmatics appear to be more at risk (? Association with exogenous steroids.)
  — Concurrent aminoglycosides may also be a risk factor.
- Peripheral neuropathies
  — Diabetes mellitus, HIV / AIDS, alcohol abuse.
- Corticosteroid myopathy
- Cervical cord pathology
  — Trauma, sepsis, vascular accident.

Marking points: There are many potential causes, and you would be expected to cite the common and important ones, including electrolyte derangements and the polyneuropathy of critical illness.

List the indications for renal support in intensive care patients. What are the principles of haemofiltration? What complications may be associated with the technique?

Haemofiltration is now a common procedure in many intensive care units where it is used to support renal function in patients in whom other organs are failing. It is frequently a mechanically cumbersome but conceptually quite simple therapy with which you are expected to be familiar.

Introduction

Acute renal dysfunction frequently complicates multi-organ failure in the critically ill. Haemofiltration provides a relatively straightforward therapy for what would otherwise be a mortal condition.

Indications

- Acute renal failure (ARF) when it is associated with one or more of the following:
  — Metabolic acidosis.
  — Hyperkalaemia.
  — High urea (vomiting, diarrhoea, pruritus, mental disturbance).
  — Volume overload.
  — Failure of drug / toxin clearance.

Principles of haemofiltration (HF)

- The filters used in HF are sometimes referred to colloquially as 'kidneys' which reflects their role as literal renal substitutes.
- In the normal kidney the glomerulus filters water, ions, negatively charged particles of molecular weight <15 000 and neutral substances of molecular weight up to ~40 000. Renal corpuscular channels have negatively charged pores which oppose the passage of negatively charged plasma proteins such as albumin (mol. wt. ~17 000).
- Normal GFR is 125 ml min^{-1} (7.5 L h^{-1}).
- Tubular reabsorption reduces the filtrate of 180 L day^{-1} to ~1 L day^{-1} and salvages many of the filtered ions and other particles (diffusion and mediated transport). Tubular secretion is the means whereby larger molecules and protein-bound substances (drugs and toxins, etc.) are eliminated.
- In the HF system, arterial pressure which may be pump assisted, can deliver a flow of up to 250 ml min^{-1} (15 L h^{-1}) to the semipermeable membrane in the filter. Water and low molecular weight substances (up to ~20 000) cross the membrane (the 'glomerulus').
- Urea and creatinine will be removed, as will electrolytes and some drugs and toxins. Plasma proteins and all formed blood components remain within the circulation.
- Tubular reabsorption is mimicked by direct infusion of balanced electrolyte solution, with concentrations adjusted as necessary. The volume infused will depend on the clinical situation. If the patient is not volume overloaded then infusion will be at the same rate as the filtration rate, plus a component for maintenance fluid. If fluid removal is indicated then negative balance is easily achieved by decreasing the infusion rate.
- HF is a good means of treating fluid overload, but is very inefficient at removing solute (when compared to the kidney). Very high volumes of ultrafiltrate (15 L day^{-1} and more) are required to remove urea, creatinine and other products of metabolism.

Complications

- **Fluid mismanagement.** Very large volumes are both filtered and infused and the scope for error is high.
- **Coagulation problems.** Blood clots in extracorporeal circulations and produces diffuse thrombi on the artificial surfaces unless the system is anticoagulated. Heparins or prostacyclin are used, and patients can be under- or over-coagulated. Undercoagulation leads to problems with the circuit and not the patient (the 'kidney' fails), whereas over-coagulation is more serious.
- **Air embolus.** Always a potential problem in relatively complex extracorporeal circuits.
- **Heat loss.**
- **Disconnection.** HF requires wide-bore dedicated arterial and venous lines.
- **Filter failure.** Can occur frequently and may threaten the efficacy of the whole haemofiltration process.

Marking points: Acute renal failure is common in the ITU and you will be expected to understand the broad principles as outlined above. You should recognise the difficulties of accurate fluid management when such high volumes are involved, and should be aware of the relative inefficiency of the technique (when compared to haemodialysis) for solute removal.

What factors influence your decision to wean an intensive care patient from mechanical ventilation?

This is an important problem in intensive care to which there is no easy answer. This question expects you to outline a logical approach based on an understanding of the principles, even though the decision, finally, may be empirical.

Introduction

At its simplest weaning from mechanical ventilation on intensive care is little more complex than doing so in theatre at the end of surgery. In a small group of patients, however, the process is much more difficult, and the sometimes empirical decision to wean should be based on a logical evaluation of the systems and the pre-morbid condition of the patient.

What is required for comfortable spontaneous ventilation?

- **Muscle power** (intercostals, accessory muscles of respiration as well as diaphragm).
  - Various criteria have been proposed.
  - Generation of negative inspiratory pressure of >25 cmH$_2$O.
  - Vital capacity >10 ml kg^{-1}.
  - Tidal volume >4 ml kg^{-1}.
  - Respiratory rate <35 (if it is greater this suggests excessive respiratory effort).
  - Index of rapid shallow breathing (V$_T$:f) <100 min L^{-1} suggests failure is likely.
  - Airway occlusion pressure >6 cmH$_2$O: predicts failure.
- **Adequate gas exchange**
  - F$_I$O$_2$ of 0.6 or less achieving a P_aO$_2$ of >10 kPa and P_aCO$_2$ of <6 kPa.
  - $P_{(A-a)}$O$_2$ gradient of <40 kPa at F$_I$O$_2$ of 1.0.
- **Adequate cough for sputum and secretion clearance**
- **Lung compliance.** Stiff lungs post ALI/ARDS/SIRS make weaning more difficult.
  - Should be >25 ml cmH$_2$O^{-1}.

Circulatory adequacy

- Inotropic suport may militate against weaning. If requirements are high then myocardial oxygen consumption must be matched by supply. Worsening gas exchange during premature attempts to wean will compromise myocardial function further.
- Cardiac failure with pulmonary oedema will impair gas exchange as above.

Pre-morbid condition

- **COPD.** Chronic obstructive pulmonary disease is a particular challenge. Exacerbations may be associated with prolonged periods of mechanical ventilation.
- **Cardiac insufficiency.**
- **Neurological disease with muscle weakness.**

Additional factors

- Adequate pain relief (upper abdominal incision, e.g. following laparotomy) is important.
- Appropriate level of consciousness.
- No drug depression of neuromuscular function.
- No drug depression of central ventilatory drive.
- Respiratory failure (ARDS) associated with non-pulmonary disease.
- Renal inadequacy with fluid overload.
- Multi-organ failure with high O$_2$ requirements militate against early weaning.

Predictive factors

- There are no tests or combination of tests which accurately predict success in weaning. It is the subjective judgement and experience of the clinician that may be the deciding factor.

Marking points: There is no single predictive test for weaning success and decisions to do so are often made intuitively. You can make this point as long as you indicate that at least some semblance of scientific assessment based on a systems approach should be attempted.

What are the indications for nutritional support in the critically ill? Outline the advantages and disadvantages both of parenteral and of enteral nutrition.

Nutrition is important in the critically ill but clinicians on intensive care units no longer have to devise regimens based upon complex estimations of nitrogen loss. You will not be expected to detail nutritional elements, but you must be aware of the compelling advantages of enteral over parenteral feeding.

Introduction

Good evidence supports the early use of nutritional support both in the critically ill patient and perioperatively, in patients who have lost body mass but who are not yet cachectic. Enteral nutrition has all but supplanted parenteral feeding for the reasons which are described below.

Indications

- Critical or prolonged illness during which a patient will be unable to maintain their nutritional requirements by mouth.

Parenteral nutrition

Advantages
- It can be used in situation of short bowel syndrome, intestinal obstruction, when there has been failure to establish enteral feeding, or when there is prolonged ileus.
- There is no evidence to support its benefit over enteral feeding in the critically ill.

Disadvantages
- Expensive: cost is 2–10× that of enteral feeding.
- Invasive: requires dedicated central venous feeding catheter.
- Catheter infection risk (and all other complications associated with central lines).
- Non-physiological: risks of electrolyte imbalance, hepatic steatosis, azotaemia.
- Hyperglycaemia: impairs immune response as well as promoting osmotic dehydration.
- Fluid overload: full nutritional replenishment cannot be delivered in volumes less than ~ 2 L.
- Lipid overload with increase in respiratory quotient (RQ) makes weaning from mechanical ventilation more difficult.

Enteral nutrition

Advantages
- Delivered via fine bore feeding tube: supplies protein, carbohydrate, lipid and some fluid requirements. Is cheaper than parenteral nutrition and is non-invasive.
- Evidence suggests that early enteral feeding improves outcome:
  — Bowel integrity and function is maintained.
  — Normal intestinal flora are preserved (antibiotics permitting).
  — Gut mucosal permeability for bacteria is unchanged and so bacterial translocation is minimised or prevented.
  — Normal gastric acidity and gastrointestinal barrier function is preserved with enhanced secretion of IgA.
  — Stress ulceration is reduced.
  — The process of nutrition is physiological and so nitrogen uptake and incorporation, carbohydrate and lipid utilisation all favour anabolism and weight retention.

Disadvantages
- **Patients require a functioning and intact gastrointestinal tract**
- **Diarrhoea**
  - — Occurs in up to 40% of patients.
- **Nausea and vomiting**
  - — Common symptoms, associated not directly with enteral feeding, but with ileus, gastric stasis, abdominal distension in the critically ill.
- **Aspiration and pulmonary injury**
  - — Concurrent drugs may decrease barrier pressure and increase reflux risk.
  - — Risk of aspiration lower with duodenal or jejunal tubes.
- **Direct pulmonary instillation**
  - — Fine bore feeding tubes can be directed into the trachea itself.
  - — Instilled feed is likely to cause significant pulmonary injury.

Marking points: Nutritional support in intensive care as well as in the perioperative period in selected patients is very common, and you should be aware of the main principles. Details of particular regimens will not be required but you should know about the broad nutritional requirements of the critically ill.

What can be measured directly and what can be derived from pulmonary artery catheters? What is the clinical value of these measurements?

PA catheters remain a widely used tool in intensive therapy despite a large study that suggested that not only was the annual cost in the USA of two billion dollars not justified, but that their use was associated with increased mortality. The papers and accompanying editorials polarised opinion and provoked much discussion, and the issue has not been resolved. In the meantime PA catheters, in theory at least, continue to provide clinically useful haemodynamic information, an understanding of which you will be expected to demonstrate.

Introduction

In recent years the safety and efficacy of the PA catheter has been called into question by studies that purport to demonstrate increased mortality in patients subjected to what in the USA is a very expensive procedure, costing some two billion dollars annually. They remain a popular tool in intensive care, however, not least because the information obtained can be used to direct rational therapy.

Direct measurements and derived values

- PA catheters measure directly:
  — Pulmonary artery systolic, diastolic and mean pressure.
  — Pulmonary capillary occlusion (or wedge) pressure (PCOP or PCWP) which is a reliable indication of left atrial and left ventricular end diastolic pressure.
  — Cardiac output (CO = stroke volume × heart rate).
  — Mixed venous blood saturation and related indices.
- Derived values which are clinically useful include:
  — Cardiac index (CI = cardiac output/body surface area).
  — Systemic and pulmonary vascular resistance (SVR and PVR) (SVR = [MAP – CVP/CO] × 80 and PVR = [MPAP – PAOP (Pulmonary artery occlusion pressure)/CO] × 80).
  — Mixed venous oxygen content.
  — Oxygen delivery (= arterial O_2 content × CO) and oxygen consumption (CI × [arterial O_2 content – mixed venous O_2 content]).

Clinical situations in which these values are useful

- Pulmonary oedema
  — Differential diagnosis is between cardiac and non-cardiac (LVF vs ARDS).
  — Cardiac failure is characterised by a high PCOP indicative of left ventricular dysfunction.
  — ARDS is characterised by pulmonary oedema in the presence of low or normal PCOP.
- Sepsis
  — Causes circulatory collapse with peripheral vasodilatation and fluid losses through deranged capillary membranes.
  — Increased cardiac index with a hyperdynamic circulation, fall in SVR, and decrease in PCOP indicative of effective hypovolaemia.
  — Hyperdynamic circulation delivers adequate O_2 to the tissues which utilise it poorly: O_2 consumption is low and mixed venous O_2 content is high (decreased extraction).
- Haemorrhage or hypovolaemia
  — Depleted intravascular volume decreases cardiac index, LVEDV and LVEDP – hence decreased PCOP, increased SVR as body tries to compensate and decreased O_2 delivery.
- Neurogenic shock following spinal injury
  — Same picture as hypovolaemia: vasodilatation with decreased SVR, decreased ventricular filling and PCOP, and reduced cardiac index.

- It can be seen that the values cited above provide both an aid to diagnosis as well as a guide to specific management. Examples might include volume replacement in hypovolaemic shock, inotropes in cardiogenic shock, norepinephrine (noradrenaline) in septic shock as a means of increasing SVR.

Marking points: You must be aware that the role of the PA catheter is a subject of particular debate, and you must also demonstrate an understanding of the variables that can help rational management of the critically ill.

What is the aetiology and pathogenesis of acute lung injury (adult respiratory distress syndrome)? How is it diagnosed? Outline its management.

The terminology of what used to be called adult respiratory distress syndrome (ARDS) has changed so that it is now referred to as 'acute lung injury' (ALI) or sometimes 'acute' respiratory distress syndrome. ALI is a spectrum, with non-cardiogenic pulmonary oedema at the mild and ARDS at the severe end. Whatever the term, the condition remains an important problem in intensive therapy, and you should know enough to provide a convincing overview of pathogenesis and management.

Introduction

Acute lung injury or acute (formerly adult) respiratory distress syndrome is a common intensive care problem whose pathogenesis is not fully understood.

Aetiology and pathogenesis

- ARDS may complicate direct lung injury (aspiration of gastric contents, pulmonary trauma, smoke inhalation) or be associated with extrapulmonary insults (pancreatitis, SIRS, fat embolism syndrome, fluid overload).
- It appears that these conditions provoke the systemic release of various inflammatory mediators, result in neutrophil and macrophage recruitment with the release into the pulmonary capillaries of oxygen free radicals, proteases and a number of leukotrienes including interleukin 6.
- This precipitates a capillary leak syndrome (non-cardiogenic pulmonary oedema) in which the alveoli are flooded initially with oedema fluid, then an inflammatory exudate, which may lead to pulmonary fibrosis.

Diagnosis

- This is clinical and is made according to the following criteria:
  — Predisposing cause (and without pre-morbid chronic lung disease).
  — Progressive hypoxaemia ($P_aO_2 : F_IO_2$ ratio of <200).
  — Bilateral infiltrates on AP or PA chest X-ray.
  — Reduced pulmonary compliance.
  — Normal LVEDP (i.e. ~ normal PCOP which excludes cardiogenic pulmonary oedema).

Management

- **Supportive.** There is no specific therapy for ARDS and so management is supportive.
- **Research therapies** include exogenous surfactant (as is used in infant RDS); leukotriene inhibitors; anti-eicosanoids, etc. Previous trials with anti-tumour necrosis factor (TNF), corticosteroids and prostaglandins have been disappointing.
- **IPPV**
  — Addition of PEEP helps maintain lung volumes, decreases shunt and reduces V/Q mismatch.
  — Lowest F_IO_2 consistent with adequate oxygen delivery (to prevent O_2 toxicity): should aim at <0.6.
  — Nitric oxide: used in some units, not universally available.
  — Ventilatory modes are contentious, options include:
      High frequency jet ventilation (minimises airway pressures).
      Low tidal volumes to minimise airways pressures.
      Normal tidal volumes to ensure recruitment of atelectatic areas.
      Inverse ratio ventilation (may be useful if compliance is markedly reduced).

Pressure control ventilation.

Ventilation in the prone position (currently has its advocates: is as good as NO).

None, however, has been shown uniformly to be superior.

Marking points: The diagnosis of ARDS is straightforward and its management is supportive. The remainder is hypothetical and speculative and so you cannot fail the question if you do not present a unifying hypothesis and treatment plan. A broad overview of the inflammatory process should be convincing enough.

What factors determine oxygen delivery? How might you optimise this prior to major surgery?

Oxygen delivery to the mitochondria for energy generation via oxidative phosphorylation is the means by which the organism survives and so the process is fundamental. There has been much interest in the concept of optimising oxygen flux both in critically ill patients and in those undergoing major surgery. Even if you are unaware of this debate, an understanding of the basic principles should allow you to deduce how the important variables can be influenced to increase oxygen delivery.

Introduction

Oxygen delivery (oxygen flux) to the tissues is governed by cardiac output (heart rate × stroke volume) and arterial oxygen content, which is determined by the product of the haemoglobin concentration × % saturation × 1.34 (O_2 carrying capacity of Hb). Dissolved oxygen (0.003 ml dl $mmHg^{-1}$ is small and effectively can be ignored, unless hyperbaric therapy is contemplated. Oxygen delivery is a sensitive index of dysfunction because it incorporates several factors that influence utilisation, all of which are amenable to manipulation.

Oxygen delivery

- Equation is commonly expressed as:
  O_2 flux = (HR × SV(L min^{-1}))/(BSA (= cardiac index) × SaO_2%)/(100 × [Hb] (g × L^{-1}) × 1.34).
- Optimisation of oxygen delivery can be undertaken by logical approach to these factors.
- Requires invasive monitoring via a pulmonary artery catheter.

Cardiac output

- Prime determinants are heart rate and stroke volume, which itself is affected by several factors including venous return and myocardial contractility.
- Can be improved by:
  — Optimising volaemic status to enhance venous return: aim at PAOP of ~12 mmHg (PAOP is a better index of left ventricular end diastolic pressure and volume than CVP).
  — Optimising left ventricular performance (contractility) by use of inotropes (dobutamine, dopexamine, epinephrine (adrenaline), enoximone).

Oxygen saturation

- May be improved by enhanced cardiac performance as above.
- May be influenced by primary pulmonary factors affecting gas exchange. Some will be amenable to treatment (chest infection, atelectasis, bronchoconstriction).
- Supplemental oxygen to increase P_aO_2.

Haemoglobin concentration

- The O_2 delivery equation confirms the importance of haemoglobin: given a CO of 5 L min^{-1} and an SaO_2 of 100%, O_2 delivery at [Hb] of 10 g dl^{-1} is 670 ml min^{-1}; at 15 g dl^{-1} it rises to 1005 ml min^{-1}.
- Oxygen flux will be enhanced, therefore, if a low haemoglobin is increased by transfusion.

Dissolved oxygen

- At atmospheric pressure breathing air the O_2 solubility coefficient (0.003 ml dl $mmHg^{-1}$) means that dissolved O_2 content is ~0.26 ml dl^{-1}. Breathing 100% oxygen it increases to 1.7 ml dl^{-1} and at 3 atmospheres in a hyperbaric chamber it reaches 5.6 ml dl^{-1}. At this level dissolved O_2 can make a significant contribution to delivery.

Optimisation

In the context of major surgery and in view of the above, an optimisation regimen could be undertaken as follows:

- Establish invasive PA monitoring in ITU.
- Fluid therapy (crystalloid, colloid or blood) to maintain PAOP at 12 mmHg.
- Blood to increase haematocrit to 37–40% (adverse rheology if too high).
- Supplemental oxygen to maximise SaO_2.
- Inotropes to optimise left ventricular output.
- These factors should be manipulated to ensure delivery of >600 ml min^{-1} m^{-2}.

Marking points: This is a very logical question based on an understanding of the determinants of oxygen delivery. If you know these determinants then a description of how they may be manipulated is straightforward.

Under what circumstances does oxygen have adverse effects? What are the symptoms of toxicity? Outline the underlying mechanisms.

One of the perennial goals of anaesthesia is the maintenance of oxygenation, but it should not be forgotten that oxygen is potentially an extremely toxic agent. This question simply tests your recognition of that reality.

Introduction

One of the fundamental tenets of anaesthetic practice is the maintenance of oxygenation, and so it is paradoxical that a molecule which is essential to life can, under certain circumstances, be lethal.

Adverse effects at atmospheric pressure

- **Oxygen toxicity is dose related.** Dose–time curves have been constructed to allow the recommendation that 100% should be administered for no longer than 12 hours; 80% for no longer than 24 hours and 60% for no longer than 36 hours. An F_IO_2 of 0.5 can be maintained indefinitely.
- **Pulmonary pathology:** changes begin with tracheobronchitis, neutrophil recruitment and the release of inflammatory mediators, impairment of surfactant production, pulmonary interstitial oedema and, after ~1 week of exposure, the development of pulmonary fibrosis. Toxicity accelerates lung injury in the critically ill, and in patients receiving certain cytotoxic drugs, particularly bleomycin and mitomycin C, ARDS and respiratory failure may supervene after 'normal' doses of O_2.
- **Absorption atelectasis.** This is an adverse effect of therapy.
- **Hypoventilation.** Will suppress ventilation in individuals who rely on hypoxaemic respiratory drive. This is another adverse effect of therapy.
- **Paediatric retrolental fibroplasia (RLF).** This is associated with relative hyperoxia (although the condition is probably multifactorial), and will develop if an infant of postconceptual age <44 weeks maintains a P_aO_2 of >10.6 kPa (80 mmHg) for longer than 3 hours.

Toxic effects under hyperbaric conditions

- Toxicity presents the major limitation of hyperbaric oxygen therapy: is dose dependent and affects the lung, the CNS, the visual system, and probably myocardium, liver and renal tract.
- Pulmonary toxicity. Oxygen at 2 atmospheres produces symptoms in healthy volunteers at 8–10 hours plus a quantifiable decrease in vital capacity (VC) which starts at ~4 hours. It persists after exposure ceases.
- Central nervous system. Oxygen at 2 atmospheres is associated with nausea, facial twitching and numbness, olfactory and gustatory disturbance. Tonic-clonic seizures may then supervene without any prodrome, although some subjects report a premonitory aura.
- Eyes. Hyperoxia may be associated in adults with narrowing of the visual fields and myopia.

Symptoms

- Initial symptoms include retrosternal discomfort, carinal irritation and coughing. This becomes more severe with time, with a burning pain that is accompanied by the urge to breathe deeply and to cough. As exposure continues symptoms progress to severe dyspnoea with paroxysmal coughing.
- CNS symptoms as described above: nausea, facial twitching and numbness, olfactory and gustatory disturbance. Premonitory aura prior to convulsions.

Mechanism of toxicity

- Complex and not fully elucidated: multisystem effects suggest interference with basic metabolic pathways and enzyme systems.
  — Hyperoxia increases production of highly oxidative, partially reduced metabolites of oxygen which include hydrogen peroxide and O_2 derived free radicals (superoxide and hydroxyl radicals and singlet oxygen).
  — These substances appear particularly to interfere with enzyme systems which contain sulphydryl groups.

Marking points: Oxygen toxicity often goes unremarked, because the processes of acute lung injury follow the same pathological course, and the main cause is sought elsewhere. Your answer must demonstrate that you are aware of the phenomenon. As with other processes in which the mechanisms are not fully elaborated, very precise and detailed knowledge will not be expected of you.

What are the indications for cricothyroidotomy and for percutaneous tracheostomy? Describe a technique for performing these procedures with reference to the anatomy involved. List the main complications.

This is a question about the anatomy of the trachea applied to two clinical techniques which have different indications but broadly similar complications. You should be familiar with both even though you should hope never to have to use emergency cricothyroidotomy.

Introduction
Cricothyroidotomy and percutaneous tracheostomy both bypass the normal translaryngeal route to secure the airway, but the circumstances and urgency of their use could not be more different.

Cricothyroidotomy
- Has been described as a 'technique of failure' because it is used when all other attempts to secure a definitive airway have failed and when critical hypoxia is imminent.
- The cricothyroid membrane spans the inferior border of the thyroid cartilage and the superior border of the cricoid cartilage and immediately overlies the subglottic region of the larynx. It is covered anteriorly by skin and by superfical and deep fascia. Immediately lateral are the sternomastoid, the sternothyroid and the sternohyoid muscles and the carotid sheath.
- The cricothyroid membrane is used for emergency access because it is readily identifiable and because it is relatively avascular.
- **Technique:**
  — Position the patient with neck extended.
  — Identify membrane and stabilise the overlying skin (which is quite lax).
  — For needle cricothyroidotomy: insert cannula or purpose-made device (typically 4.0 mm internal diameter) through the membrane at angle of ~45° caudally (aspirating during needle advancement).
  — For surgical cricothyroidotomy: make small vertical skin incision followed by transverse incision in the membrane.
  — Insert spreader (or use scalpel handle) to open the airway and insert the appropriate tube under direct vision.

Percutaneous tracheostomy
- This is an elective, not an emergency procedure, which has become a well-established alternative to definitive surgical tracheostomy. It is an intensive care technique whose indications are the same as for formal tracheostomy in the critically ill: typically to simplify airway management in a patient who otherwise would face the problems of long-term tracheal intubation.
- There are variations in approach, but all are based on a modified Seldinger technique for placing a tracheostomy tube.
- **Technique**
  — A skin incision is made to allow a needle and guidewire to be placed through the fibro-elastic tissue that joins the tracheal rings.
  — The isthmus of the thyroid gland covers the second to fourth tracheal rings. A higher approach avoids the isthmus but is associated with greater incidence of tracheal stenosis. The technique can be performed through the subcricoid membrane or below any of the accessible tracheal rings. Many intensivists prefer to go low, below the second or even third ring.
  — Progressively larger dilators enlarge the diameter of the hole until it will accept a definitive tracheostomy tube.

— It is usual for a second anaesthetist to monitor this procedure from within by using a fibreoptic bronchoscope. The posterior wall of the trachea may be so ragged and friable that it can easily be perforated.

Complications

- Bleeding (immediate).
- Bleeding (delayed – erosion into vessels): not a problem with cricthyroidotomy because it is usually only a temporising measure before a definitive surgical or other airway is established.
- Creation of false passage.
- Oesophageal perforation.
- Barotrauma.
- Subcutaneous emphysema.
- Accidental decannulation.
- Subglottic stenosis: much more common after cricothyroidotomy because of the anatomical site of insertion.

Marking points: If these procedures are performed incorrectly the results can be disastrous. The applied anatomy is not complex but you should give a simple authoritative account of the techniques, particularly in relation to the potentially life-saving manoeuvre of cricothyroidotomy. If the techniqes that you describe put the patient in jeopardy then you will fail this question.

Obstetric anaesthesia and analgesia

A woman complains of persistent headache following a regional anaesthetic for obstetric delivery. What are the distinguishing clinical features of the likely causes?

Postpartum headache is common and is sometimes related directly to the anesthetic technique that has been used. It may be trivial or it may herald serious intracranial problems. Anaesthetists are asked frequently to review such patients and knowledge of the differential diagnosis is vital for all those who cover labour wards.

Introduction

Postpartum headache is common and is frequently, but not always trivial. For this reason a complaint of headache should always be taken seriously until its cause can be shown to be benign. The differential diagnosis includes:

- **Postdural puncture headache (PDPH)** after inadvertent, unrecognised or deliberate dural puncture. Onset is variable: usually after 24 hours but may occur earlier or later. May be frontal or occipital rather than global. It is typically postural and relieved by recumbency or abdominal pressure. Associated with photophobia, visual disturbance, neck and shoulder stiffness, tinnitus, anorexia, nausea and vomiting. The patient may feel systemically very unwell. Presentation is not always typical.
- **Headache associated with pregnancy-induced hypertension (PIH).** Generalised headache. No postural component. May be associated with visual disturbances ('eclampsia' comes from the Greek and means 'to flash forth'). Other findings may include epigastric pain, proteinuria, oliguria, thrombocytopenia.
- **Subarachnoid haemorrhage (SAH) (associated with PIH).** Severe headache of sudden onset. Photophobia. Decrease in conscious level (not invariable).
- **Cortical vein thrombosis (CVT).** Sudden onset. Similar clinical picture to SAH and may require CT/MR scanning to diagnose. May have focal neurology.
- **Migraine:** protean in its manifestations. May range from mild to very severe headache which is associated with transient focal neurological abnormalities. Patient history will be crucial to diagnosis.
- **Non-specific:** patient history useful. It may be related to caffeine withdrawal.
- **Space-occupying lesion:** rare but may masquerade as PDPH. Headache is usually dull and is associated with signs of raised ICP. Fitting may be misdiagnosed as eclampsia (44% of fits occur postpartum without prodromal signs). Needs CT scan.

155

- **Meningitis:** chemical or infective. Pyrexia, leucocytosis, meningism. Lumbar puncture should not be contemplated until other intracranial pathology has been excluded.

Marking points: Failure to diagnosis correctly the major causes of postpartum headache can be catastrophic and so a clear account of the clinical features of the important causes is essential.

What are the anaesthetic options for manual removal of retained placenta?

The incidence of retained placenta can be as high as 2% of all vaginal deliveries. It does carry potential hazards and this question is looking for the considered management of a common problem.

Introduction
Retained placenta occurs in up to 2% of all vaginal deliveries and anaesthetic assistance is usually required for its manual removal. In most cases the procedure is straightforward, but it can be associated with massive postpartum haemorrhage. There is always the potential for haemodynamic instability in this situation and the procedure should be viewed as urgent.

Risks of the procedure
- **Haemorrhage prior to manual removal:** quantitative assessment of blood loss is notoriously inaccurate in obstetrics and full assessment of volaemic status and circulatory adequacy must precede any anaesthetic. Good intravenous access is essential.
- **Intraoperative haemorrhage:** may be difficult to assess, and may be dramatic in some cases, e.g. of placenta accreta.
- **Uterine inversion:** a risk if umbilical cord traction is not counteracted by pressure on the uterus: the resulting shock results both from vagal stimulation and from bleeding.

Surgical requirements
- **Anaesthesia:** either general or regional: requirement is for sensory loss from T10 to S5.
- **Cervical relaxation** (the uterus may contract firmly round the placenta)
  — Pharmacological maneouvres have included the use of nitroglycerin (GTN) and beta$_2$-agonists such as salbutamol. If under general anaesthesia uterine relaxation by volatile inhalational agents is dose dependent.

Anaesthetic options
- General anaesthesia: advantages
  — Preferable (arguably) in a hypovolaemic or potentially hypovolaemic patient.
  — Allows adequate cervical relaxation as above.
- General anaesthesia: disadvantages
  — Generic problems associated with peripartum general anaesthesia (risk of aspiration of gastric contents).
  — Uterine atony: relaxation by volatile anaesthetics.
  — Polypharmacy: a patient receiving an obstetric GA will receive at least seven drugs and the patient may already have received prepartum opioids.
- Regional anaesthesia (existing epidural or subarachnoid block): advantages
  — Effective, rapid, simple.
  — Minimal drug load, no loss of contact with baby, no hangover effects.
- Regional anaesthesia: disadvantages
  — Sympathetic block may exacerbate hypotension in hypovolaemic mother.
  — Has no effect on uterine relaxation (but other drugs can be used to effect this as above).
  — Generic complications such as postdural puncture headache.

Marking points: This is a straightforward safety question and the candidate is expected to give a balanced view of the anaesthetic options in view of potential problems associated with this condition.

A fit primigravida suffers inadvertent dural puncture with a 16G Tuohy needle during attempted epidural insertion for analgesia in the first stage of labour (cervix 4 cm dilated). What is your management?

Inadvertent dural puncture is the most significant complication of lumbar epidural analgesia in obstetrics and every anaesthetist should have a strategy for its management.

Introduction

Inadvertent dural puncture rates of 1% or less mean that it is a relatively rare complication. Dural puncture, however, may albeit rarely have disastrous sequelae and the complication must be taken seriously. Immediate management varies between units but the broad approaches are described below.

- **Conduct of labour.** A 'dural tap' does not commit a mother to an instrumental delivery and so labour can proceed normally. It used to be held that the Valsalva manoeuvre which mothers use during the second stage increased CSF leak and increased the likelihood of PDPH. Increasing intra-abdominal pressure in fact is known to decrease CSF leak.
- **Re-siting.** Some units recommend that the epidural catheter is sited in another interspace. Other units believe that this approach is illogical and argue that it both risks another dural puncture and may also be associated with an abnormally high block. The advantage of having a catheter in the epidural space is that it can be used post-delivery to infuse normal saline; a manoeuvre which reduces the incidence of postdural puncture headache (PDPH).
- **Continuous spinal.** Other units recommend continuous subarachnoid anaesthesia. This provides several advantages: it provides certainty about catheter position; it removes the risk of further breaches in the dura, particularly if the procedure has been technically challenging; it minimises the likelihood of a high block; it ensures good analgesia for labour, normal delivery or operative delivery should it prove necessary; and it may – although this is contentious - reduce the incidence of PDPH.
- A typical regimen for bolus doses through an intrathecal epidural catheter might be 2.0 ml of a standard low dose solution (bupivacaine 2 mg and fentanyl 4 μg).
- In both cases top-up doses must be given by an anaesthetist.
- It is vital that the catheter is clearly marked as being in the intrathecal space.
- Some anaesthetists perform an immediate autologous blood patch in these circumstances. The evidence, such as it is, suggests that early blood patching in this way is less effective.
- A consultant obstetric anaesthetist should be informed.

Marking points: There is no consensus and so examiners will expect you to justify your own management of a significant complication.

A fit multigravida complains of a typical postdural puncture headache 24 hours after inadvertent dural puncture with a 16G Tuohy needle during attempted epidural insertion for analgesia. What is your management?

Inadvertent dural puncture will result in a severe headache in the majority of mothers. It is the most significant complication of lumbar epidural analgesia in labour and may rarely have disastrous sequelae. Prompt and effective management is of utmost importance.

Introduction

Inadvertent dural puncture with a 16G Tuohy epidural needle will result in a severe headache in about 80% of mothers. It may rarely have disastrous sequelae and mandates prompt and effective management. There is, however, no national consensus, and over 50 different treatments have been described. One approach to the management of PDPH is outlined below.

- **Confirm the diagnosis.** The classic PDPH develops at 24–48 hours, is postural in nature, may affect any part of the cranium, radiates to the neck and shoulders and is disabling. It may be associated with photophobia, tinnitus, dizziness, anorexia, nausea and vomiting. PDPH is due probably to traction on intracranial pain sensitive structures (tentorium and blood vessels) which become unsupported by CSF.
- **Assess the severity.** If the PDPH is moderate or improving then this may suggest more conservative management. If systemic symptoms supervene – nausea, anorexia, lethargy and profound malaise – this is an indication that there is significant sagging of intracranial contents with pressure on the brain stem at the foramen magnum. How disabling is the headache?
- **Assess the social circumstances.** Is the mother keen to return home to her other children? Are there other domestic factors which require her to be fit and mobile? It is inevitable that these considerations will have some effect upon management.
- **Drug treatment.** Assuming moderate severity and no urgency to leave hospital, initial treatment can be conservative: recumbency when headache supervenes and simple analgesia. Patients are advised frequently to overhydrate. This has no influence on CSF production. The only agents which increase it are corticosteroids: ACTH analogues such as tetracosactide ('Synacthen') are used by some anaesthetists. Benefits are anecdotal. Other drugs which have been used include sumatriptan and caffeine. Both are cerebral vasoconstrictors and address the symptoms but not the cause.
- **Blood patching.** If the headache is very disabling then the only technique that is likely to provide immediate relief is an extradural blood patch (EBP). This will abolish symptoms in almost all patients but in at least 30% of mothers the procedure may need to be repeated. It should only be carried out after thorough and documented discussion with the patient. EBP has been associated with a lumbovertebral syndrome and this risk must be weighed against those of persistent long-term headache, or neurological disaster (subdural haemorrhage) if PDPH is left untreated.

Marking points: PDPH is an important complication of a routine anaesthetic procedure. You must be able to diagnose the problem and describe safe and considered management.

What are the advantages of retaining motor power in a woman having an epidural for normal labour? How can this be achieved? What checks should be made before allowing the woman to get out of bed?

Ambulatory epidurals are increasingly popular and you may not even be familiar with 'traditional' high dose local anaesthetic administration for labour pain. There remains some disagreement about just how much walking a mother should do. Your answer should critically appraise the technique and demonstrate that checks of motor function are important.

Introduction

Ambulatory epidurals in labour are supplanting traditional high dose local anaesthetic epidurals. They are popular because their advantages as described below are evident to mothers and midwives alike.

Advantages

- Maternal satisfaction. Most dislike the motor paralysis associated with traditional epidurals which is accompanied by a sense of loss of control.
- Upright position is independently associated with swifter labours and less pain.
- Infusions of fluid are not usually necessary, and crystalloid infusions of 1 L have been shown to act as tocolytic agents for 20–30 min.
- Mobility allows cooperation with the midwife as labour proceeds (paralysed mothers are a heavy nursing problem).
- Ability to push during second stage of labour is retained.
- The influence of epidurals, both traditional and ambulatory, on the progress of labour is contentious. The latter is multifactorial and latest evidence suggests minimal influence by epidural blocks.

Methods of retaining motor power

- Rely either on low dose local anaesthetic alone (typically bupivacaine 0.625–0.1%, given by infusion or as bolus top-ups) or more commonly low dose plus an opioid. Fentanyl, alfentanil and diamorphine are used in the UK.
- Infusion pumps may restrict mobilisation, although they provide steady state analgesia.
- Avoid test doses (which contribute significantly to motor block should they be used). This makes some anaesthetists apprehensive. Intrathecal doses of low dose local anaesthetics, however, are not associated with total spinal anaesthesia.
- Combined spinal-epidural anaesthesia reduces the total amount of local anaesthetic agent delivered (the first dose of bupivacaine 2.5 mg, e.g., will last ~90 minutes).
- Ropivacaine. The claims that this drug produces differential sensory block are dubious. The agent is less potent than bupivacaine and at low doses motor sparing is not obviously better.

Checks prior to ambulation

- **Routine checks** should include maternal cardiovascular status (including presence of iv access) and fetal well-being (CTG monitoring).
- **Specific checks of motor power.** Scales such as that described by Bromage are impractical in late pregnancy. Proprioception will be impaired and the mother must not walk unaccompanied. Some weakness of quadriceps (which may be progressive with repeated top-ups) is likely, but if the mother can support her weight on one leg slightly bent then she will be able to move from the bed.

Marking points: Ambulatory epidurals in labour are popular but this must not be at the cost of maternal or fetal safety. Your answer should make this clear.

A fit primigravida is undergoing elective caesarean section for breech presentation under subarachnoid anaesthesia and suffers amniotic fluid embolism. What is the pathophysiology? How may it present and what is the differential diagnosis?

Amniotic fluid embolism is a rare but frequently fatal condition that may occur in normal pregnancy. Treatment is supportive and not specific, but immediate and effective management is crucial to survival and it is a problem with which anaesthetists should be familiar.

Introduction

Amniotic fluid embolism (AFE) is diagnosed rarely, but in the triennial maternal mortality report covering 1994–96 there were 17 deaths attributed to this cause, and it remains one of the most lethal, yet unpredictable, complications of pregnancy.

Predisposing factors

- Long-held belief that AFE is associated with factors such as overstimulation, placental abruption, increasing maternal age, difficult labour has not been supported by any well-designed study. The relationship is anecdotal.
- Access to the circulation occurs via disruption of normal barriers between amniotic fluid and the maternal venous circulation. How? Rupture of fetal membranes, open uterine or cervical veins (caesarean section, abruption) and a positive pressure gradient.

Pathophysiology

- The cause is not clear: access to the circulation of clear amniotic fluid is associated with less catastrophic sequelae than meconium-containing fluid. The clinical picture is similar to anaphylactoid reactions and septic shock. Pathophysiology may be the same: amniotic fluid contains arachidonic acid metabolites, prostacyclins, thromboxane, leukotrienes, prostaglandins. Amniotic fluid may enter circulation earlier in pregnancy and sensitize a mother. It may not be an embolic phenomenon but an immunological one.
- Haemodynamic changes supervene, plus pulmonary capillary injury and coagulopathy. Right heart failure secondary to pulmonary vasospasm is rarely severe: left ventricular dysfunction is the problem (confirmed in all human cases that have been monitored invasively) which may in turn elevate right-sided pressures.
- Biphasic response has been described:
  - Initial phase: transient pulmonary hypertension and fall in cardiac output due to physical obstruction by embolism in the pulmonary system. Is temporary (15–30 minutes), associated with V/Q mismatch and may lead to profound hypoxaemia.
  - Secondary phase: right-sided pressures decrease and LVF supervenes.
- Coagulopathy
  - Ranges from mild dysfunction to disseminated intravascular coagulation (DIC). May be the presenting feature in ~15%.

Clinical presentation

- Sudden and unexplained dyspnoea, patient may be restless and confused.
- Bronchoconstriction and cough.
- Rapid desaturation and cyanosis: may be profound enough to obtund cerebration and lead to coma.
- Hypotension, tachycardia, arrhythmias.
- Cardiorespiratory arrest.

- Coagulopathy may appear early: widespread oozing from wound and puncture sites, also massive vaginal bleeding (amniotic fluid causes uterine atony).

Differential diagnosis

There is no single clinical or laboratory finding that alone can confirm AFE and many other conditions may have a similar presentation. In this situation of caesarean section under spinal these would include:

- Pulmonary embolus.
- Anaphylaxis.
- Sepsis (likely to have been some prodrome).
- Air embolism.
- Cerebrovascular accident.
- Eclampsia.

Marking points: There is too much information in this answer for one question, but an outline of the pathophysiology may inform your description of the clinical presentation. The differential diagnosis is very broad and a sensible selection of possibilities will suffice.

What is the aetiology of pre-eclampsia? List the clinical features of severe pre-eclampsia and outline the relevance of the condition for anaesthesia.

Pre-eclampsia is a common complication of pregnancy which rarely can prove fatal. For this reason the disorder is taken very seriously on labour wards and anaesthetists must be aware of its potential problems.

Introduction

Pre-eclampsia complicates up to 7% of all pregnancies and is the second commonest cause of maternal death after thromboembolic disease. Its aetiology remains elusive, although there is no shortage of theories.

- Uteroplacental inadequacy. This stimulates production of endogenous vasoconstrictors as a means of ensuring uteroplacental perfusion. The resulting hypertension is mediated via humoral substances (vasoactive compounds have been identified in blood, placenta and amniotic fluid).
- Increased thromboxane A_2 (vasoconstrictor) and decreased prostacyclin (vasodilator) production results from a process of primary endothelial damage. This provides the rationale for treatment with aspirin, which has not, however, proved to be of benefit.
- Vascular damage results from circulating immune complexes. These are produced because of a maternal antibody response to the foreign fetal allograft that is inadequate.
- Primary disseminated intravascular coagulation (DIC): due to the formation and deposition of microvascular thrombin in all vascular beds, hence the multisystem nature of the disorder.
- More than one of these processes may be involved in the development of pre-eclampsia.

Clinical features of severe pre-eclampsia

- Hypertension: SBP >160 mmHg and DBP (Diastolic blood pressure) >110 mmHg.
- Proteinuria >5 g in 24 hours.
- Oliguria <500 ml in 24 hours.
- Headache and visual disturbances.
- Epigastric and hypochondrial pain.
- Hyperreflexia and clonus.
- Pulmonary oedema.
- Thrombocytopenia (<100 000).
- HELLP syndrome.
- Convulsions (= eclampsia).

Anaesthetic implications

- Coagulopathy may preclude neuraxial blockade.
- Treatment may include antihypertensive agents which may influence response to epidural and subarachnoid block.
- Hypotension associated with subarachnoid block may be difficult to control accurately (sensitivity to exogenous vasopressors is enhanced).
- Treatment may include $MgSO_4$ (may potentiate neuromuscular blocking drugs if GA needed).
- May be effectively hypovolaemic (vasoconstricted hypertensive circulation).
- May be easily overloaded with fluid and develop pulmonary oedema secondary to leaky pulmonary capillaries.
- Laryngoscopy, tracheal intubation and extubation can provoke pressor response with extreme surges in systolic blood pressure (>250 mmHg).

- May be associated with laryngeal and upper airway oedema.

> **Marking points:** When the aetiology of a particular condition is disputed it is hard to mark rigorously: as long as you demonstrate some basic knowledge of possible causation you should pass that part of the question. The clinical features are straightforward and the main anesthetic implications should be familiar, and so you will be expected to cover most of the major points.

You have sited a lumbar epidural catheter for pain relief in the first stage of labour but the midwife tells you that it is ineffective. Why might it have failed and what is your management?

The epidural that is inadequate either initially or throughout labour is a problem which every anaesthetist on the labour ward encounters. This question aims to test your knowledge of the important causes and to assess your clinical management.

Introduction
The inadequate epidural is a familiar problem for labour ward anaesthetists. Some workers have reported an incidence of patchy sensory analgesia that is initally as high as 35%. While the final percentage of epidurals that are unsatisfactory is in low single figures, it has to be acknowledged that there are some mothers for whom it is impossible to provide adequate analgesia because of anatomical or technical factors beyond anaesthetic control.

- **Problem: It is completely ineffective**—the mother claims to have had no relief at all (continued use of Entonox is a useful guide).
  - May not be in the extradural space at all. Was there difficulty in insertion? Was loss of resistance equivocal? It will need to be resited, after discussion with the mother, or alternative analgesia used.
  - Solution may be incorrect (unlikely but worth checking).
  - Solution may be inappropriate for the stage of labour and level of pain. If contractions rapidly become severe, either naturally or with augmentation of labour, the initial dose(s) of epidural anaesthesia may be unable to catch up. It may be useful to give a single dose of high concentration local anaesthetic solution before reverting to the typical low dose/opioid mixture.
- **Problem: It is one-sided**
  - Epidurograms have confirmed that catheters readily escape through intervertebral foramina and can remain unilateral even when only 2–3 cm remain in the space.
  - Some mothers do appear to have a dorsomedian fold (its composition remains disputed) which can effectively separate the two sides of the extradural space.
  - Withdrawal of the catheter is worth trying: it sometimes works.
  - Position: top-ups with the mother lying on the unblocked side is rarely helpful. A mother who remains in the decubitus position for 30 minutes will have a sensory block only one to two segments higher on the dependent side, and so the influence of posture is not great.
  - A 'standard' top-up of plain bupivacaine 0.25–0.50% may be worth trying, although it will prevent mobility.
- **Problem: There is rectal pressure or perineal discomfort**
  - This can be a significant problem in which analgesia is often satisfactory until the descent of the baby's head.
  - Extradural opioids attenuate but do not abolish the problem.
  - Caudad spread to the sacral roots may be slow, and may also be inhibited by a large S1 nerve root.
  - Spread to the sacral segments is optimised if a top-up is given with the patient sitting (or lying) at a head-up angle of 25°.
  - In cases in which the perineal pain is intolerable some anaesthetists advocate performing a sacral extradural block. Great care is needed because of the proximity of the baby's head to the sacrum (assuming cephalic presentation).

- **Problem: The block is atypical, high and patchy**
  - — An epidural catheter may inadvertently have entered the subdural space.
  - — Subdural block is often patchy, it may be extensive and unilateral, may extend very high (the subdural space extends into the cranium), and usually spares the sacral roots. Because the dura and arachnoid are more densely adherent anteriorly there may be a relative sparing of the motor fibres. Sympathetic block may be minimal and analgesia may be delayed. Horner's syndrome may be apparent.
  - — The use of a multi-holed catheter may further confuse the picture. It may lie partly within the epidural and partly within the subdural space. Slow injection will favour emergence of the solution from the proximal epidural holes; more vigorous injection will favour dispersal through the distal subdural hole.
  - — Should an atypical block raise the suspicion of subdural placement then the catheter should be removed and the epidural resited (if desired).
- **Problem: There is a 'missed segment'**
  - — 'Missed segments' are very rare: this complaint is usually revealed on formal sensory testing to be a unilateral block.
  - — May occur following LOR (Loss of Resistance) technique to air in decubitus position. Injected air rises to the upper part of the epidural space and may prevent access of local anaesthetic to the nerves. Commonest dermatome affected is L1.
  - — Can try stronger solutions, change of position, or if necessary resite.
- **Problem: There is a dense block in one segment: minimal elsewhere**
  - — Catheter may be in the paravertebral space (rare complication).
  - — Withdrawal of catheter may help. May need resiting.

Marking points: This is a common clinical problem for which even some large specialist textbooks do not provide very clear guidance. Your own clinical experience will be relevant in your answer which will gain more credibility if you convey some sense of having dealt with this situation.

What clinical features would alert you to the fact that a woman undergoing caesarean section under subarachnoid anaesthesia was developing a high block? Describe your management.

This is a question about a significant clinical problem in obstetric anaesthetic practice which requires accurate diagnosis and safe management.

Introduction

Although the final height of a subarachnoid block is determined mainly by the mass of drug that is injected, there are some patients in whom spread is unpredictable and to a much higher level than the dermatomal level of T5 which is necessary for pain-free caesarean section.

Clinical features

- **Onset.** The development of a high block may be sudden or insidious. The latter is more usual.
- **Respiratory symptoms.** It is common for intercostal paralysis from the mid-thoracic level to cause subjective dyspnoea. If the block ascends higher the patient will complain of increasing difficulty in breathing to the point at which they become unable to cough or speak in more than a whisper. If the block renders them apnoeic it has reached C3 and affected diaphragmatic function.
- **Sensory loss.** As the block ascends there will be paraesthesia in the upper limbs. Sensory testing must take note of the fact that in the thorax the dermatomal level immediately above T1 is C5. The skin of the lower face and jaw is supplied by the trigeminal nerve, numbness of which indicates sensory block at brain stem level.
- **Motor weakness.** Lags behind sensory loss by ~two dermatomes. Weakness of hand grip is a reliable sign of a block that has reached the level of the cervical roots.
- **Circulatory effects.** A high block may be associated with hypotension, although it is the lumbar sympathetic block which makes the greatest contribution. It is often written that paralysis of the cardiac accelerator fibres (sympathetic outflow from T1 to T4) gives rise to a marked bradycardia. In practice high blocks and total spinals do not consistently cause this effect.
- **Conscious level.** A very high block, or 'total spinal' will be accompanied by loss of consciousness.

Management: depends on rapidity of onset and height of spread

Total spinal (high block affecting diaphragmatic function and conscious level)

- Maintain left lateral tilt to minimise aortocaval compression.
- Oxygen via bag and mask.
- Tracheal intubation with cricoid pressure.
- Anaesthetic induction agents and muscle relaxants should not be necessary, although some would advocate a very small dose of induction agent or a benzodiazepine.
- Ephedrine 6 mg or phenylephrine 50–100 μg boluses (repeated as needed) for hypotension, plus fluid administration.
- The block will take some time to regress to the point at which comfortable respiration will be possible: maintain anaesthesia throughout with nitrous oxide, oxygen and low concentration volatile agent.
- Reassure the relatives and keep them informed at all times.
- One or more postdelivery visits will be essential.

High block

- Maintain left lateral tilt to minimise aortocaval compression (if predelivery).
- Ensure that the shoulders (and cervical spine) are kept higher than the thoracic spine.
- Oxygen via facemask.
- Ephedrine 6 mg or phenylephrine 50-100 μg boluses (repeated as needed).
- Fluid administration.
- Consider a small dose of benzodiazepine (e.g. midazolam 1 mg increments).
- Reassure mother and partner if present.
- Intubate if necessary (this may not always be so – a characteristic of these high blocks is that they regress quickly), but maternal distress may make this inevitable.
- Ensure that you make, at the very least, one postdelivery visit.

Marking points: Your answer must make clear that you can diagnose rapidly an ascending block and that you can manage the situation safely and appropriately, given the emotional implications of the operation that is being performed.

A woman undergoing caesarean section under subarachnoid anaesthesia complains of pain. Describe your management. How may this situation be prevented?

This is an important problem. Litigation which relates to the perception of 'pain' during caesarean section performed under regional block is now more common than litigation relating to awareness during general anaesthesia. You must have a strategy for dealing with the situation.

Introduction
A potential problem of the otherwise very successful technique of spinal anaesthesia for caesarean section is the complaint of pain or discomfort during parts of the procedure. A block of dubious efficacy provides particular difficulties for the anaesthetist.

Assessment
The patient must be believed and the complaint of pain taken seriously. At any stage the nature of the sensation must be identified: is it sharp pain or is it the discomfort of pressure that is worsened by apprehension, or is it visceral discomfort associated with uterine or peritoneal traction?

Timing
- **At incision**
  - Was the performance of the block uneventful and the intrathecal administration of local anaesthetic (+/– adjunct) unequivocal?
  - Has the patient lost motor power in the lower limbs?
  - If the answer is 'Yes': wait – the block may be slow in onset.
  - If the answer is 'No': it is probable that the block will fail. Options are to repeat the block in the decubitus position while maintaining sterility (it has been done, but is not a favoured option for obvious practical reasons) or to proceed to general anaesthesia. The mother should be involved in any decision and the discussion documented.
- **After incision but during stretching of the muscle layers prior to delivery**
  - Is it pain or discomfort, or apprehension of pain?
  - Symptoms must be elucidated and additional analgesia offered.
  - Options: entonox, intravenous opioids (paediatrician should be warned about neonatal depression), intravenous clonidine (the drug is not used widely in the UK), or infiltration with local anaesthetic. Benzodiazepines cause amnesia, which is undesirable in the emotional context of chidbirth.
  - Clinical findings and the actions taken must be documented.
  - If the mother complains of severe pain then general anaesthesia should be offered, despite the fact that delivery may be imminent.
- **After delivery but during uterine exteriorisation or peritoneal traction**
  - As before symptoms must be elucidated and additional analgesia offered as above. Atropine or glycopyrrolate may attenuate vagally mediated symptoms.
  - Treatment or proceeding to GA must be discussed with the mother and documented.
- **During closure**
  - The operation is near its end and it is unfortunate to have to resort to general anaesthesia with the administration of another six or seven drugs and the attendant risks, but the block may be regressing rapidly.
  - Management must be guided by assessment of the patient's symptoms and after discussion with her. The same analgesic options are available but general anaesthesia may still be necessary. Five minutes of untreated severe pain constitutes awareness under anaesthesia and is not defensible.

Prevention

- **Appropriate anaesthetic technique**
  — Adequate volume of local anaesthetic.
  — Must lie patient supine (tilted) rapidly after use of hyperbaric solutions in the sitting position lest they fix rapidly in the lower lumbar and sacral areas.
  — Appropriate positioning using tilt if the block is slow to ascend.
- **Use of adjuncts**
  — Opioids (fentanyl, morphine, diamorphine).
  — Alpha$_2$ adrenoceptors agonists such as clonidine.
  — These agents at least double the duration of effective analgesia and reduce the problems of visceral discomfort.
- **Appropriate assessment of block height**
  — Surgery should not proceed until the block has been assessed.
  — Ideally a block to T5 is required, using light touch as the sensory modality. Testing sensory levels to pinprick or temperature are much less effective at predicting visceral discomfort.

Marking points: This is a core area of obstetric anaesthetic practice and you must demonstrate that you can manage the problem of pain during caesarean section rationally and pragmatically.

What are the pathophysiological and clinical features of HELLP syndrome? What are the diagnostic laboratory findings and the priorities in management?

HELLP is an uncommon but important variant of pre-eclampsia which can be perilous. Although its diagnosis and management are largely obstetric, anaesthetic input extending to critical care may be needed and a broad acquaintance with the problems is expected.

Introduction
HELLP syndrome was first described in 1982 and is seen in a subset of patients with pre-eclampsia. The acronym stands for *H*aemolysis, *E*levated *L*iver enzymes and *L*ow *P*latelets.

Pathophysiology
- The cause of pre-eclampsia remains unknown, but a simplification of the pathophysiology is summarised below. It is a disease of potentially widespread organ ischaemia.
- Normal vasodilatation of vessels in the placental bed after the first trimester does not develop: the vessels instead become constricted and may develop atherosclerosis.
- Simultaneously there may be evidence of endothelial abnormality and increased vascular reactivity.
- Increased thromboxane A_2 (vascoconstrictor) and decreased prostacyclin (vasodilator) production results from this process of primary endothelial damage, which manifests as an increase in SVR. There may be an increase in platelet turnover, together with abnormal cytokine release that may precipitate intravascular coagulation.
- The clinical manifestations of pre-eclampsia are hypertension, proteinuria and IUGR. At worst the ischaemia leads to multi-organ failure. Fatal cases demonstrate fibrinoid ischaemic necrosis in placenta, kidneys, brain and liver. Microvascular thrombin is found in all vascular beds.
- HELLP syndrome is a variant of this parent disorder. It is characterised by hepatic ischaemia with periportal haemorrhage and even necrosis. There is microangiopathic haemolytic anaemia plus thrombocytopenia (not necessarily associated with other derangements of coagulation).

Clinical features
- Hypertension and proteinuria may initially be mild.
- Epigastric pain (90%), malaise (90%), nausea and vomiting (50%).
- Right upper quadrant (RUQ) pain (liver surface may have multiple petechial haemorrhages which can coalesce and rupture. The clinical features are of RUQ pain and hypovolaemia.)
- RUQ pain may splint the right hemi-diaphragm leading to atelectasis.

Diagnostic laboratory findings: consistent with the acronym
- Thrombocytopenia: particularly important is a rapid downward trend.
- Haemolytic anaemia.
- Hepatic dysfunction: elevated transaminases: AST, ALT, GTT and other enzymes.
- Renal impairment: rising urea and creatinine, haemoglobinuria (haemolysis).

Management priorities
- The underlying condition is reversible upon delivery: the main priority is to deliver the fetus.

- HELLP is an ischaemic disorder and so part of its management includes haemodynamic manipulation by plasma volume expansion and vasodilatation to increase O_2 delivery.
- Vasodilatation reduces SVR and improves perfusion. Drugs used include hydralazine, labetalol (best in those with hypertension associated with high cardiac output), GTN (in cases with pulmonary oedema).
- Complications may require critical care: although delivery initiates reversal of the disease, platelets may continue to fall for up to 72 hours.

Marking points: This is a large question, so do not spend excessive time on the as yet unelucidated pathophysiology of the condition. Broad principles should suffice to inform your account of the clinical features and laboratory findings (which the acronym should help you to recall). Pre-eclampsia and all its variants are diseases of pregnancy and are treated by delivery. Assume the worst case scenario for postdelivery intensive care and you may well pass a question on which you thought you might struggle.

Describe the anaesthetic management of major intrapartum haemorrhage requiring emergency operation.

There were 12 deaths in the 1994–96 triennium directly attributed to haemorrhage: three were associated with placenta praevia, four with placental abruption and five with postpartum haemorrhage following caesarean section. Although the absolute numbers remain small, for every fatality there will be an unquantifiable, but much larger number of near misses, and the trend suggests that management of maternal bleeding is suboptimal. Life-threatening haemorrhage is reported as occurring in 1 in every 1000 deliveries. It is a very important area of obstetric anaesthetic practice.

Introduction

There were 12 deaths reported in the maternal mortality report for the 1994–96 triennium which were attributed directly to haemorrhage. There were almost certainly many more near misses and suboptimal management may result in renal failure, disseminated intravascular coagulation or multi-organ failure. Effective management is crucial.

Assessment

The blood supply to the uterus at term can reach 800 ml min^{-1} and so acute antepartum haemorrhage is usually recognised. The slow loss of blood volume over a number of hours postpartum is arguably even more dangerous because patients may compensate until the point almost of irreversible circulatory collapse.

- Assessment should be made without delaying resuscitation. It should include assessment of the source of the bleeding as well as of the fetal gestation and viability.
- Assessment should include heart rate and blood pressure (but note that SBP may not drop until decompensation occurs at 30–40% loss of blood volume), capillary refill time, pulse pressure (this is a subtle sign: it narrows during early phase of blood loss, and MAP may increase), respiratory rate, urine output and mental state. Significant derangements of any of these denote substantial blood loss.

Resuscitation phase

- High flow oxygen via face mask.
- Left uterine displacement using right pelvic wedge, or left decubitus position.
- Intravenous access with two short 14 G cannulae.
- Restore circulating volume aggressively with colloid, crystalloid, O-negative blood.
- Blood for cross-match (at least 6 units) and baseline investigations.
- Alert laboratory to possible need for FFP, platelets, cryoprecipitate.
- Minimal monitoring should include SpO$_2$, blood pressure, ECG, urine output.

Anaesthetic phase

- Consider upgrading monitoring: CVP and intra-arterial BP, temperature, and have transducers available.
- Upgrade fluid delivery apparatus to include blood warmers and pressure infusors. Filters are not necessary. Recent work questions the traditional teaching that blood salvage devices cannot eliminate amniotic fluid and should not be used, but experience is very limited and so this advice should probably stand.
- Maintain uterine displacement and high flow oxygen administration (unless the mother has delivered).
- Induce anaesthesia with an intravenous dose appropriate to the assessment of the circulation. A well-resuscitated mother may require 4 mg kg^{-1} thiopental: a moribund patient requires nothing. Other agents that can be used include ketamine 0.5–1.0 mg kg^{-1} and etomidate 0.1–0.3 mg kg^{-1}.

- Suxamethonium; cricoid pressure and tracheal intubation.
- Oxygen; nitrous oxide and volatile agent should be given in appropriate proportions: sick mothers will require only 100% O_2 and 0.5–0.75 MAC of volatile.
- Continue postdelivery resuscitation with blood/blood products according to coagulation, seek advice of consultant haematologist.
- Consider inotropic agents: dobutamine; dopamine; epinephrine (adrenaline); dopexamine (to improve renal and splanchnic blood flow).
- Beware circulatory overload (but remember that a drop in blood pressure may indicate a reduction in blood volume of up to 30–40%).
- Consider stabilising the mother postoperatively on the intensive care unit.

Marking points: This answer contains a lot of detail, but the important principles are in rapid simultaneous assessment and resuscitation, and anaesthesia in the hypovolaemic pregnant patient. Your overall management must be safe and effective, even if there is not time to include all of the points above.

Describe the management of emergency caesarean section for cord prolapse in a fit 21-year-old primagravida.

Cord prolapse is an obstetric emergency which is managed, perhaps too frequently, by caesarean section under general anaesthesia. This question, however, is not simply asking you to rehearse your standard obstetric GA technique, but seeks a considered discussion of the possible options.

Introduction

Cord prolapse defines the situation in which the umbilical cord passes through the cervix before the presenting part of the fetus. It is an obstetric emergency for which the only management is caesarean section.

- Speed is essential, but this need not militate against reasoned consideration of the options, which will depend on the status of the fetus, and particularly whether or not the midwife or obstetrician can keep the cord free by manual upward pressure on the presenting part.
- Labour should be stopped. Vigorous uterine contractions make it more difficult to keep the cord clear and can be diminished by use of a tocolytic: ritodrine (may be impractical as it needs to be given by infusion), salbutamol, glyceryl trinitrate or $MgSO_4$.
- If the fetal blood supply is at risk then general anaesthesia is the only realistic option (unless the mother refuses) and a standard technique with usual safety precautions can be used.
- The urgency of the situation should not prevent a calm but swift preoperative assessment, which must include the anaesthetic and drug history, and airway assessment. Cord prolapse is not associated with cervical 'shock' or other cardiovascular disturbance.
  — Oral antacid (0.3 molar Na citrate typically): ranitidine iv will be ineffectual.
  — Pre-oxygenation with 3 vital capacity breaths (~ as effective as 5 minutes and speed is vital).
  — Mother should be wedged or tilted to avoid aortocaval compression.
  — Rapid sequence induction via adequate intravenous access.
  — Tracheal intubation and IPPV with N_2O/O_2 at least 50 : 50, and volatile (e.g. isoflurane using an overpressure technique to minimise likelihood of awareness: the surgeon will be in a hurry).
  — Revert to standard technique after cord clamping, opioid analgesia.
- If the cord is free from compression by the presenting part and the situation is stable, there is no reason why regional anaesthesia should not be used. Its advantages are numerous but the anaesthetist is likely to come under pressure from both obstetrician and midwives to proceed to general anaesthesia. The experience and seniority of the anaesthetist will be of importance here.
- **Extradural anaesthesia.** There is no place for initiating an epidural de novo, but a working epidural may be in place.
  — Top-up using e.g. lidocaine (lignocaine) 2% × 20 ml plus epinephrine (adrenaline) 1 in 200 000 plus $NaHCO_3$ 8.4% × 2 ml. This reduces the onset time by at least 50%.
  — This option should only be used if the anaesthetist is very confident that analgesia will be satisfactory: an epidural that has been less than perfect during the preceding labour should be abandoned.
- **Subarachnoid anaesthesia**
  — After removal of the epidural catheter. Some anaesthetists fear that spinal superimposed upon epidural anaesthesia will result in an excessively high block. With low dose/opioid epidural mixtures this is not a problem, and as long as the shoulders and cervical spine are kept higher than the curve of the

thorax at T5/6 the block height can be controlled.

— De novo. Standard subarachnoid block can be performed in the decubitus position using all usual precautions, including those to prevent hypotension. Analgesia adequate to begin surgery usually develops within 5–6 minutes of subarachnoid injection (with bupivacaine 0.5% in glucose 8%).

- **Maternal consent.** This situation can be very fraught and it is important that the anaesthetist represents a centre of calm focus. If the cord is free from compression then the situation is urgent but not extreme, and the anaesthetic options can be discussed. This conversation may have to take place in theatre or even on the way to theatre, but it is essential to involve the mother (and partner if appropriate) in the anaesthetic decsions that are made.

Marking points: Your answer will make clear whether you are simply following the standard party line (GA at all costs) or whether you appreciate the options in this situation. Your answer should include a discussion of those other options, even if you reject them, and you must emphasise the importance of involving the mother.

Paediatric anaesthesia

How does the physiology of an infant aged 6 months differ from that of an adult?

This is a standard question which is orientated towards basic science and which aims to test your understanding of the important physiological differences in paediatric patients.

Introduction
Anatomical and physiological differences between adults and children are most marked at birth and converge with increasing age. At 6 months of age the physiological differences are best described by reference to the individual systems.

Surface area to mass ratio
- The smaller the child the larger is the ratio of surface area to mass. This is probably the most important single factor and it explains a number of the physiological differences.
- A large surface area is associated with increased heat loss, and all infants are at greater risk than adults or larger children of hypothermia.
- The need to maintain body temperature via heat production results in a higher metabolic rate and higher tissue oxygen demand. Desaturation occurs quicker.
- The higher BMR is associated with higher resting heart and respiratory rates.

Cardiovascular
- In the cardiovascular system the capacity of the heart to increase cardiac output by increasing stroke volume is limited. Cardiac output increases predominantly by increasing heart rate.
- The limbs are smaller in relation to the body. This means that there is less blood volume to mobilise from the periphery in response to hypovolaemia. Infants have less reserve.

Respiratory
- Respiratory compensation occurs via an increase in respiratory rate more than by increases in tidal volume. Infant ribs are more horizontal and respiration is predominantly diaphragmatic. Intercostal and accessory muscles are relatively weak. (Deficient in type 1 muscle fibres until ~2 years old.)
- Closing capacity exceeds FRC (up to about the age of 6 years) and infants generate physiological CPAP (~4 cmH$_2$O) by partial adduction of the cords during expiration.

Renal

- Infant kidneys have a reduced glomerular filtration rate, diminished tubular function and sodium excretion and a decreased concentrating ability. The excretory load is diminished by the fact that 50% of the nitrogen is incorporated into growing tissue. Complete maturation of renal function occurs at about 2 years of age.
- Neonates are certainly more sensitive to opioids (causes include blood–brain barrier immaturity and decreased hepatic clearance). By 6 months the response to morphine is probably the same as in adults.
- Total body water content is proportionately higher in infants, who have a larger volume of distribution for water soluble drugs. (Need higher initial dose to achieve blood level.) Fat content is lower: lipid soluble drugs whose effect is terminated by redistribution will have enhanced effects. Lower protein binding increases the amount of free drug.

Marking points: This is a large topic and so a broad overview is adequate, provided that the main safety points (temperature control, opioid sensitivity) are covered.

What are the anatomical differences of relevance to the anaesthetist between an infant aged 6 months and an adult?

This is a variation on the previous question but which again is orientated towards basic science and which aims to test your understanding of the important anatomical differences in paediatric patients.

Introduction
Anatomical and physiological differences between adults and children are most marked at birth and converge with increasing age. At 6 months of age the anatomical differences are best described by reference to the individual systems.

Surface area to mass ratio
- The smaller the child the larger is the ratio of surface area to mass. This results in a higher metabolic rate and makes infants more prone to hypothermia and desaturation. (This, strictly speaking, is physiology, but it is a consequence of the anatomy.)

Airway
It is in the airway that anatomical differences are significant for the anaesthetist:

- Head size is greater in relation to the body.
- Angle of the jaw is greater (140° vs 120°).
- Dimensions of the upper airway are effectively narrowed by large tongue, lymphoid tissue, narrow nares and pharynx.
- Epiglottis is 'infantile': longer, stiffer and U-shaped. It makes an angle of 45° with the anterior pharyngeal wall (in adults it lies closer to base of the tongue).
- Larynx is higher: C3/4 (C5/6 in adults); lies more anteriorly and is also tilted anteriorly.
- Cricoid ring is the narrowest part of the upper airway. Important to avoid trauma. Circumferential oedema is significant if structure is small.
- Trachea is short (4–5 cm) and narrow.
- Peripheral airways (<2 mm) account for ~50% of total airways resistance. Significant in diseases such as laryngotracheobronchitis and bronchiolitis.
- Infant ribs are more horizontal and respiration is predominantly diaphragmatic.

Cardiovascular system
- In the CVS the left and right ventricles have attained the adult ratio by 6 months. Limbs are smaller in relation to the body. Less blood volume is available to mobilise from the periphery in response to hypovolaemia. Infants have less reserve.

Nervous system
- **In the CNS** the spinal cord ends at ~L4 at birth, is at the adult level by the end of the second year of life. There is less fibrous connective tissue in the sacral epidural space than in adults and so local anaesthetic spread is greater.
- **Myelination.** Not complete until at least 6 months.
- **Sympathetic effects.** Hypotension following epidural analgesia in children up to about the age of 6 years is rare. This suggests some delay in maturation of the sympathetic autonomic system.

Marking points: Your answer should include the key safety points associated with common procedures: temperature loss, problems with intubation, the lower spinal cord level.

Describe the anaesthetic management for a 5-year-old patient who requires re-operation for haemorrhage an hour after tonsillectomy.

This is a serious emergency which is relatively common and which presents problems enough for it to be of considerable importance to anaesthetists. It is also a favourite examination topic to which every candidate should have given some thought.

Introduction

The child who is bleeding following tonsillectomy may be gravely unwell, and the anaesthetic management of these patients is challenging. Although there is agreement among anaesthetists about the problems, there is some divergence of opinion about the optimum anaesthetic technique.

Main problems

- **Haemorrhage.** The main problem is that of hypovolaemia.
- Blood loss may be occult: although the child who has been bleeding from the tonsillar beds may lose a significant proportion of their blood volume, they may swallow rather than vomit or cough out the blood.
- The child may be agitated and very distressed. This may be compounded by disorientation and hangover from the anaesthetic if recent (as in this scenario).
- The child will have a stomach full of blood.
- There is likely to be continuing bleeding into the airway.
- The child will have undergone recent tracheal intubation (usually, although some anaesthetists use laryngeal mask airways).
- There may be an underlying bleeding diathesis (e.g. von Willebrand's disease or abnormalities of platelet function).

Management

- **Fluid resuscitation** must be initiated, although in a severe case it may be impossible to restore volaemic status before resorting to surgery. Depending upon assessment of blood loss (remembering that most will be invisible) give blood or colloid. Crystalloid restores circulating volume less effectively.
- **Premedication.** Atropine is favoured by some. Opioids or benzodiazepines are inappropriate if not dangerous in this situation.
- **Induction of anaesthesia.** Traditional teaching recommended inhalation induction in the left lateral and head-down position, followed by tracheal intubation under deep volatile anaesthesia. There are disadvantages to this approach, even when performed by senior and experienced clinicians.
  - Inhalation induction may be difficult in the lateral position with a distressed and uncooperative child who is continuing to bleed.
  - Anaesthesia deep enough to allow smooth tracheal intubation is likely to compromise the circulatory reflexes of a child who is probably hypovolaemic.
  - Intubation in the left lateral postion in a child who continues to bleed into the airway is potentially difficult.
- **Induction of anaesthesia.** The alternative technique is rapid sequence induction with cricoid pressure.
  - Less fraught although still potentially difficult in the distressed child.
  - Potential problems with hypotension remain, but less than with inhalation.
  - Rapid control of the airway is more certain.
- **Maintenance of anaesthesia**
  - Endotracheal tube should be smaller than predicted (check previous anaesthetic record and go one size down to avoid laryngeal oedema).

- — Standard anaesthetic technique; maintenance of CVS stability with continuing fluid resuscitation.
- — Nasogastric tube to try to empty the stomach (do not leave it down).
- **Postoperative care**
  - — Fluids; oxygen; cautious analgesia (remember the child has received two anaesthetics and hypovolaemia is still a risk).
  - — Beware continued bleeding.
  - — Oxygen if tolerated.
  - — Later investigation of possible cause if indicated.

Marking points: This is one of the standard paediatric emergencies and you should be very clear about the potential problems and be able to justify your choice of anaesthetic technique.

A 6-week-old child presents for pyloromyotomy (for pyloric stenosis). Describe the management of this case.

This is one of the commonest surgical conditions seen in infants. The question tests your knowledge of its pathophysiology and the principles of resuscitation of dehydration.

Introduction

Congenital pyloric stenosis presents typically with projectile vomiting in a lusty male infant in the early weeks of life. Persistent vomiting means that babies are dehydrated, alkalotic, hypochloraemic and hypokalaemic.

Preoperative management

- This is not a surgical emergency, and surgery should be deferred until the biochemistry is returning to normal with HCO_3 <30 mmol L^{-1} and Cl^- >90 mmol L^{-1}.
- Assess the degree of dehydration (mild ~5%; moderate ~10%; severe ~15%) and calculate deficit. This is more difficult than it sounds and likely to be quite inaccurate.
- Clinical features include: weight loss, decreased skin turgor, sunken fontanelles and eyes, listlessness and oliguria.
- Rehydrate. Dextrose infusion will replace the intracellular water deficit: and NaCl is required to resuscitate the ECF (Extracellular fluid) volume. Replacement regimens vary between units, but a dehydrated child may require as much as 10–12 ml kg h^{-1}, given as a combination of dextrose, saline and replacement potassium. Solutions include NaCl 0.45%/glucose 2.5% (may contain insufficient glucose for a neonate); NaCl 0.45%/glucose 5% (hypertonic) and NaCl 0.18%/glucose 4% (adequate glucose but may contain insufficient sodium).
- If the child is severely dehydrated to the point at which the peripheral circulation is compromised they may require an initial fluid bolus of NaCl 0.9% of 20 ml kg^{-1}.
- Nasogastric tube and washouts will empty the stomach (which may contain residual barium).

Anaesthetic management

- Generic problems of anaesthesia in the neonate:
  — Small size and high surface area : mass ratio, with consequences for heat loss.
  — Limited cardiovascular reserve.
  — Limited respiratory reserve.
  — (*Do not spend overlong on these general problems.*)
- Traditional teaching insists on a rapid sequence induction. This is probably the safest technique although arguably the NG tube and washouts should have emptied the stomach. Awake intubation is not acceptable (risk of intracranial haemorrhage, particularly if premature).
- Technique should rely on minimal doses of muscle relaxants.
- Care is needed in the prescription of opioids for postoperative analgesia: it is better to infiltrate the wound with local anaesthethic and encourage rapid restoration of feeding. Infants are more susceptible to opioid effects, particularly if premature, and any such child whose postconceptual age is less than 60 weeks should be nursed in a special high dependency area because of the risk of postoperative apnoea.
- This procedure can be done under local anaesthesia.

Marking points: This is a standard paediatric question which combines physiology and anaesthetic management. It is a safety question: you will not pass if your fluid resuscitation is inadequate or if you cannot justify your anaesthetic technique.

What are the problems associated with anaesthetising patients with Down syndrome?

This question tests your knowledge of a well-known syndrome which can present significant anaesthetic challenges.

Introduction
More children with Down syndrome (which has an incidence of 0.15% of all live births) are now surviving into adult life and they can present for a wide range of surgery. The anaesthetic problems which they may pose can be described using a systems approach.

Central nervous system
- Down's patients have learning difficulties, but the degree of mental retardation covers a wide spectrum. The approach should be tailored to their level of understanding. Communication may be difficult. Premedication may be needed in a patient who is very anxious and uncooperative. Rapport with parents is important.

Cardiovascular system
- Cardiac anomalies
- Occur in over 50% of patients: these include AV septal defect, the tetrad of Fallot, patent ductus arteriosus, ASD (Atrial Fibrillation) and VSD (Ventricular septal defect). Patients with these lesions (corrected or uncorrected) will require antibiotic prophylaxis.
- Any patient with a direct communication between right and left circulations is at risk of paradoxical embolus (including air from intravenous infusions or injection).

Drugs
- These patients are said to be sensitive to the vagolytic effects of atropine.

Respiratory system and airway
- Dysmorphological features and their consequences include:
  - Short neck, small mandible and maxilla, a small mouth and large tongue.
  - Salivation may be excessive.
  - Up to 20% will have abnormalities of the upper cervical spine including the atlanto-axial joint.
  - The trachea may be smaller than predicted for the age of the patient, and there may be a degree of subglottic stenosis.
  - Obstructive sleep apnoea is common and may compound the right heart problems associated with cardiac defects.
  - Patients may be more sensitive to narcotic analgesics.

Immune system
- An unspecified defect or defects increases the risks of infection. Institutionalised patients have a higher than expected risk of hepatitis B, and acute leukaemia has a higher incidence.

Marking points: Down syndrome is common. It is particularly important to cover all the airway problems and to be aware of the significance of corrected or uncorrected cardiac defects.

Describe your procedure for cardiac life support of a child aged 5 years.

This question is very straightforward if you have completed an APLS or PALS course and/or are familiar with paediatric resuscitation algorithms. It is more difficult if you have to stop to think. The required answer is the APLS-type cardiac arrest algorithm.

Introduction

There is little solid evidence to support the current recommendations for cardiac life support, but most clinicians have accepted that the algorithm approach to resuscitation is probably the most practical and the most effective.

Weight and endotracheal tube (ETT) size

A child aged 5 years will weigh approximately 18 kg ([2 × age] + 8, or [age + 4] × 2) and will require an endotracheal tube of internal diameter 5.0 mm (age/4 + 4), but note that advanced life support is based on immediate and effective basic life support (BLS):

- **Approach:** safe approach; check response; summon help.
- **Airway:** head tilt, chin lift (not if cervical spine trauma), jaw thrust.
- **Breathing:** look, listen and feel for 10 seconds. If none give 5 rescue breaths.
- **Circulation:** carotid pulse (10 seconds): if absent begin chest compressions (one finger breadth above xiphisternum) at rate of 100/min in ratio of 5 compressions to 1 breath. Go for help after 1 minute of BLS.
- Advanced life support: attach defibrillator/monitor and assess rhythm.
- There are three main abnormalities: ventricular fibrillation; asystole and pulseless electrical activity (PEA formerly known as EMD).
- **Ventricular fibrillation** (or pulseless ventricular tachycardia)
  - DC shock 2 J kg^{-1}; 2 J kg^{-1} and 4 J kg^{-1}.
  - Ventilate with O_2; intubate; intravenous or intraosseous access.
  - Epinephrine (adrenaline) 10 μg kg^{-1} iv or io.
  - DC shock 4 J kg^{-1}; 4 J kg^{-1} and 4 J kg^{-1}.
  - Adrenaline 100 μg kg^{-1} iv or io.
  - 20 cycles of CPR (1 minute) and repeat sequence as above.
  - Consider alkalinising agents and antiarrhythmics after 3 cycles.
  - Note that VF is an unusual rhythm in children without cardiac disease.
  - Drugs can be given via the ETT at 10× the iv dose. The value of this route of administration is debated.
- **Pulseless electrical activity (EMD)**
  - Ventilate with O_2; intubate; intravenous or intraosseous access.
  - Adrenaline 10 μg kg^{-1} iv or io.
  - Fluids: 20 ml kg^{-1} iv or io.
  - Consider causes: hypovolaemia, cardiac tamponade, pulmonary embolism, tension pneumothorax, electrolyte distrurbance. Treat as appropriate.
  - Adrenaline 100 μg kg^{-1} iv or io.
  - 60 cycles of CPR (3 minutes) and repeat sequence as above.
- **Asystole**
  - Ventilate with O_2; intubate; intravenous or intraosseous access.
  - Adrenaline 10 μg kg^{-1} iv or io.
  - 60 cycles of CPR (3 minutes).
  - Consider fluids (20 ml kg^{-1}) and alkalising agents (NaHCO$_3$ 1 mmol kg^{-1}).
  - Adrenaline100 μg kg^{-1} iv or io.
  - 60 cycles of CPR (3 minutes).
  - Adrenaline 100 μg kg^{-1} iv or io.
  - 60 cycles of CPR (3 minutes) and repeat high dose adrenaline.

— Evidence suggests that if there is no response to the second dose of epinephrine the outlook is very poor.
- Postresuscitation care. If resuscitation is successful the child must be transferred to a PICU (Paediatric intensive care unit) for continued monitoring and further supportive care.

Marking points: This is quite a difficult question to organise unless you are able to construct the main points of the cardiac algorithm. The criterion the examiner will use is whether or not your management as described would pass an APLS test scenario. If you are anaesthetising children then it should, and the answer will be marked rigorously.

You are called to A&E to see a 3-year-old child with stridor: what are the principal differential diagnoses?

Paediatric airway problems are amongst the most alarming that an anaesthetist can face. It is important to be aware of the diverse conditions that may present in this way, because their management may be very different.

Introduction

The paediatric airway is narrow and so there are many potential causes for the upper airway obstruction of which stridor is characteristic. Some may be life threatening: all are alarming because of the rapidity with which children can deteriorate. They may be classified as follows:

- **Infection**
    - Acute epiglottitis. Rare since the introduction of HiB vaccine. Cases which do present are even more dangerous because anaesthetists have less experience in their management.
    - Acute viral laryngotracheobronchitis (croup): a common winter condition.
    - Other upper airway infections: tracheitis, diphtheria (both rare).
    - Retropharyngeal abscess or peritonsillar abscess.
    - Retropharyngeal or peritonsillar haematoma.
- **Trauma**
    - Direct injury. Should be obvious from history and clinical findings.
    - Burns (fire or steam) and/or smoke inhalation injury. Obvious clinically.
- **Inhaled foreign body**
    - Very common cause of stridor. More likely in younger children and infants who are unable to give a clear history. Toys, food, tools, batteries, coins and various other objects have all found their way into the airway.
- **Allergic**
    - Angioneurotic oedema.
    - Oedema due to sensitivity to insect stings.
- **Congenital**
    - Laryngomalacia. Not a cause of acute stridor unless upper airway infection is superimposed. Usually not a problem after ~18 months of age.

Marking points: This question has simply asked for a list of the causes of stridor and not for your management. It tests, therefore, whether the candidate has a system for classifying the possible causes of an important symptom that the anaesthetist may have to manage.

A 3-year-old child presents to A&E with a presumptive diagnosis of acute epiglottitis. List the differential diagnoses. How would you manage this condition?

Acute epiglottitis is much less common following the introduction of haemophilus influenzae B vaccination. It does, however, remain a life-threatening condition in which anaesthetic and airway management can be crucial.

Introduction

The child with acute epiglottitis is usually very toxic, with a bacterial septicaemia associated with pyrexia and peripheral circulatory failure. Superimposed on this is acute airway obstruction which can rapidly become total in the face of any provocation. It is a life-threatening illness, and any suspicion of the diagnosis mandates early involvement of a senior anaesthetist, ENT surgeon and paediatrician.

Differential diagnosis

- Croup
  - Croup and epiglottitis account for 98% of all cases of acute upper airway obstruction in children.
- The remaining 2%
  - Inhalation of a foreign body.
  - Trauma.
  - Acute tonsillitis.
  - Tonsillar enlargement (glandular fever).
  - Retropharyngeal abscess.
  - Angio-oedema.
  - Smoke inhalation.
  - Diphtheria.

Management

The child with acute epiglottitis is toxic and very unwell, with a precarious airway that may obstruct with minimal provocation.

- Disturbance must be minimal. If the child is maintaining its airway by leaning forward in an exaggerated posture, or is sitting on the parent's lap they must be allowed to remain so. Any attempt to interfere by examining the throat, by moving the child or seeking iv access may precipitate immediate airway occlusion. Humidified oxygen from a short distance may be feasible.
- Airway control is the first priority. Inhalation induction using sevoflurane in oxygen 100% (case reports have confirmed that sevoflurane is an acceptable alternative to traditional halothane), carried out in whichever position the child is least distressed. ENT surgeon must be immediately available for emergency tracheostomy.
- Full monitoring as soon as child is unconscious (in a safe environment).
- Deep sevoflurane anaesthesia is necessary before attempting tracheal intubation. A tube much smaller than predicted may be necessary, but as the oedema fluid is compressed away it is usually possible to change it for a larger size once the child has been stabilised.
- Intravenous access: blood cultures, FBC, electrolytes, glucose, fluids (20 ml kg^{-1} bolus repeated according to response) and antibiotics (e.g. cefotaxime 100 mg kg^{-1}).
- Transfer to PICU or comparable high-intensity nursing area. Child will require sedation sufficient to prevent deliberate extubation. May require IPPV (sepsis and multi-system involvement) but usually such children respond very rapidly to treatment: extubation is possible within 2–3 days, with full recovery by 5–7 days.

Marking points: The disease is now rare, but swift recognition and appropriate safe management is crucial. For this reason the examiner will wish to see a safe and solid management plan. If you fail the child you will fail this question with a '1'.

A 10-year-old boy is brought into A&E unconscious, having been found at the bottom of an outdoor swimming pool. His rectal temperature is 30°C and his heart rate is 25 bpm. Describe your management.

This is a question about near drowning, which is defined as occurring when there is any recovery, however temporary, following submersion in a fluid. Such patients can be retrieved and the question seeks an orderly approach to an uncommon, but important problem.

Introduction
This clinical scenario exemplifies the problems associated with near drowning, which is said to have occurred when there is any recovery, however slight, following submersion. Resuscitation should follow logical advanced life support guidelines: overall survival of those who receive full CPR in hospital is around 15%, 70% of whom will survive intact.

Primary survey
● Assume other injuries until they are excluded. An unconscious swimmer may have sustained a cervical spine (diving) injury. Neck immobilisation is mandatory.

Airway
● Secure by tracheal intubation in order to protect lungs from gastric contents (including swallowed water).

Breathing
● IPPV with warm gases: 100% O_2.

Circulation
● Inadequate: hypoxia and hypothermia likely contributors, occult hypovolaemia possible, arrhythmias probable, refractory ventricular fibrillation at 28–30°C.

Treatment of hypothermia
● Active rewarming (at temperatures <32°C):
  — Radiant heat, radiant blanket, intravenous fluids at 39°C.
  — Warmed inspired gases.
  — Gastric and/or bladder lavage with saline at 42°C.
  — Peritoneal lavage with dialysate at 42°C.
  — In extremis and if facilities available: extracorporeal warming (using cardiopulmonary bypass pump).
● Beware lest vasodilatation on rewarming unmasks significant hypovolaemia.
● Core temperature has to increase to at least 32°C before discontinuation of resuscitation can be considered.
● Transfer to ICU/PICU for further supportive management.

Poor prognostic features
● Immersion time >10 minutes (depends on temperature of water).
● Core temperature on admission >33°C (cerebral protective effect of rapid hypothermia).
● Persistent acidosis (pH <7.00).
● Persistent hypoxia (P_aO_2 <8.0 kPa on 100% O_2).
● Persistent coma.
● Prognosis is probably no better after immersion in salt water than fresh.

Marking points: Key management features of this situation are to presume other injuries (particularly cervical spine) until proven otherwise, to be aware of the prognostic significance of hypothermia and to manage active rewarming appropriately.

A 5-year-old girl is brought into A&E, having been rescued from a house fire. An estimated 20% of her body surface area has been affected and she has burns to face, neck and torso. Describe your management.

Burned patients present several challenges to the anaesthetist, and some 6000 children annually are admitted to hospital. This question invites you to demonstrate a systematic approach, and to show that you recognise the particular problems caused by thermal injury.

Introduction
If the age of a burn victim added to the percentage area burn exceeds 100 then mortality approaches 100%. A 5 year old, therefore, should have a very good chance of survival. But that survival depends crucially on a systematic approach which takes account of the specific problems which are presented by facial and truncal burns.

Primary survey
- Assume other injuries until they are excluded. Burns victims may have suffered blast injury, deceleration and other injuries (motor accidents), been damaged by falling structures in a house fire, or injured as they attempt to escape. Neck immobilisation is important where indicated.

Airway
- The airway may be compromised by the direct burns, as well as by the inhalation of hot smoke. The presence of inhalational injury would be indicated by blackened sputum or carbonaceous deposits around the mouth.
- Burns cause oedema and so airway obstruction in this child may supervene. Early tracheal intubation is indicated if there is any airway compromise, or if there is any suspicion that later airway problems are likely. The child should meanwhile receive high flow humidified oxygen.

Breathing
- This may be compromised by other injuries or by circumferential burns. Injured tissue becomes completely inelastic and may severely restrict chest wall movement. Escharotomy may be necessary.

Circulation
- **Early.** Although burns cause massive fluid loss, this process occurs later on. Burns are not the cause of immediate hypovolaemia: a child who has features of hypovolaemic shock immediately on admission is almost certainly bleeding from additional injuries. Resuscitation should proceed along conventional lines, with the administration of blood and recourse to surgery if indicated.
- **Late.** Fluid losses through injured tissues are huge. Various formulae are used to calculate fluid requirements due to burns. One example is [weight (kg) × %burn × 4 ml 24 h^{-1}]. Half of this should be given in the first 8 hours, calculated from the time of the burn. This 5 year old, of weight approximately 18 kg would need 18 × 20 × 4 = 1440 ml in 24 hours. The fluid used is usually human albumin solution 4.5%. Additonal fluid is required to cover normal maintenance. Urine output (2 ml kg h^{-1}) is a useful guide to resuscitation.

Assessment of burn
- **Percentage area:** either use chart or use child hand size (palm and adducted fingers of the child = 1% BSA).
- **Thickness:** superficial, partial thickness, full thickness.

Other management

- Expose for secondary survey and then cover. Burned children lose heat very rapidly.
- Analgesia: full thickness burns are painless. Mixed picture is common and the child should receive iv morphine (or other strong opioid) titrated against response.
- Definitive care in specialist burns unit.

Marking points: Major problems in this case are the airway (which must be managed safely), the exclusion of other injuries, and the large fluid losses which accompany a 20% burn in a small child. The specific formula that you use does not matter, but you should give some indication of the volumes that will be needed.

A 2-year-old child is believed to have inhaled a foreign body 2 days ago, although there are no signs of upper airway obstruction. The child requires bronchoscopy: outline your anaesthetic management.

This is a specialised paediatric procedure for a relatively common condition and you should be aware of the basic principles of safe management.

Introduction

Many foreign bodies find their way past the upper airways of young children and because the clinical signs may be deceptive or absent proper investigation is mandatory.

Preoperative assessment

- **Retain a high index of suspicion:** foreign bodies in the airway are notoriously deceptive. After an initial cough as the object passes the larynx there may be either no signs or minimal symptoms or signs.
- **Airway and breathing:** if no upper airway obstruction then inspect chest and auscultate. Seek hyperinflation, decreased air entry and wheeze (signs may vary according to nature of the foreign body: organic matter may excite inflammatory reaction, whereas plastic or glass will be inert).
- **CXR:** foreign bodies are often radiolucent. If a main or lobar bronchus is occluded then may get hyperinflation of the lung or zone beyond the obstruction. There may be signs of infection or inflammation (organic oils released by peanuts, for example).

Premedication

- Atropine as drying agent (20 μg kg^{-1} im or iv; 50 μg kg^{-1} orally) plus EMLA or Ametop gel for topical analgesia prior to venepuncture.

Anaesthetic technique

Any technique used must ensure good surgical access, anaesthesia and optimal oxygenation during a procedure which exemplifies the shared airway.

- **Induction.** Positive airways pressure must be avoided lest the foreign body is driven deeper into the bronchial tree. A relaxant technique is less suitable, as is one in which induction may be associated with apnoea necessitating bag and mask ventilation. Optimal technique is (probably) calm inhalation induction with oxygen and sevoflurane.
- Laryngeal mask airway allows anaesthesia to be deepened prior to bronchoscopy. Topical anaesthesia to the upper airway can be used (lidocaine (lignocaine) spray: do not exceed 5 mg kg^{-1}).
- **Maintenance.** Technique will be dictated by surgeon and equipment.
  - **Rigid bronchoscope** (Negus). This device is tapered and the view can be poor. It may be easier to retrieve material using long fine forceps. An anaesthetic breathing system cannot be attached: a patient either breathes spontaneously (air plus insufflated oxygen) or is ventilated via an injector at the proximal end which entrains air by the venturi principle. The injector is potentially dangerous: it may force a foreign body deeper or may cause barotrauma. With either technique anaesthesia must be maintained intravenously.
  - **Ventilating bronchoscope** (Storz) plus Hopkins telescope. This is optically superior and allows anaesthetic gases to be delivered via a side arm. Foreign body retrieval may be more difficult, but it is a much safer system which ensures both oxygenation and anaesthesia. Spontaneous ventilation is preferable to IPPV, although movement of the airway with respiration may interfere more with surgical access.

Postoperative care

- Depends on the nature of the foreign body, but at 48 hours there will be, at the least, residual oedema.
    — Observation in specialised area.
    — Humidified oxygen if tolerated.
    — Antibiotics if indicated.
    — Corticosteroids +/– nebulised epinephrine (adrenaline) for oedema if indicated.

> **Marking points:** It is crucial to ensure that this child remains oxygenated and that you minimise the risks of other complications. If your suggested management does not do this then you will fail the question. If you endanger the child you will receive a '1'.

What are the choices for postoperative analgesia for a child aged 4 years presenting for repair of inguinal hernia as a day case? State briefly the advantages and disadvantages of each method.

The principles of pain control in children are no different from those in adult practice and this question explores your understanding of 'balanced analgesia' in children in the context of day-case surgery.

Introduction

Herniotomy and herniorrhaphy can be surprisingly painless. There is at least one series of patients less than 6 years of age in which 50% of children had no apparent pain despite having received no analgesia. Anaesthetic management should not be predicated upon that assumption, however, and the main analgesic options are described below.

Options for pain control

Just as in the treatment of adult pain, children should receive where appropriate a 'balanced' analgesic technique (local anaesthetic +/- opioids +/- NSAIDs +/- paracetamol or paracetamol-compound analgesics).

- Opioid
  - Intraoperative fentanyl 1 μg kg^{-1}. Effective short lasting analgesia. Longer acting morphine is unnecessary if local anaesthesia is effective and as severe pain is unlikely.
- NSAIDs
  - Perioperative and postoperative diclofenac 1–3 mg kg^{-1} or ibuprofen 5 mg kg^{-1}. NSAIDs have an opioid sparing effect and when given simultaneously with paracetamol will have a useful additive effect. NSAIDs can be used in children who have asthma, but should be discontinued if there is any associated deterioration in respiratory function (which occurs in ~10%).
- Paracetamol
  - Perioperative and postoperative paracetamol 20 mg kg^{-1}. It has an established safety record in all age groups, can be given in daily doses up to 90 mg kg^{-1}. It does have anti-inflammatory, analgesic and antipyretic actions.
- Codeine phosphate
  - Perioperative and postoperative codeine phosphate 1 mg kg^{-1}. Effective against moderate to severe pain. Sedation, respiratory depression are complications if doses are high, constipation is not a particular problem following short-term use in children.
- Local anaesthesia
  - Infiltration of the wound with bupivacaine 0.25% is as effective as ilioinguinal and iliohypogastric combined nerve block.
  - Direct block by the surgeon of the ilioinguinal and iliohypogastric nerves while also infiltrating the hernial sac. Reliable, but will wear off after ~4–6 hours (this is variable).
  - Sacral extradural (caudal) anaesthesia using bupivacaine 0.25% × 1 ml kg^{-1}, with or without adjuncts: clonidine 2 μg kg^{-1} (doubles the duration of analgesia, but may cause sedation) or preservative-free ketamine 0.5 mg kg^{-1} (quadruples the duration of action). A caudal provides very effective analgesia at the expense of motor weakness and urinary retention. Their use is probably inappropriate in the context of day-case surgery for only moderate pain.

Marking points: Principles of pain relief in children are the same as those in adults, but do not give a generic answer in which you simply cite all the options available. You must focus your answer on the specific problems of a day-case procedure.

Outline the circulatory changes that take place at birth. What problems may congenital heart disease present to the anaesthetist?

Congenital heart disease occurs in approximately 1 in 250 live births. Most lesions are identified early and the problems can be left to the paediatric cardiac anaesthetists. This is not always the case, however, and so an understanding of the consequences of the lesions and the principles of rational management is important.

Introduction

Congenital cardiac anomalies complicate some 0.4% of all live births and may have implications for anaesthesia both during infancy, and in some uncorrected cases, into adulthood. Successful management depends on recognition of the pathological cardiovascular changes that may follow.

Circulatory changes at birth

- In utero the right and left hearts pump in parallel. There are connections between the systemic and pulmonary circulations via the ductus arteriosus (pulmonary artery to the aorta) and the foramen ovale (left and right atria). The pulmonary circulation has high resistance and the right and left ventricular pressures are equal, although the RV ejects 66% of the combined ventricular output.
- With clamping of the umbilical cord there is a sudden rise in systemic vascular resistance and aortic pressure.
- Respiration expands the lungs, and pulmonary vascular resistance decreases in response to expansion, respiratory movements, increased pH and increased oxygenation. (PVR continues to decrease with recruitment of small arteries and the reduction over weeks of pulmonary vascular smooth muscle). Pulmonary blood flow increases. Enhanced pulmonary venous return into the left atrium raises left atrial above right atrial pressure and the foramen ovale closes by a flap valve effect.
- The increase in left-sided, and fall in right-sided pressures decreases, or even reverses, shunting through the ductus arteriosus.
- The ductus closes in response to O_2, prostaglandins, bradykinin and acetyl choline. The process takes up to 14 days to complete.

Cyanotic congenital heart disease

- Exists when there is:
    - Right to left shunt with pulonary oligaemia, as in the tetrad of Fallot (VSD, overriding aorta, pulmonary stenosis and right ventricular hypertrophy (RVH)).
    - Parallel left and right circulations (transposition of the great arteries).
    - Mixing of oxygenated and deoxygenated blood without decreased pulmonary blood flow (double outlet RV, single ventricle, TAPVD (total anomalous polmonary venous drainage), truncus arteriosus).
- Chronic hypoxia stimulates polycythaemia. Suboptimal rheology which worsens with dehydration (sludging and thrombosis is possible): risk of CVA at haematocrit >65%.
- Risk of paradoxical emboli: scrupulous care to avoid injection of any air is vital, should use in-line filters.
- Risk of bacterial endocarditis (as with any cardiac structural abnormality).
- If there is pulmonary oligaemia inhalation induction is delayed.

Acyanotic congenital heart disease

- The main problem is pulmonary hypertension which develops as the circulation attempts to 'protect' itself from high pulmonary blood flows caused by intracardiac left to right shunting (e.g. through a septal defect) by developing hypertrophy of the media of vascular smooth muscle.

- With progressive disease the resistances in the left and right circulations become finely balanced so that an increase in PVR or a decrease in SVR may reverse the shunt (from left to right to right to left). This is Eisenmenger's syndrome.
- Anaesthesia must therefore avoid anything that will:
  — Increase the resistance in the hyperreactive pulmonary vascular tree: hypoxia, hypercapnia, acidosis, nitrous oxide, pain-stimulated catecholamine release.
  — Decrease systemic vascular resistance: particularly by drug-induced vasodilatation.
- Left ventricular function is also impaired by chronic hypoxia, by increased pulmonary venous return and because mechanical efficiency is impaired by loss of some of the stroke volume through a VSD.
- Risk of paradoxical emboli and bacterial endocarditis as above.

Marking points: There is more than one question here because there is too much detail for a short answer. The key to success is to understand the basic pathophysiology associated with the lesions and to identify the particular anaesthetic influences that may prove dangerous.

An 8-week-old male infant weighing 3.0 kg is scheduled for inguinal hernia repair. He was delivered prematurely at 34 weeks. List the risk factors and state how these can be minimised.

This is the kind of case that increasingly is being carried out only in specialist paediatric hospitals, but this question tests your theoretical knowledge about the very risks which explain why this should be so.

Introduction

This type of case exemplifies certain safety issues which increase the pressure to operate on very young children only in specialist paediatric centres.

Potential problems

There are the generic problems associated with all neonatal anaesthesia:

- The smaller the child the larger is the ratio of surface area to mass.
- A large surface area is associated with increased heat loss, and neonates are very vulnerable to rapid hypothermia. They generate heat via non-shivering thermogenesis: by utilising brown fat.
- The need to maintain body temperature via heat production results in a higher metabolic rate and higher tissue oxygen demand. Desaturation occurs very quickly.
- In the cardiovascular system the capacity of the heart to increase cardiac output by increasing stroke volume is limited. Cardiac output increases predominantly by increasing heart rate.
- Respiratory compensation occurs via an increase in respiratory rate more than increases in tidal volume. Neonatal and infant ribs are more horizontal and respiration is predominantly diaphragmatic. Intercostal and accessory muscles are relatively weak. (Deficient in Type 1 muscle fibres until ~2 years old.)
- The incidence of neonatal gastro-oesophageal reflux is high (coordination of swallowing with respiration does not mature until ~4–5 months) but this is rarely a clinical problem.
- Closing capacity exceeds FRC and neonates are at risk of hypoxia. Risk is reduced by tracheal intubation with IPPV and modest PEEP.
- Neonatal kidneys have a reduced glomerular filtration rate, diminished tubular function and sodium excretion and a decreased concentrating ability.
- Neonates are very sensitive to opioids (causes include blood–brain barrier immaturity and decreased hepatic clearance), and are at risk of grave respiratory depression.

There are in addition specific problems associated with prematurity: the premature neonate has been described as functioning 'on a marginal basis' so that any type of stress, especially thermal stress, is very poorly tolerated.

- **Hypothermia**
  - Premature infant is very susceptible to cold: thin skin and limited fat stores. Heat loss must be minimised (particularly from the head). Anaesthesia affects thermoregulation more in neonates.
- **Hypoglycaemia**
  - Premature neonatal liver has minimal glycogen stores and cannot handle large protein loads. They are at risk of hypoglycaemia and acidaemia.
  - Prolonged fasting must be avoided.
  - Glucose increases hypoxic brain damage: neonates should receive balanced crystalloid solution for third space losses and dextrose 5% with NaCl 0.45% for maintenance.

- **Fluid overload/underload**
  — Renal maturation is further delayed in premature infants. They cannot handle free water and solute loads. Excretion of drugs/metabolites that undergo renal excretion delayed.
  — High insensible losses are further increased by radiant heaters.
- **Drug effects**
  — Plasma proteins are low in prematurity: low albumin binding increases free drug levels.
  — Immature hepatic and renal function delay metabolism and excretion.
  — Total body water is high in the premature neonate: so water soluble drugs have high volume of distribution and require higher initial dose. Fat soluble drugs have longer clinical effect (less redistribution because of lower body fat).
  — MAC is lower in the premature: must avoid overdose.
- **Retinopathy**
  — Must avoid hyperoxia. SpO_2 should be kept at 93–95% because retinopathy of prematurity is a risk until 44 weeks postconceptual age.
  — P_aCO_2 also influences retinopathy of prematurity and should be kept at 4.5–6.0 kPa.
- **Postoperative apnoea**
  — The risk of apnoea occurring without warning in the postoperative period does not decrease to 1% until 54 weeks postconceptual age when delivered at 34 weeks.
  — Apnoea may still occur after regional anaesthesia alone.
  — Infants less than ~60 weeks, therefore, require special postoperative monitoring.
  — (The problem is exacerbated in the presence of anaemia with Hb < 10 g dl^{-1}.)

Marking points: Many of the problems are generic and some are very specialised (such as the influence of P_aco_2 on retinopathy). The most important point is the risk of postoperative apnoea, and you should also mention the susceptibility to thermal stress and the probability of hypoglycaemia.

How does the common cold influence fitness for anaesthesia in children?

Upper respiratory tract infections present some difficulty for anaesthetists. Viral infections are common, but it is sometimes difficult to judge their significance and data are lacking. This question assesses whether you are aware of such evidence as is available and whether you are likely to be able to make a judgement in a particular case.

Introduction

The clinical features of coryza, the common cold, may range from local rhinorrhoea alone to a febrile viral illness with predominant upper respiratory tract symptoms and signs. The condition is endemic but the absence of robust data can make it difficult to make decisions about anaesthesia that are based on good evidence.

Pathophysiology of coryza

- Causation is diverse: typical pathogens include rhinovirus, myxovirus and respiratory syncitial virus, with adenoviruses also causing upper respiratory tract infection (URTI). In general the clinical features of infection with different organisms are similar.
- Viral URTIs alter the volume and quality of airway secretions.
- Increase airflow obstruction that may persist for up to 5 weeks.
- Compromise bacterial defence mechanisms.
- Cause marked bronchial and upper airway reactivity for 3–4 weeks: sensitise airway reflexes to mechanical, chemical and other irritant stimulation (with risks of laryngospasm and bronchoconstriction, and hypoxia).

Risks of anaesthesia and surgery

- The risk of adverse respiratory events is ~10× greater up to 2 weeks after URTI, and lower levels of risk may persist for 6–7 weeks.
- Children who are intubated for surgery within 5 weeks of URTI have higher incidence of respiratory morbidity (postoperative chest infection, wheeze, cough).
- Cardiac sequelae. This is more difficult. There is evidence that respiratory complications persist for some weeks, and it is clear that systemic malaise is associated with a viraemia. It is possible, therefore, that this may cause a subclinical myocarditis. Myocarditis is one of the causes of Q-T prolongation which may degenerate into torsade de pointes (a malign type of ventricular tachycardia) and thence to fibrillation. Anecdotal speculation attributes sudden death in individuals exercising during, or soon after viral infection to this process. The hypothesis is plausible, although the evidence in children is not available. It is obvious, therefore, that anaesthesia in such children should be accompanied by full ECG monitoring with the instant availability of clinicians trained in paediatric cardiac resuscitation.

Practical considerations

- All that coughs and sneezes is not viral URTI. Children may have chronic rhinorrhoea due to vasomotor rhinitis, teething infants exhibit similar symptoms and children with adenotonsillar hypertrophy (the very condition for which they are admitted for surgery) frequently look as though they have colds.
- If the recommendation to defer surgery for 5–6 weeks is accepted then the operation may never be done, because children average between 5 and 8 URTIs annually and so a 6-week symptom-free interval may not transpire.
- Ideally, however, the evidence suggests that if an elective procedure does involve tracheal intubation then it should be deferred for 5 weeks. Adenotonsillectomy within this time is more likely to be associated with haemorrhage and with infection.

- Differential diagnosis. A practical distinction should be made between uncomplicated URTI without systemic upset (in essence the child with a runny nose), and a febrile (>38°C) illness with systemic symptoms, malaise and lower respiratory tract signs.
- Additional factors. Any decision should also take into account the nature of the surgery planned and any coexisisting medical condition, such as asthma.

Marking points: The commonest form of surgery in chiildren is ENT, and the nature of their conditions means that they frequently present with URTI-like clinical features. For the reasons cited above, they cannot all be deferred. In your answer you should adopt a practical approach to the difficulty while demonstrating that you understand the safety considerations that mandate surgical cancellation in a smaller group of individuals whom you can identify as being at risk.

Neuroanaesthesia

What are the causes of raised intracranial pressure? Describe the clinical features and explain the underlying pathophysiological mechanisms.

Head injury is common and there are many other disorders which cause raised intracranial pressure. Knowledge of the basic underlying mechanisms is important both for diagnosis and for rational management.

Introduction

The skull of an adult is in effect a rigid box which contains brain tissue, blood and CSF. There is very limited scope for compensation and an increase in the volume of one component invariably results in an increase in ICP unless the volume of another component decreases.

Causes

- Intracranial contents comprise: brain tissue ~1400–1500 g, blood ~100–150 ml, CSF ~110–120 ml and ECF <100 ml.
- ICP is raised by mass lesions which increase brain, bone or meningeal tissue volume.
  — Neoplasms (of brain, meninges or bone).
  — Infection with formation of brain abscess.
- ICP is raised by conditions which impede drainage of CSF (produced at 0.4 ml min^{-1}) and increase its volume.
  — Hydrocephalus: congenital, due to blocked shunt, caused by trauma, tumour or infection.
- ICP is raised by conditions which increase non-CSF fluid volume.
  — Blood: intracranial haemorrhage (trauma, aneurysm, AV malformation, etc.).
  — Oedema: following trauma, infection, metabolic disorder, hypoxia, venous obstruction, hydrostatic pressure (steep or prolonged Trendelenburg).

Clinical features

- **Symptoms** (will depend on time course of the rise).
  — Headache, nausea and vomiting (worse in the morning), changes in level of consciousness, visual disturbances (see below).
- **Signs**
  — Neurological signs caused by brain distortion or by one of the brain herniation syndromes (see below), including pupillary changes and failure of upward gaze.

— Papilloedema, hypertension, bradycardia and abnormal respiration (Cushing's triad – a late sign).
- ICP can rise without accompanying signs.

Pathophysiology
- **Decreased cerebral perfusion**
  — Cerebral perfusion pressure (CPP) = mean arterial pressure (MAP) – cerebral venous pressure. In presence of ICP which is raised: CPP = MAP – ICP.
  — Perfusion is maintained until CPP is <50 mmHg. Ischaemia and death may follow.
- **Focal ischaemia**
  — May get local ischaemia in region of a mass lesion.
- **Vasomotor paralysis**
  — Cerebral blood flow loses autoregulation and passively follows MAP.
- **Cerebral herniation** (several syndromes described)
  — **Central:** brain is pushed downwards through foramen magnum ('coning') as cerebellar tonsils herniate and compress the medulla.
  — **Cingulate:** cingulate gyrus and part of hemisphere are displaced beneath the falx cerebri. Anterior cerebral vessels are affected.
  — **Uncal:** uncus (part of hippocampal gyrus) herniates through and is compressed against the tentorium.

Specific clinical signs
- **Cushing's reflex:** is a late sign as carotid body receptors attempt to mediate an increase in perfusion pressure that is doomed to fail.
- **Pupillary signs:** may follow uncal compression or kinking of the oculomotor nerve by distorted vessels. Get ipsilateral dilatation followed by motor paralysis of extraocular muscles (not lateral rectus or superior oblique).
- **Eye signs:** failure of lateral gaze (lateral rectus) due to displacement of the 6th cranial nerve which has a very long intracranial course.

Marking points: Your answer should demonstrate an understanding of the reasons why ICP may rise and the salient clinical features. It should be based on first principles.

A young adult requires intramedullary nailing of a femoral fracture 18 hours after an accident in which he was knocked unconscious. What are the anaesthetic options in this case?

This is a question which explores your safe management of an important problem. It is common enough for most anaesthetists to have encountered it early in their careers and you will be expected to demonstrate that you understand the need for an assessment of the anaesthetic risks against the need to proceed.

Introduction
The risks of anaesthesia in a patient with a recent significant head injury have to be balanced against the urgency of the surgical procedure. The decision should be informed, but is inevitably one on which the anaesthetist has to make some compromise.

- A patient who is knocked unconscious has received a significant head injury and is at risk of extradural or subdural haematoma as well as evolving cerebral oedema. General anaesthesia may mask these signs.
- Significant head injury together with a major long bone fracture suggests the possibility of other injuries. These should be excluded and the cervical spine should be assessed.
- It would be ideal to wait for at least 48 hours until the likelihood of cerebral derangement had passed. A serious femoral fracture, however, requires early fixation.

Anaesthetic options
- **General anaesthesia**
  - Technique should avoid increasing ICP.
  - Spontaneous ventilation is not optimal: it is hard to keep CO_2 in the normal range and high concentration volatile agents increase cerebral blood flow and compromise autoregulation.
  - Intubation and IPPV: must attenuate pressor response to laryngoscopy, maintain normocapnia, avoid head-down tilt, avoid coughing and straining.
  - Must allow rapid recovery to allow continued assessment of conscious level.
- **Fluid resuscitation**
  - Avoid glucose-containing solutions (hyperglycaemia is bad for injured brain).
- **Regional anaesthesia**
  - Extradural block: good perioperative analgesia, sensorium unaffected. Dural puncture is dangerous in presence of raised ICP. Extradural fluid injection may also increase ICP (although this risk is minimal).
  - Subarachnoid block: provides good intraoperative analgesia and sensorium unaffected (cannot use adjuncts such as opioids or alpha$_2$ agonists because of potential sedation). No opportunity to prolong analgesia. CSF loss through dural puncture may be significant.
- **Peripheral nerve block**
  - Femoral nerve block is unlikely to be dense enough to allow femoral nailing. It would, however, provide good postoperative analgesia and obviate the need for opioids.
- **Postoperative care**
  - Should be nursed in an area (HDU or ITU) where careful surveillance of neurological status can be undertaken.

Marking points: You will have to anaesthetise this patient earlier than you would wish. Your anaesthetic technique must do nothing to make that compromise more hazardous than it already is.

A young adult is admitted with an acute head injury. What are the indications for tracheal intubation, ventilation and transfer to a neurosurgical unit?

Minor head injury is common and major head injury accounts for ~1% of all deaths in the UK. Primary brain damage following head injury may be exacerbated by hypoxia, hypercarbia and hypotension. All these are avoidable and so it is crucial to protect patients against these secondary insults by rapid assessment and management. Your answer should demonstrate a decisive approach.

Introduction

Primary brain damage following severe head injury may be worsened by secondary insults such as hypoxia, hypercarbia or hypotension. These are largely avoidable and so the head-injured patient requires rapid asessment and decisive management in order to minimise that risk.

Assessment

Initial assessment will include a Glasgow Coma Score (GCS), which should be done more or less simultaneously with assessment of Airway and Breathing.

The GCS is a 15 point scale (minimum score 3; maximum 15) which sums the totals from 3 areas of assessment (eye opening, verbal response and motor response) to give a numerical assessment of conscious level.

Criteria for intubation and ventilation

GCS
- A score of 8 or less (= 'severe' head injury) mandates immediate tracheal intubation (to protect the airway) and IPPV.

Airway
- Obstruction or other inability to maintain airway (increases ICP further).

Breathing
- Hypoventilation or hyperventilation.
- Arterial gases: hypoxia, hypercapnia, hypocapnia.

Circulation
- No specific criteria for intubation/ventilation, although oxygen delivery in presence of failing circulation is likely to be improved by a secure airway and IPPV.

Disability
- Focal neurological signs, including pupillary abnormalities.
- Convulsions.

Associated injuries
- Chest injury with rib fractures; major orthopaedic or other injury for which urgent surgery is likely.

Criteria for transfer
- Injury which is amenable to intracranial surgery: mainly extradural and subdural haematoma.
- Neurosurgical units will not accept such patients without CT scan evidence: a patient who shows cerebral irritability and is too restless to cooperate will need intubation and ventilation even if other criteria are not met.

Marking points: There is one straightforward criterion for transfer: will the regional unit accept them after viewing the CT scan? Criteria for intubation and ventilation can be deduced from the basic tenet of head injury management, which is to prevent the secondary insults provoked by hypoxia, hypercarbia, and everything that may raise ICP or compromise cerbral perfusion pressure. Decisive management based on these principles is what is expected.

How would you manage the transfer of a patient to a regional neurosurgical unit for evacuation of an extradural haematoma?

It is the minority of head injuries which are accepted by neurosurgical units: most diffuse injuries are managed in district general hospitals. But where there is a mass lesion which is amenable to surgical intervention the quality of transfer is crucial. Many of the principles are generic and apply to each of the 12 000 transfers that take place in the UK annually, but this question requires some additional focus.

Introduction

Transfers to neurosurgical units for emergency surgery after head injury trauma make up only a very small propoportion of the 12 000 critically ill patients who are transferred each year in the UK. They are a group, however, in whom urgent and efficient transfer is crucial to outcome.

- **The decision to transfer: do the benefits outweigh the risks?**
  - Urgent evacuation of extradural haematoma is the only feasible treatment: they must be transferred.
- **Is the condition of the patient optimised?**
  - This general principle of transfer cannot always apply because of the pathophysiology of intracranial bleeding.
  - Transfer conditions must be such that the effects of any deterioration can be attenuated (by trying to reduce ICP, for example).
  - Should be intubated and ventilated prior to transfer.
- **Who should tranfer the patient?**
  - Ideally it should be a senior clinician, usually an anaesthetist. At the least it should be an individual who has received adequate training.
  - Trained assistance must also be available.
- **What should be the mode of transport?**
  - General rule is: road if total transfer time <2 hours, air ambulance if longer. A 2 hour delay before surgery is likely significantly to worsen outcome.
  - Transfer should be urgent but smooth: rapid acceleration and deceleration forces may increase ICP in supine patients, as may steep gradients. Ambulance should not have to stop and will need blue light and police escort.
- **Communication**
  - Vital to inform the receiving centre about progress, including departure and estimated arrival time.
- **Equipment**
  - **Airway:** full (re-) intubation equipment, adjuncts, cricothyrotomy set, portable suction.
  - **Breathing:** means of delivering O_2 manually and via ventilator with appropriate alarms, and for head-injured patients in particular, $ETCO_2$ monitoring. Adequate O_2 supply (some ventilators are O_2 driven).
  - **Circulation:** fluids, cardiac arrest drugs, intravenous access ×2 sites; mannitol for the emergency treatment of rising ICP (temporary measure but buys some time before decompensation).
  - Infusion pumps: sedation and neuromuscular block are better delivered continuously.
- **Monitoring**
  - ECG, NIBP, IABP (intra-arterial blood pressure), CVP, ICP (if available), temperature, urine output, $ETCO_2$.
- **Other**
  - Take hard copies of relevant medical notes; all scans and X-rays.
  - Take any blood that has been cross-matched .

Marking points: There are generic principles which apply to any transfer of a critically ill patient. As long as the small number of points specific to transfer of an acute neurosurgical case are also addressed, this approach will be satisfactory.

A patient is admitted to ITU with a severe closed head injury. There is no focal lesion requiring neurosurgical intervention. What principles govern your management during the first 24 hours?

This is a common scenario. Only a small proportion of head-injured patients undergo neurosurgical decompression: most are admitted to general intensive care units. Your answer should demonstrate that you understand the importance of avoiding secondary damage.

Introduction
A minority of patients with head injury require neurosurgical intervention. Most have diffuse brain injury and so in these the management is supportive, but with the prime objective of avoiding secondary insults: hypoxia, hypercarbia and hypoperfusion.

Management
- Cerebral perfusion
  - Cerebral perfusion pressure (CPP) is given by the formula: CPP = MAP – ICP.
  - This can be modified to CPP = MAP – (ICP + CVP) (especially with IPPV and PEEP).
  - An appropriate CPP in an adult is ~70 mmHg, although quantification of this will require direct ICP monitoring.
  - In the absence of monitoring clinical signs of raised ICP must be sought.
- Maintenance of CPP (control of BP and ICP)
  - Adequate blood pressure: volume expansion if indicated by low CVP, plus inotropic support if this proves insufficient.
  - Sedation and analgesia to prevent surges in ICP.
  - Muscle relaxants to prevent fighting against the ventilator (cerebral irritability).
  - Moderate hyperventilation to achieve $P_a CO_2$ of ~4.0–4.5 kPa.
  - Osmotic therapy: mannitol or hypertonic saline. May get rebound hypertension and repeated therapy may be ineffective. The issue is contentious.
  - Barbiturates: may lower ICP but at expense of hypotension requiring inotropes .
  - Nimodipine or other calcium antagonists, steroids and hypothermia currently have no role, although hyperthermia will increase cerebral metabolic rate ($CMRO_2$) and should be avoided.
- Maintenance of oxygenation
  - Early tracheal intubation with cricoid pressure will protect the airway, but aspiration may have occurred around the time of injury.
  - IPPV with different ventilatory modes and supplemental oxygen is usually sufficient to ensure that the perfusing blood is adequately oxygenated.
  - Convulsions, should they occur, should be treated to prevent increased $CMRO_2$.
- Management in face of deterioration
  - Cannot assume that this is due to cerebral oedema alone.
  - Patient will need CT scan to exclude bleed amenable to surgical intervention.
  - Should keep in contact with neurosurgical unit for further assistance.

Marking points: ITU management should be directed towards the avoidance of secondary damage by maintaining cerebral perfusion and cerebral oxygenation. The concepts are not complex but you should show that you would be decisive in their employment.

What are the pathophysiological insults which exacerbate the primary brain injury following head trauma? How can these effects be minimised?

This is a more direct form of the previous question and aims to test your understanding of the pathophysiology of cerebral decompensation. If your basic management is flawed then the outcome may be gravely affected.

Introduction

As much damage may ensue from secondary insults to the brain as are due to the primary head injury. It is crucial, therefore, to attend to all the factors which may compromise cerebral oxygenation.

- Airway and Breathing: maintenance of oxygenation
  - Early tracheal intubation with cricoid pressure to protect the airway (aspiration may have already occurred).
  - Laryngoscopy and intubation must be preceded by adequate anaesthesia (to prevent inevitable ICP rises).
  - IPPV as indicated with supplemental oxygen to maintain normal $P_a o2$ (~12–13 kPa).
- Circulation: inadequate cerebral perfusion
  - Cerebral perfusion pressure (CPP) is given by the formula: CPP = MAP – ICP.
  - This can be modified to CPP = MAP – [ICP + CVP] (especially with IPPV and PEEP).
  - An appropriate CPP in an adult is ~70 mmHg (needs ICP monitoring to quantify).
  - Compromised by hypotension and raised ICP.
- Prevention: maintenance of CPP: control of BP
  - Adequate blood pressure: volume expansion if indicated by low CVP.
  - Inotropic support as necessary.
- Prevention: maintenance of CPP: control of ICP
  - Hypertension in the presence of impaired autoregulation will increase ICP.
  - Sedation and analgesia to prevent consequent surges in ICP.
  - May need muscle relaxants to prevent fighting against the ventilator (cerebral irritability).
  - Moderate hyperventilation to achieve $P_a co2$ of ~4.0–4.5 kPa.
  - Osmotic therapy: mannitol or hypertonic saline. (May get rebound hypertension: the issue is contentious.)
  - Barbiturates: may lower ICP but at expense of hypotension requiring inotropes.
  - Prevent venous engorgement; nurse with head-up tilt (15°).
  - Treat fits effectively (increase $CMRO_2$).
  - Avoid hyperthermia (increases $CMRO_2$).
- Monitoring for signs of decompensation
  - Neurological signs (pupils; GCS – If appropriate).
  - Invasive ICP if available.
  - Repeat CT scan if unexplained deterioration.

> **Marking points:** The single vital pathological insult is failure of cerebral oxygenation. Your answer should manifest a methodical approach which demonstrates your understanding of the causes of secondary damage.

What particular problems may occur during lower abdominal surgery in a patient who suffered a traumatic transection of the spinal cord at the level of C6 four weeks previously? How would you prevent them?

Two individuals a day in the UK are paralysed after traumatic spinal cord injuries. The chances of an individual anaesthetist outside a specialist centre, therefore, encountering a patient who requires such surgery is not high, but should they do so there are significant anaesthetic implications.

Introduction

On average two individuals in the UK will be paralysed each day following traumatic spinal cord injury and such patients may present a significant anaesthetic challenge for many months following the insult.

Airway
- Tracheal intubation may be necessary.
  - Within about 48–72 hours after the acute inury there is increased production of acetylcholine receptors by denervated muscle.
  - Administration of suxamethonium results in a large efflux of potassium into the circulation. This dangerous hyperkalaemic response may persist for 6 months or more.

Breathing
- A lesion at C6 spares the diaphragm (C3,4,5).
  - Breathing is still affected: expansion of the rib cage via the intercostals and accessory muscle of respiration is responsible for ~60% of normal tidal volume.
  - Lung capacities are reduced (TLC and VC) although FRC is unchanged.
  - Cough may be impaired leading to sputum retention and chest infections.
  - In the spontaneously breathing tetraplegic patient it is the supine position that is associated with the greater diaphragmatic excursion (up and down).

Circulation
- After the resolution of the initial haemodynamic instability ('~~spinal~~' or 'neurogenic' shock – which may last for up to 3 weeks) the major concern is the autonomic hyperreflexia which appears following the return of spinal cord reflexes.

Autonomic hyperreflexia
- Massive reflex sympathetic discharge which occurs in response to stimulation below the level of the spinal lesion. The autonomic nervous system below the level of transection is not subject to any inhibitory influences.
- Visceral (particularly associated with bladder distension or other genitourinary stimulus, but also bowel disorders) or cutaneous stimuli can provoke the mass sympathetic response. This is confined to the area distal to the lesion: proximally there is compensatory parasympathetic overactivity.
- **Clinical features.** Muscle contraction and increased spasticity below the lesion, vasoconstriction. Severe hypertension may be accompanied by tachycardia or a compensatory bradycardia. Arrhythmias may occur. Diaphoresis and flushing (above the level of the lesion). The more distant is the dermatome stimulated from the lesion the more emphatic is the sympathetic response.
- Autonomic hyperreflexia is more pronounced with higher cord lesions (such as in this case) in which the capacity for parasympathetic compensation is limited.
- **Prevention.** Reliable prevention is by neuraxial block, although if an epidural is used it is important to ensure that the sacral segments are blocked. Dense

subarachnoid anaesthesia will prevent hyperreflexia completely. Deep anaesthesia or the use of vasoactive drugs to treat developing hypertension are less successful techniques.

Marking points: For most anaesthetists this will be a theoretical rather than an encountered clinical problem, but you will be expected to comment on the dangers of suxamethonium and the problems of hyperreflexia.

Describe how cerebral blood flow is regulated. How may it be influenced by general anaesthesia?

This is a standard question which has obvious relevance for general anaesthesia, for head injury, for techniques such as induced hypotension and for anaesthesia in patients with hypertensive disorders, including pre-eclampsia.

Introduction

The brain weighs some 2% of the human organism yet receives 15% of the cardiac output: figures which confirm the central importance of the structure and the mechanisms which ensure its continuous oxygenation.

Regulation

- **Cerebral blood flow (CBF)** is linked to cerebral metabolic rate ($CMRO_2$) by a mechanism that has not yet fully been elucidated. There is a short lag time of 1–2 minutes.
- **Cerebral perfusion pressure**
  — Cerebral perfusion pressure (CPP) is given by the formula: CPP = MAP – ICP.
  — This can be modified to CPP = MAP – (ICP + CVP).
- **Autoregulation** maintains CBF and perfusion over a wide range of arterial pressure.
  — Normal blood flow is ~50 ml 100 g^{-1} min^{-1}.
  — Autoregulation maintains this at MAP between 60 and 130 mmHg.
  — Mechanisms are myogenic (stretch receptors in vascular smooth muscle) and metabolic.

Anaesthetic factors

- **Anaesthetic drugs**
  — CBF is increased by all volatile inhalational anaesthetic agents.
  — These attenuate cerebral autoregulation (isoflurane at >1 MAC; others at <1 MAC) and uncouple CBF and $CMRO_2$.
  — Response to P_aCO_2 is maintained.
  — CBF, $CMRO_2$ and ICP are increased by ketamine.
  — Intravenous barbiturates and propofol decrease $CMRO_2$ and CBF.
  — Mannitol (as used, e.g. as free radical scavenger in aortic surgery) reduces CBF/ICP.
- **Anaesthetic associated factors**
  — P_aCO_2: The most important influence on CBF (mediated by H^+ ions). Between 4 and 8 kPa an increase in P_aCO_2 increases CBF in a relationship that is linear. Below 2 kPa there is no further decrease but CBF will continue to rise to its maximal level at ~20 kPa.
  — P_aO_2: CBF increases with relative cerebral hypoxia, so that at 4.0 kPa it is doubled. Hyperoxia is associated with decreases in CBF.
  — **Blood pressure:** Chronic hypertension shifts the autoregulatory curve to the right; drug-induced hypotension shifts it to the left.
  — **Temperature:** changes influence $CMRO_2$ and CBF accordingly.
  — **Venous pressure:** any factors which increase it (position; coughing; straining against ventilator; decreased drainage from head and neck; volume overload; IPPV and PEEP) decrease CPP and CBF.

Marking points: This is a basic science-orientated question and you should be able to apply the underlying principles to anaesthesia. Do not get diverted into raised ICP and the loss of autoregulation after brain injury: these are not part of the question.

Acute and chronic pain

What methods of pain relief are available following abdominal hysterectomy?

This is a very straightforward type of question in which 'abdominal hysterectomy' could be substituted by 'laparotomy', 'total hip replacement' or 'thoracotomy'. Some of your answer can be a generic account of postoperative pain management, but you must focus also on the particular operative procedure that is cited.

Introduction

Abdominal hysterectomy is a common surgical procedure that is usually performed via a transverse subumbilical abdominal incision. In general the postoperative pain is moderate to severe, and it is complicated in as many as 70% of cases by nausea and vomiting. It is interesting that patients who have identical abdominal wounds following caesarean section are frequently mobilising on simple analgesics within 24 hours.

Analgesia options

- Patients undergoing abdominal hysterectomy are typically ASA I or II and may be well informed. The range of options, therefore, is wide and should be discussed in full with the patient. This is particularly important if regional analgesia is considered.
- **Extradural analgesia via infusion or PCEA (patient controlled epidural analgesia)**
  - Low dose bupivacaine plus opioid represents (arguably) the optimal analgesic technique with reliable, flexible and continuous pain relief.
  - Disadvantages include complications of the technique, reliance on expensive technology, increased immobility, and requirement (according to some authorities) for nursing in a high dependency area.
- **Ilio-inguinal blocks (bilateral)**
  - Appear to reduce opioid requirements in some patients undergoing total abdominal hysterectomy (TAH).
- **Intrathecal opioid**
  - Intrathecal diamorphine, for example, will provide 16–24 hours good analgesia.
  - Disadvantages include complications of subarachnoid block plus those associated with the opioid: nausea, vomiting and pruritus. Nausea is already a problem (up to 70%) after TAH. Delayed respiratory depression is also of concern. It is a single shot technique and transition to parenteral opioids may be unsatisfactory.

- **Patient-controlled analgesia**
  - — Good for visceral pain with advantages of immediate availability for patient.
  - — Disadvantages: nausea and sedation associated with opioids, need for secure pumps. Problems again with nausea in gynaecological surgery.
- **Parenteral opioids (im or sc)**
  - — Good for visceral pain, simple and familiar.
  - — Disadvantages: opioid side effects, peak and trough effects, unpredictable absorption, and likelihood of inadequate dosing and inappropriate timing of administration.
- **Non-steroidal anti-inflammatory drugs**
  - — Effective morphine-sparing adjuncts.
  - — Disadvantages: side effects of NSAIDs, patients may not tolerate oral form (PONV) so may require suppository (e.g. diclofenac) or wafer (e.g. piroxicam).
- **Paracetamol and co-drugs**
  - — Paracetamol in regular adequate doses is also an effective adjunct.
  - — Co-drugs should not be administered concurrently with other opioids.

Marking points: This is part of almost every anaesthetist's regular practice and you will be expected to be aware of all the main options. It is hard to avoid a generic type of answer to this question, hence the need for references to gynaecological surgery.

What is meant by 'neuropathic' pain? What symptoms does it produce? Outline with brief examples the major causes.

This is potentially a large question and you should not be expected to have more than a broad theoretical overview of an important cause of disability.

Introduction

Neuropathic pain is defined most simply as pain whose source is neural injury or irritation. It can be either acute or chronic but it does usually outlast the normal healing process. Neuropathic pain is due partly to abnormal central sensitisation.

Symptoms

- Pain
  - Usually described as burning or stabbing, may be lancinating (as in trigeminal neuralgia).
  - May be provoked by innocuous stimulus (allodynia).
  - May complain of exaggerated response to a normally painful stimulus (hyperalgaesia).
  - May have increased perception of a non-painful stimulus (hyperaesthesia).
  - May have abnormally intense painful response to repetitive stimuli (hyperpathia).
  - May be described as unlike any pain previously experienced.
- Focal deficits
  - May have weakness.
  - May exhibit focal autonomic changes related to circulation: swelling, colour changes, temperature alteration (vasomotor instability).
  - May show trophic changes: loss of normal healthy appearance of skin, nails, underlying tissue.

Causes

- **Direct nerve damage**
  - Phantom limb pain, trauma (e.g. avulsion of nerve roots: classically brachial plexus injury in the neck), postherpetic neuralgia.
- **Nerve entrapment**
  - In scar or other compressing tissue (e.g. in mechanisms which produce carpal tunnel syndrome) or by aberrant blood vessels (may cause some cases of trigeminal neuralgia).
- **Central**
  - Central pain may accompany many deafferentation syndromes. Examples include CVA producing thalamic pain, spinal cord injury (trauma, demyelination or other cord pathology).
- **Peripheral neuropathy**
  - Painful neuropathy can be caused by many conditions which include: diabetes mellitus, chronic alcoholism +/– nutritional deficiency, specific vitamin deficiency (e.g. B_{12} and thiamine), toxins, Guillain–Barré syndrome (acute demyelination).
- **Complex Regional Pain Syndrome Type 1 (Reflex Sympathetic Dystrophy)**
  - (Type 2 is due to overt neurological trauma.)
  - May complicate sometimes minor injury to bone or soft tissue, and can be of spontaneous onset.

Marking points: You are expected to recognise the characteristics of neurogenic pain because this may complicate normal anaesthetic practice. A broad understanding of the different causes is required but not the small print detail of major chronic pain textbooks.

List with brief examples the causes of neuropathic pain. What treatments are available?

This is a variation on the previous question and emphasises treatment rather than diagnosis.

Introduction
Neuropathic pain is defined as pain whose source is neural injury or irritation. It can be either acute or chronic but it usually outlasts the normal healing process. It is due partly to abnormal central sensitisation.

Causes
- **Direct nerve damage**
  - Postamputation stump pain, trauma (e.g. avulsion of nerve roots: classically brachial plexus injury in the neck), postherpetic neuralgia.
- **Nerve entrapment**
  - In scar or other compressing tissue (e.g. in mechanisms which produce carpal tunnel syndrome) or by aberrant blood vessels (may cause some cases of trigeminal neuralgia).
- **Central**
  - Central pain may accompany many deafferentation syndromes. Examples include CVA producing thalamic pain, spinal cord injury (trauma, demyelination or other cord pathology), phantom-limb pain.
- **Peripheral neuropathy**
  - Painful neuropathy can be caused by many conditions which include: diabetes mellitus, chronic alcoholism +/– nutritional deficiency, specific vitamin deficiency (e.g. B_{12} and thiamine), toxins, Guillain–Barré syndrome (acute demyelination).
- **Complex Regional Pain Syndrome Type 1 (Reflex Sympathetic Dystrophy)**
  - (Type 2 is due to overt neurological trauma.)
  - May complicate sometimes minor injury to bone or soft tissue, and can be of spontaneous onset.

Treatment
- **Analgesia during acute phase**
  - Simple analgesics; co-drugs.
  - NSAIDs.
  - Opioids can be used.
- **Topical analgesia**
  - Local analgesia (EMLA, lidocaine (lignocaine) 10%, and 'Ametop'): practical only for smaller areas.
  - NSAID creams/gels (little evidence for benefit).
  - Capsaicin (depletes peptide neurotransmitters from primary afferents) can be effective.
- **Systemic analgesia**
  - Adjuvants such as: triyclics, carbamazepine and other membrane stabilisers, gabapentin, phenytoin, clonidine, calcium channel antagonists. Intravenous lidocaine (lignocaine).
  - Corticosteroids may benefit some patients.
- **Other analgesia**
  - Infiltration with local anaesthetics +/– corticosteroids.
  - Sympathetic blockade.
- **Other measures during chronic phase of post-herpetic neuralgia**
  - TENS, dorsal column stimulation.
  - Behavioural therapy.

The large number of therapeutic modalities suggests that none is uniformly reliable in the management of these difficult symptoms.

Marking points: A broad understanding of the different treatment options is expected but not the fine details.

What are the clinical features of post-herpetic neuralgia? How may it be treated?

Post-herpetic neuralgia is one of the common pain syndromes and a reasonable breadth of theoretical knowledge is expected.

Introduction

Post-herpetic neuralgia (PHN) is defined by the persistence of pain following the resolution of acute herpes zoster infection. The infection produces inflammation of peripheral nerves (usually in the dermatome supplied by a single dorsal root ganglion where the virus has lain dormant), of the ganglia and sometimes of the spinal cord. PHN is characterised by chronic inflammation together with some axonal and myelin loss in the peripheral nerve affected.

Clinical features

- Herpes zoster erupts in thoracic dermatomes in 50% or more of cases. Eruption in the distribution of the ophthalmic branch of the trigeminal nerve is the second commonest site.
- Pain is neuropathic, and is described as burning and lancinating. Patients may also describe itching, aching, allodynia (pain provoked by an innocuous stimulus) and hyperpathia (abnormally intense painful response to repetitive stimuli). Some are hyperaesthetic so that touch by garments is very uncomfortable.
- In many patients the natural history of PHN is benign, but in the elderly (>70 years) almost 50% may have persistent pain at 1 year.

Treatments

- **Prevention by treament during acute phase**
  - Antiviral agents (famcyclovir is promoted for this purpose). Some evidence of benefit.
  - Tricyclics (amitryptiline) during the acute phase may also be of benefit.
- **Analgesia during acute phase**
  - Antiviral agents; corticosteroids; sympathetic block.
  - NSAIDs.
  - Opioids have been used in the acute phase.
- **Topical analgesia during chronic phase of PHN**
  - Local analgesia (EMLA, lidocaine (lignocaine) 10%, and 'Ametop'): practical only for smaller areas.
  - NSAID creams / gels (little evidence of benefit).
  - Capsaicin (depletes peptide neurotransmitters from primary afferents) very effective in a small group of patients.
- **Systemic analgesia during chronic phase of PHN**
  - Generic approach as for any neuropathic pain.
  - Adjuvants such as: triyclics, carbamazepine and other membrane stabilisers, gabapentin, phenytoin, clonidine. Intravenous lidocaine (lignocaine) has been used.
  - Standard analgesics (co-drugs, NSAIDs and opioids) may benefit some patients.
- **Other analgesia during chronic phase of PHN**
  - Infiltration with local anaesthetics +/− corticosteroids.
  - Sympathetic blockade, extradural steroid, cryotherapy.
  - Adjuvants such as: triyclics, carbamazepine and other membrane stabilisers, phenytoin, clonidine.
- **Other measures during chronic phase of PHN**
  - TENS, dorsal column stimulation.
  - Behavioural therapy.

The large number of therapeutic modalities suggests that in the small number of patients in whom PHN is refractory there is no single treatment that will reliably treat all.

> **Marking points:** Post-herpetic neuralgia may be common but the list of treatments demonstrates that all the resources of an experienced clinician in chronic pain may be required. You will be expected only to have a theoretical understanding of the pathophysiology of the condition and some knowledge of the scope of therapeutic options.

A 62-year-old man is to undergo an above-knee amputation. What can be done to relieve any pain he may experience thereafter?

This is not simply a question about phantom limb pain, but invites you to consider all the possible causes of postamputation pain. An orderly and structured approach will help.

Introduction
Above-knee amputation is a procedure that not only may be preceded by severe pain but is also likely to be associated with different types of postoperative pain, including phantom limb pain, which can be difficult to treat.

Pain management
- Immediate postoperative pain
  — Will require the standard resources of the acute pain team.
  — Options include epidural analgesia (PCEA), intrathecal opioids (at time of surgery), intravenous opioids (PCA), tramadol, adjuvant pain control with NSAIDs and co-drugs.
- Immediate postamputation stump pain
  — Standard resources of the acute pain team.
  — Additional options include treatment of ischaemia and infection, and the use e.g. of baclofen to relieve spasm of quadriceps.
- Delayed stump pain
  — Strong association with development of phantom limb pain.
  — Peripheral neuropathic pain due to neuroma formation at stump site.
  — May be treated with injection into neuroma or surgery.
- Phantom limb pain
  — Deafferentation pain (pain in an area of sensory loss).
  — Specific mechanisms not elucidated.
  — Occurs initially in nearly all amputees (not young children).
  — Declines over time in >50%; persistent and resistant in some cases.
  — Pre-emptive regional anaesthesia may benefit some (especially if pre-amputation pain is severe).
  — Sympathetic block sometimes useful.
  — Sensory block may worsen symptoms (neurolysis is worse still).
  — Neurostimulatory treatments are better: TENS, acupuncture and dorsal column stimulation (have mixed results).
  — Adjuvants such as: triyclics, carbamazepine and other membrane stabilisers, gabapentin, phenytoin.

Marking points: This question aims to assess your appreciation of the global pain problems which an amputee may face, and requires as much information about the immediate pain management as about the later phantom limb pain.

What are the clinical features of trigeminal neuralgia and what is its pathogenesis? Describe the main treatments that are available.

Trigeminal neuralgia is a condition seen quite frequently in the chronic pain relief clinic, and classically it is described as one of the most severe pains in human experience, one which is said to have driven some patients to suicide. It is, therefore, a dramatic condition, and one that is amenable to dramatic treatments. You should be familiar with it.

Introduction

Trigeminal neuralgia has a reputation as a neuropathic pain which is amongst the most severe in human experience; one – it is said - which has driven some patients to suicide.

Clinical features

- Peak onset is in middle age.
- Pain is intermittent, lancinating and extremely severe.
- Attacks last for seconds and patients are pain free in the interim, but attacks may be very frequent.
- Pain is limited usually to one (occasionally two) of the branches of the trigeminal nerve: ophthalmic (least common ~5%), maxillary or mandibular divisions, which supply sensation to the face. The distribution is always unilateral.
- Trigger points around the face may react to the lightest stimulus (breeze, touch, chewing) by precipitating paroxysmal pain.

Pathogenesis (remains speculative)

- **Central hypothesis**
  — Abnormal neurones in the pons exhibit spontaneous and uncontrolled discharge in the nerve.
- **Peripheral hypothesis**
  — Demyelination: trigeminal neuralgia in younger patients may herald multiple sclerosis.
  — Compression: aberrant blood vessels in the posterior fossa.

Treatments

- **Pharmacological**
  — Carbamazepine: is effective in >90% with true trigeminal neuralgia (100 mg bd up to maintenance of 600–1200 mg day^{-1}) FBC must be monitored for marrow suppression.
  — Phenytoin: is effective in ~60% and can be given iv for acute intractable pain (starting dose ~ 300–500 mg/day).
  — Baclofen: GABA analogue binds to GABA$_B$ (up to 80 mg/day).
- **Destructive**
  — Radiofrequency ablation. Needle is passed percutaneously and under X-ray control through the foramen ovale to the Gasserian (trigeminal) ganglion. Chemical ablation may also be used.
- **Surgical decompression**
  — Very invasive. Requires posterior fossa exploration to identify aberrant vessel(s) which are compressing the nerve near its emergence from the pons.

Marking points: This condition is relatively common and can be very severe. Precise details of treatment will not be expected but you should convey the important clinical features and the broad scope of its management.

Outline the causes and the clinical features of the 'Complex Regional Pain Syndrome'? How may it be managed?

Complex Regional Pain Syndrome Types 1 and 2 (previously known as Reflex Sympathetic Dystrophy and Causalgia) are important examples of neuropathic pain which may affect a wide range of age groups. The conditions appear more commonly in the examination than they do in clinical practice.

Introduction

Complex Regional Pain Syndromes (CRPS) Types 1 and 2 are the names given to what formerly were known respectively as Reflex Sympthetic Dystrophy and Causalgia. In some, but not every case, sympathetically maintained pain may be a prominent feature.

Causes

- The pathophysiology of the disorders is unknown, but where there is a sympathetic component it is postulated that nociceptive impulses from visceral afferents travel with efferent sympathetic fibres.
- **CRPS Type 1** (formerly Reflex Sympathetic Dystrophy) is associated with injury to tissue: bones, joints and connective tissue, but not necessarily nerves. The injury may be relatively trivial, and is most commonly precipitated by an orthopaedic injury to a distal extremity (lower leg and ankle, wrist, etc.).
- **CRPS Type 2** (formerly Causalgia), by contrast, is characterised by significant nerve injury without transection. It is more commonly associated with proximal nerves in the upper leg and upper limb. Most frequently affected are the sciatic, tibial, median and ulnar nerves.

Clinical features

- Both are examples of neuropathic pain which are distinguished only by the nature of the injury and the fact that in type 1 there is more diffuse pain whereas in Type 2 there is more discrete localisation to the distribution of a single nerve.
- Symptoms include burning pain, allodynia (provoked by an innocuous stimulus), hyperpathia (abnormally intense painful response to repetitive stimuli) and hyperalgesia (exaggerated pain response to a noxious stimulus).
- The pain is accompanied by signs of failure of autonomic regulation in the region affected. These include: swelling, temperature changes (vasomotor instability), colour changes, abnormal sudomotor activity.
- There may be associated weakness and trophic changes with loss of normal healthy appearance of skin (becomes thin and translucent), hair and nails, focal atrophy of underlying tissue including muscle. Focal osteoporosis may also develop.

Management

- **Sympathetic block (diagnostic).** If this is effective it will both diagnose the presence of sympathetically mediated pain and initiate its treatment, although the evidence for benefit is disputed. Procedures include stellate ganglion block, lumbar sympathectomy, plexus blocks, or more commonly, guanethidine blocks. Treatment regimens vary.
- **Sympathetic block (therapeutic).** A series of blocks may confer benefit which increases in duration after each one or may confer only temporary relief which finally disappears. Some patients may be considered for a permanent neurolytic procedure.
- If a patient shows little or no response to sympathetic blockade their chronic neuropathic pain is treated accordingly:
  — Simple analgesics; co-drugs; NSAIDs; opioids.

- Topical analgesia is rarely effective; capsaicin (depletes peptide neurotransmitters from primary afferents) may help symptoms.
- Systemic analgesia with adjuvants: tricyclics, carbamazepine and other membrane stabilisers, gabapentin, phenytoin, clonidine, calcium channel antagonists. Intravenous lidocaine (lignocaine).
- TENS and dorsal column stimulation.
- Behavioural therapy: pain management programmes.

Marking points: A generic management plan, which includes sympathetic blockade, for the treatment of neuropathic pain is appropriate in this answer, but you will also be expected to identify the (modest) differences between the two syndromes in your description of the salient clinical features.

What are the principles of the management of cancer pain?

Palliative care, of which pain management is a large part, is a large subject. This question expores whether you appreciate both the important differences from, as well as the similarities to, acute postsurgical or traumatic pain.

Introduction

The pain of cancer is complicated by the emotional context and by the fact that it may well be destructive and progressive. The whole range of generic treatments, up to and including neuroablative techniques, can be used, but management must take place within the broader framework of multidisciplinary supportive care. The overall objectives of management must be to optimise pain control while minimising side effects, so as to enhance functional abilities and the patient's quality of life.

Diagnosis

- It must not be assumed that the pain is necessarily associated with the diagnosed malignancy. It may well be, but thorough physical examination and further investigation may be needed. 10% of patients with cancer have pain related to another cause.
- Once diagnosed there must be a clear understanding of the aetiology and pathophysiology of the pain to allow rational treatment.
- The patient should be believed: cancer pain is not psychogenic, but there may be contributory pyschosocial factors including reactive depression.

Evaluation

- Complete pain history: quality and nature, intensity, duration, precipitants, relieving factors, associated features.
- Where is the site? Cancer pain is due to tumour involvement in pain sensitive structures.
  - Most common is bony metastasis. Particularly painful is vertebral involvement (commonly from primary in breast, lung, prostate).
  - May also be neuropathic due to invasion of lumbosacral or brachial plexus.
  - Post-herpetic neuralgia is more common (due to immunocompromise, the age of the population and sensitivity of irradiated areas).
  - Peripheral neuropathy (can be drug-induced: cisplatin, vinca alkaloids, procarbazine) and phantom limb pain can occur.
  - Visceral pain (pancreas, liver, colon).
  - Headache due to mass lesion.
  - Pain in a scar that has been pain free suggests tumour recurrence.

Management

- Will vary with the patient's status: different groups have been identified.
  - The patient with acute cancer pain (with possible contributions from surgery, radiotherapy or chemotherapy).
  - The patient with chronic cancer-related pain (+/− treatment contribution) and associated with disease progression.
  - The dying patient with cancer-related pain in whom palliative surgery or radiotherapy may yet be indicated (e.g. spinal stabilisation for vertebral collapse).
- The generic WHO analgesic ladder can be used: non-opioids +/− adjuvant medication; weak opioids +/− non–opioids +/− adjuvants; strong opioids +/− non-opioids +/− adjuvants. Adjuvants will be important in the treatment of neuropathic pain.
- Indwelling neuraxial drug delivery systems may be appropriate.
- Intractable pain can be treated with neurodestructive techniques such as

intrathecal phenol for sacral invasion in a patient who is already incontinent, or percutaneous cordotomy for the pain of a unilateral lesion. These are only appropriate for patients with a short life expectancy, because pain can reappear within months.

- Associated adverse effects must be treated: constipation, sedation, nausea and vomiting, mental clouding, myoclonus, pruritus, urinary retention.

Marking points: The management of cancer pain can be complex. Your answer need not include the detail above but you should emphasise proper diagnosis and evaluation, a multidisciplinary approach and the fact that the whole range of analgesic options can be invoked.

A 62-year-old man presents for major gastrointestinal surgery. How may the choice of pain management influence his recovery from surgery?

This is a question about the role of good analgesia, and specifically epidural analgesia, in accelerating hospital discharge after major surgery. The issue is topical, but although neither proven nor universally accepted, is a subject about which you should have some thoughts. If you are struggling, then start by identifying the consequences of unrelieved pain and work backwards.

Introduction

Severe and inadequately relieved pain following major surgery is likely to delay mobilisation and discharge from hospital. The converse hypothesis is that by providing optimal analgesia the opposite may apply and patient outcome may be improved. Further evidence is needed but the underlying principles can be outlined as follows.

Adverse effects of postoperative pain

- Respiratory
  - Inhibition by muscle and diaphragmatic splinting decreases FRC, VC and leads to alveolar hypoventilation and atelectasis.
  - If cough reflex is inhibited by pain, secretion retention may precipitate pneumonia.
  - Impaired oxygenation is potentially deleterious to wound healing and myocardial oxygenation.
- Cardiovascular
  - Catecholamine release: tachycardia, hypertension, peripheral vasoconstriction, increased myocardial work.
- Gastrointestinal
  - Stress response, in particular the sympathetic component, impairs gut motility and prolongs postoperative ileus.

Pre-emptive analgesia

- Aim is to attenuate central sensitisation (spinal cord 'wind-up')
  - Analgesia initiated prior to surgical trauma should minimise the sympathoadrenal and neuroendocrine stress response, as well as modulating the pain processing that takes place in the dorsal horn of the spinal cord.
  - It reduces opioid consumption, but there is as yet no consistent evidence that morbidity and mortality are improved.

Influence of analgesia on recovery

- Opioids. PCA with opioids, and the concept of 'balanced analgesia' using other agents, improves the overall pain experience of the patient. It has only a modest effect in modifying the stress response and may contribute to alveolar hypoventilation and postoperative ileus.
- Epidural analgesia (local anaesthetic/opioid mixtures).
  - No consistent evidence of beneficial effect on mortality or cardiac morbidity.
  - Convincing evidence that effective epidural anaesthesia has other benefits:
    Extensive extradural block ablates adrenocortical and glycaemic responses to surgery.
    Reduces thromboembolic complications.
    Reduces pulmonary complications (atelectasis, hypoxaemia, infection).
    Reduces time to restoration of gut function. Reduces sympathetically mediated inhibition of peristalsis.

Decreases time to extubation and ITU discharge in gastro-oesophagectomy patients.

Decreases time to ambulation after major surgery.

Consensus increasingly secure that targeted and sustained regional anaesthesia has a beneficial effect on surgical outcome.

Marking points: This issue is topical and there are multicentre trials under way that may in due course provide more evidence. If you have experience of using epidurals for pain relief then you will have intuitive knowledge of the likely benefits, but do not make exaggerated claims based on anecdotal experience. The bald answer to this question is fairly thin, so base your arguments on the underlying principles.

9

Trauma and emergency anaesthesia

What fluids are available for the restoration of circulating volume in a patient suffering from acute blood loss? Discuss the advantages and disadvantages of each.

Arguments about optimal resuscitation of the intravascular compartment continue, the role of albumin remains controversial, and there are persistent concerns about the safety of homologous blood transfusion. This question examines your knowledge of these areas while also testing one of your emergency skills.

Introduction

There are three main groups of fluids which are used to resuscitate the intravascular compartment folllowing acute blood loss: crystalloid solutions, colloids and blood. Solutions such as perfluorocarbons and stroma free haemoglobin may offer some future promise in terms of oxygen carriage but are not available and will not be discussed. There is no consensus about the optimum regimen but the main arguments for and against each can be summarised as follows.

Crystalloid solutions

- **Crystalloid.** A crystalloid solution is defined chemically as one which contains a water soluble crystalline substance capable of diffusion through a semipermeable membrane.
- **Examples.** Include Hartmann's solution (Compound Sodium Lactate Intravenous Infusion or Ringer-Lactate Solution for Injection), Ringer's Solution for Injection (NaCl 0.9%), Hypertonic Saline (NaCl 3.0%), Dextrose (4%)/Saline (0.18%) and Glucose (5%).
- **Crystalloid advantages**
  — Readily available and cheap.
  — Balanced salt solutions approximate ECF composition.
  — Simple to infuse large volumes.
- **Crystalloid disadvantages**
  — Duration in circulation is very short: 50% in ECF/ICW after 20 minutes.
  — Hartmann's is contraindicated in diabetes (lactate is gluconeogenic).
  — Large sodium and water load.
  — Potential for overinfusion, pulmonary oedema, subsequent ARDS.
  — Glucose distributes throughout body water: minimal effect on intravascular volume.
  — No oxygen carrying capacity.

Colloids

- **Colloid.** A colloid is defined chemically as a dispersion, or suspension of finely divided particles in a continuous medium.
- **Examples.** Macromolecular substances include gelatins (Gelofusine and Haemaccel), plasma protein and albumin solutions, hydroxylethyl starch (hetastarch, hexastarch, pentastarch) and dextrans (polysaccharides classified according to molecular weight: 40, 70 and 110×10^3). (Blood is also a colloid but is discussed separately.)
- **Gelatins**
  — Effective: $t_{1/2}$ in circulation 3 hours.
  — Risk of allergic reactions (Haemaccel > Gelofusine).
  — No oxygen carrying capacity.
- **Starch**
  — Effective: $t_{1/2}$ in circulation 24 hours.
  — Uptake by reticuloendothelial system and may remain for > a year.
- **Dextrans**
  — Effective: $t_{1/2}$ in circulation 3 hours upwards.
  — Risk of allergic reactions.
  — May interfere with blood cross-matching (70).
  — May cause renal problems (40).
- **Plasma protein fraction (PPF) and albumin**
  — Effective: $t_{1/2}$ in circulation 24 hours.
  — Expensive.
  — Risk of cross-infection.
  — Controversy about role in rescuscitation: may cross leaky capillary membranes (lung, damaged brain, etc.) and worsen outcome. No consensus.

Colloids are theoretically more effective in resuscitation but there is as yet no evidence to support its superiority over crystalloids.

Blood

- Blood is also a colloid, but it is convenient to discuss it separately .
  — In acute blood loss whole blood is the ideal replacement: has oxygen-carrying capacity and expands the intravascular volume.
  — Red cell concentrate (e.g. SAG-M) supplies O_2 carriage, but each unit is only ~300 ml.
  — Numerous potential disadvantages of homologous transfusion must be set against urgency of optimal intravascular resuscitation.
  — Autologous transfusion is ideal but impractical in unexpected major blood loss.
  — Expensive.

Marking points: Volume replacement is an important part of anaesthetic practice. You will be expected to demonstrate knowledge of the main categories of fluids above.

A 25-year-old man is admitted with a fracture of the cervical spine at C5/6 with spinal cord trauma. There are no other injuries. Describe the management of this patient in the first 48 hours after injury.

Two individuals a day in the UK are paralysed after traumatic spinal cord injuries. The chances of an individual anaesthetist outside encountering such patients are not high, but should they do so there are significant anaesthetic implications. Many patients, moreover, arrive in A&E with the suspicion of cord injury and so the principles of early management are important.

Introduction
On average two individuals in the UK will be paralysed each day following traumatic spinal cord injury and it is vital that their immediate management both ensures survival while preventing any secondary cord damage. Over half of these injuries (55%) affect the cervical spine.

Management
Manage according to standard trauma care principles: Airway, Breathing and Circulation with cervical spine control. Should exclude other injuries (none here).

- **Cervical spine**
  - Control with collar or manual in-line stabilisation prior to surgical traction or halo.
- **Airway**
  - No acute problem in this scenario, unless acute respiratory distress is apparent. Respiratory function tends to worsen with cord oedema and haemorrhage over the first 2–3 days.
  - If intubation is required there are two options:
  - Rapid sequence induction with manual in-line stabilisation (denervation hyperkalaemia does not appear until ~48 hours after injury, and so suxamethonium can be used in the acute situation).
  - Awake fibreoptic intubation under local anaesthesia: this allows neurological evaluation to be maintained throughout.
- **Breathing**
  - Cervical lesions at C5 or C6 largely spare the diaphragm, but accessory muscles of respiration are affected, including intercostals, and these may contribute as much as 60% of tidal volume in the healthy individual.
  - Acutely the effect of a lesion may extend for several segments rostral and caudad from the site of the lesion (due to local oedema and inflammatory response to injury), and so diaphragmatic respiration may be affected.
  - Neurogenic pulmonary oedema may supervene: is more common in cervical spine injury (mechanism probably related to increased SVR and afterload associated with massive sympathetic activity).
  - Oxygen by face mask if breathing spontaneously; IPPV if indicated.
- **Circulation**
  - Acute spinal cord injury is associated with 'neurogenic shock' (sometimes known as 'spinal shock', which term is now used to describe the flaccidity and arreflexia following cord damage).
  - More pronounced in cervical than in thoracolumbar cord damage.
  - Loss of vascular tone causes profound hypotension (may persist for up to 3 weeks after injury): attempts to treat with fluid alone are mainly ineffective and risk pulmonary oedema.
  - Accompanied by cardiac arrhythmias ranging from sinus bradycardia (commoner in cervical injuries due to vagal tone unopposed by T1–4

sympathetic cardiac accelerator input) to complete AV block. Atrial and ventricular tachyarrhythmias.

— Patients in spinal shock compensate poorly for hypo- or hypervolaemia, for changes in position and for the circulatory and cardiodepressant effects of anaesthetic drugs.

Other systems
- **Gastrointestinal and renal**
  - Acute gastric dilatation and ileus.
  - Requires decompression by nasogastric tube.
  - Bladder catheterisation.
- **Haematological**
  - Total immobility, circulatory instability, catecholamine surge all predispose to venous thrombosis. Requires prophylaxis.
- **Drug treatment**
  - High dose corticosteroids (methyl prednisolone 30 mg kg^{-1}) may reduce final neurological deficit, but must be given within 8 hours of the injury to confer benefit. Their use is contentious.
  - Prophylaxis against stress ulceration.
  - Prophylaxis against DVT.
- **Specialist care**
  - Spinal injuries unit must be contacted: this patient will require specialist care when clinical condition permits transfer.
- **Pastoral care**
  - This is a devastating injury for patient and for the family. Prognosis is very uncertain in the early stages, but empathetic communication is vital at all times.

Marking points: Acute cord injury has some key treatment points: cervical spine stabilisation, maintainance of oxygenation and awareness of circulatory instability. You will be expected to convey the importance of these aspects.

Describe the anaesthetic management of a patient with a perforating eye injury who had a large meal about an hour before the accident.

This is another question whose popularity is not matched by its frequency in clinical practice. This is a question which requires some discussion of the risks and benefits of particular techniques, based upon an understanding of the underlying principles relating to intraocular pressure. There is no consensus, so be confident in your clinical views.

Introduction
Penetrating eye injury in a patient with a full stomach presents an anaesthetic challenge in which the risks of pulmonary aspiration of gastric contents are set against the risks of ocular loss. There is no consensus about management and it is possible that the risks which perturb some anaesthetists may be more theoretical than actual.

The ocular problem
- Normal IOP is between 10 and 22 mmHg. As soon as the globe is entered the IOP becomes atmospheric, so any sudden increase can result in extrusion of the contents.
- IOP is affected by changes in the volume of intraocular compartments: choroidal blood volume, aqueous volume (anterior and posterior chambers) and vitreous volume.
- IOP is also affected by external pressure, compression by actions of the extraocular muscles (as stimulated by suxamethonium).
- Hypercapnia, hypoxia and impaired venous drainage increase IOP (and may be under anaesthetic control).
- Anaesthetic induction agents generally reduce IOP (exception is ketamine).

Risk of aspiration: minimise if possible

Preoperatively
- Defer the procedure to allow gastric emptying. Largely impractical: eye injury if severe may cause gastric stasis and the operation is usually urgent.
- Empty the stomach using a prokinetic drug such as metoclopramide (while hoping that the drug does not excite an oculogyric crisis).
- Reduce gastric acidity by H_2 antagonist such as iv ranitidine.
- Neutralise gastric contents with non-particulate antacid such as 0.3 molar Na citrate.

Perioperatively
- Tracheal intubation is unavoidable in presence of full stomach and rapid sequence induction is indicated. Laryngoscopy increases IOP (can attenuate with opioids).
- Suxamethonium: raises IOP acutely (returns to baseline within 6 minutes), although some have found that after adequate dose of induction agent and after pretreatment with a non-depolarising agent the rise in IOP is minimal and there is no evidence from case reports that this technique is associated with ocular loss.
- Can perform RSI with a non-depolarising drug. Rocuronium will give reliable intubating conditions within 60–90 seconds. Pre-oxygenation should ensure several minutes of O_2 reserves (unless the patient is a child or pregnant). Coughing will increase IOP by 40 mmHg and so it is imperative to wait until intubating conditions are optimal.
- Smooth eduction of anaesthesia and extubation are also important.
- There is in addition the practical fact that penetrating eye injury is an unpleasant injury that is frequently associated with vomiting and which will raise IOP more than suxamethonium (and will partly empty the stomach).

Marking points: There is no definitive answer to the problem of a perforating eye injury in a patient with a full stomach, but you will be expected to offer an informed appraisal of the risks and benefits of your management.

Describe the diagnosis and immediate assessment of a patient with smoke inhalation injury.

Smoke inhalation is an important factor in thermal injury and because it involves the airway is of immediate relevance to anaesthetists. This question tests your recognition of the need for early intervention if indicated. To a lesser extent it tests your appreciation of the importance of systemic effects of substances that have been inhaled.

Introduction
Smoke inhalation injury occurs when hot gases, including toxins and reactive smoke particles, reach the bronchial tree. It is the most common cause of death in the first hour following thermal injury and increases dramatically the mortality associated with body surface burns.

Diagnosis
- History: exposure to smoke or fumes in a confined space.
- Carbonaceous or other deposits around the nose and mouth.
- Signs of burns to neck or face.
- Carbonaceous sputum.
- Evidence of intraoral thermal injury. Gases disperse heat rapidly to the oropharynx (gas at 142°C at the mouth cools to 38°C before it reaches the lungs) causing erythema and blistering, and later desquamation and necrosis.
- Evidence of immediate airway embarrassment: stridor, dyspnoea, wheeze.

Assessment
- The composition of smoke may be complex: commonly it includes carbon monoxide (CO), also may contain dioxides of nitrogen and sulphur, and acids including hydrocyanic. Depending on the toxin, systemic effects (decreased O_2 carriage and cellular toxicity associated with COHb or CN (Cyanide)) may occur before the local effects, and are largely responsible for early mortality.
- Hypoxia. May be present due to asphyxiation.
- Signs of CO poisoning. Pulse oximetry is inaccurate: requires direct measurement by co-oximeter, symptoms and signs are those of tissue hypoxia.
- Airway assessment: oedema, local direct damage.
- Breathing: stridor, tachypnoea, wheeze, pulmonary oedema, excessive sputum (inhalation may destroy cilia), crepitations (oedema and intraluminal reactive fluid), decreased air entry.
- Many of these features may not be apparent immediately after inhalation injury but may develop over succeeding hours. Respiratory deterioration may be rapid: there should be a high index of suspicion because it is better by far to intervene too early than too late.

Marking points: This is a safety question. Can you recognise when smoke inhalation is likely to have occurred and are you aware of the probable need for airway intervention? This is of more immediate importance than the possible systemic effects of inhalation, but you must be aware of the problems associated with carbon monoxide poisoning.

Outline the key points in the management of a patient with massive haemorrhage.

Every anaesthetist will encounter massive haemorrhage and every anaesthetist should have a system for its assessment and a strategy for its management. This is a question about the safe conduct of an acute serious problem.

Introduction

There are alternative definitions for 'massive haemorrhage' which include the loss of one blood volume within 24 hours, the loss of 50% of blood volume within 3 hours, or continuing loss at the rate of 150 ml min^{-1}. The clinical features of these would be somewhat different, but the outcome if mismanaged would be the same. Survival of such patients requires early and accurate assessment, and effective and considered action.

Assessment

- Key points in initial management:
  - — Suspect massive haemorrhage if the clinical situation renders it possible.
  - — Blood loss is frequently underestimated (particularly in obstetrics).
  - — Recognise the symptoms.
  - — Treat early and vigorously.
- The clinical picture results from the normal compensatory mechanisms which are manifest mainly in the cardiovascular and respiratory systems. Mental state is also affected.
- **<25% loss.** At blood volume loss of up to 25% the system compensates. Tachycardia is one of the first signs, even in low volume loss, but blood pressure may be normal (although pulse pressure will narrow and MAP may even increase). Capillary refill will be at upper end of normal (<2 seconds) or prolonged. Respiratory rate increases and the patient may be restless.
- **25–40% loss.** At blood volume loss of 25-40% the system decompensates, with increasing tachycardia, decreasing arterial pressure, prolonged capillary refill, tachypnoea, oliguria and confusion.
- **>40% loss.** At a loss of >40% circulating volume the system risks irreversible shock with bradycardia, profound hypotension, prolonged capillary refill, periodic respiration, anuria and coma.

Key points in management

- **Circulatory access:** at least two large bore cannulae, at worst a PA catheter sheath (8G) may be necessary. CVP monitoring may only be possible to initiate when the circulation has been at least partly restored.
- **Arrest the bleeding.** This is likely to require surgical intervention, which will form part of the resuscitation. It may be inevitable that the patient will require anaesthesia while still hypovolaemic.
- **Fluid replacement:** warm crystalloid, colloid, and blood as soon as it is available. (Hypothermia increases the risks of disseminated intravascular coagulation (DIC).) O negative un-crossmatched if necessary (2 units only), then type specific and finally fully cross-matched units until one blood volume has been lost. Once this has been replaced then further cross-matching becomes unnecessary. Cell salvage may be appropriate in major visceral trauma or ruptured aortic aneurysm. Probably inadvisable in obstetrics (presence of amniotic fluid) although it has been used.
- **Specialist help.** It is essential to involve a senior haematologist as soon as the clinical picture becomes clear.
- **Blood components.** Replacement should be based on laboratory investigations: FBC, PT, APTT, fibrinogen. These should be repeated after blood component therapy.

- **Fresh frozen plasma.** FFP should be given to maintain PT and APTT at <1.5× control. Should be based on laboratory results rather than given by formula. Most blood, however, e.g. SAG-M, has minimal coagulation activity so FFP should be started after the loss of one blood volume. Likely to require at least 4–8 units (4 units = ~1 L).
- **Cryoprecipitate.** Fibrinogen may fall to <1.0 g L^{-1} after loss of ~1.5 blood volumes. Request 1–1.5 packs per 10 kg body weight.
- **Platelets.** Crucial for coagulation. Order early because delivery time from the blood centre may be significant. By the time that platelets have fallen to 50 × 10^9 L^{-1} up to two complete blood volumes will have been lost. Haematological advice about volumes needed.
- **General points.** Blood components may be delayed by distance from the transfusion centre to the hospital. It is preferable to overestimate requirements for blood and blood products, because although some may end up wasted, that is preferable to allowing a patient to develop disseminated intravascular coagulation because of inadequate resuscitation with the appropriate blood products.

Marking points: This is an important safety topic, and although your answer need not contain every detail above, it will gain much credibility if you can convey some sense of the organised urgency that should attend the resuscitation of such a case. If you do not have a structured template ready in your mind for this sort of question, do not struggle to recall what you read in the protocol book but simply remember the last time that you managed such a situation. If the patient survived intact then you must have done something right.

What is the physiological response to the rapid loss of 1 litre of blood in the adult?

Blood loss is commonplace in anaesthetic practice. It may frequently be negligible and sometimes obvious and overwhelming. In other cases, however, blood loss may be more insidious and it is only by understanding the normal physiological mechanisms of compensation that anaesthetists can recognise the signs. It is an important topic.

Introduction

Blood volume comprises approximately 7% of body weight, so a 1 litre blood loss in a 70 kg individual represents about 20% of total blood volume. Healthy subjects will compensate for this loss by mounting a physiological response which is described below.

- **Blood loss**
  - Decreased venous return, right atrial pressure and cardiac output.
- **Baroreceptor reflex activation (immediate)**
  - Decrease in discharge rates of baroreceptors: sensitive stretch receptors in the carotid sinus and aortic arch.
  - Decreased afferent input to medullary cardiovascular centre: results in decreased parasympathetic and increased sympathetic activity.
  - Tachycardia (an important sign, even in lower volume loss), increased myocardial contractility, sympathetically mediated arteriolar constriction.
  - Also stimulation of vasopressin secretion because of fewer discharging afferents to the hypothalamus.
- **Immediate effect**
  - Decrease in effective venous reservoir and so decreased VR (venous return) and CO.
  - The factors changed as a direct result of haemorrhage: SV, CO and MAP are restored by baroreceptor reflexes towards, but not to, normal.
  - The factors changed indirectly as part of the reflex response: HR and SVR are increased above pre-haemorrhage values.
- **Hypothalamic–pituitary–adrenal response (slower)**
  - Reduced renal blood flow stimulates intrarenal baroreceptors with renin release from the juxta-glomerular apparatus. This in turn leads to the conversion of circulating angiotensinogen to angiotensin I and then angiotensin II (in the lung).
  - Angiotensin II is a powerful arteriolar vasoconstrictor and also stimulates aldosterone release from the adrenal cortex and arginine vasopressin (ADH) release from the posterior pituitary.
  - ADH release is also stimulated by decreased extracellular volume (atrial receptors).
  - These enhance Na^+ and H_2O reabsorption at the distal renal tubule.
- **Starling forces**
  - Hypovolaemia encourages movement of fluid into capillaries: BP fall and arteriolar constriction decrease capillary hydrostatic pressure and so favour absorption of interstitial fluid with an increase in plasma volume and restoration of arterial pressure towards normal. These mechanisms are efficient (particularly if blood loss is slow).
- **Other factors**
  - Sympathetically mediated catecholamine and cortisol secretion.
  - Redistribution of CO from skin, muscle and viscera to heart and brain.
  - Compensation explains the clinical signs of cold periphery, pallor, cyanosis, reduced capillary refill.
- **Carotid chemoreceptors**
  - Respond to changes in P_aO_2, P_aCO_2 and H^+ to stimulate hyperventilation.

Marking points: It is the basic physiological responses which explain the clinical features of hypovolaemia and which should guide its rational management. You will be expected, therefore, to have a grasp of the fundamental points.

Explain, with examples, the mechanisms by which a pneumothorax may occur.

Pneumothorax is an important complication in anaesthesia and trauma. Rapid recognition and prompt management are the keys to a successful outcome but they must be based on an understanding of the mechanisms by which pneumothorax can occur.

Introduction

A pneumothorax is present when there is air in the pleural space. The presence of air will diminish lung volume on the affected side and this may be relatively innocuous. If, however, the intrapleural gas is under tension this can develop rapidly into a life-threatening emergency.

Mechanisms

- At the end of expiration there is no pressure differential between intra-alveolar and atmospheric pressure. The intrapleural, or transpulmonary pressure, however, is subatmospheric, and the slight negative pressure of ~4–6 cmH$_2$O (caused by opposing elastic recoil of lung and chest wall) keeps the lungs expanded. This pressure differential also opposes the tendency of the thoracic wall to move outwards.
- When air gains access to the intrapleural space the negative transpulmonary pressure is lost and the stretched lung collapses while the chest wall moves outwards.
- Air can gain access to the intrapleural space via a breach in the parietal or visceral pleura (or both) or via the mediastinal pleura as a consequence of intrapulmonary alveolar rupture.
- **Damage to the parietal pleura**
  - Open penetrating chest trauma.
  - During operative procedures: nephrectomy, spinal surgery, tracheostomy, laparoscopy (gas gains access via the mediastinal pleura).
  - Tracheal, oesophageal or mediastinal perforation.
- **Damage to the visceral pleura**
  - Commonly iatrogenic and caused by needle punctures or vascular cannulation.
  - Vascular access: subclavian and internal jugular puncture.
  - Nerve blocks: supraclavicular, interscalene, intercostal.
- **Intrapulmonary alveolar rupture**
  - Gas esapes from alveolus, dissects towards hilum and ruptures the mediastinal pleura.
  - Causes include barotrauma from mechanical ventilation (excessive pressures) or high pressure gas delivery systems (injectors); chronic obstructive pulmonary disease with bullous emphysema. Is also caused by blast injury. Can occur in asthmatics.
  - May occur if the alveolar septa are weakened or distorted by infection, collagen vascular disease or connective tissue disorders (e.g. Ehlers–Danlos and Marfan's syndromes).
  - Severe hypovolaemia has also been implicated as a risk factor for the same reason.

Marking points: It is relatively simple to compile a list of the many tens of causes of pneumothorax, and so this question explores whether you understand the principles which underlie the clinical phenomenon. You will be expected to know the basic science.

List the important causes of pneumothorax. What are the diagnostic features and what is the immediate management?

This is an extension of the previous question which concentrates on diagnosis and management, but which again places emphasis on your understanding of the principles of treatment.

Introduction

There are many causes of pneumothorax, which is caused when air gains access to the intrapleural space via a breach in the parietal or visceral pleura, or via the mediastinal pleura as a consequence of intrapulmonary alveolar rupture. The presence of air will diminish lung volume on the affected side and this may be relatively innocuous. If, however, the intrapleural gas is under tension this can develop rapidly into a life-threatening emergency.

Causes

- **Traumatic:** penetrating injury, rib fracture, blast injury, etc.
- **Iatrogenic (surgical):** during operative procedures such as nephrectomy, spinal surgery, tracheostomy (especially in children), laparoscopy (gas gains access via the mediastinal pleura), or as consequence of oesophageal or mediastinal perforation.
- **Iatrogenic (anaesthetic):** during attempted subclavian and internal jugular puncture, supraclavicular, interscalene or intercostal nerve blocks. Barotrauma from mechanical ventilation at excessive pressures or in patients with chronic obstructive pulmonary disease with bullous emphysema. Use of high pressure gas delivery systems (injectors).
- **Miscellaneous:** may occur if the alveolar septa are weakened or distorted by infection, severe hypovolaemia or connective tissue disorders (e.g. Ehlers–Danlos and Marfan's Syndromes). Is associated with many diseases, including asthma.

Diagnosis of pneumothorax in the awake patient

- Predisposing clinical conditions as above.
- Typical features (which are not invariable and which will depend on the size of the pneumothorax and whether or not it is expanding) include:
  — Chest pain, referred shoulder tip pain, cough, dyspnoea, tachypnoea, tachycardia.
  — Diminished movement of the affected hemithorax, hyperresonance, diminished breath sounds, decreased vocal fremitus, and sometimes a postive coin test (*bruit d'airain*), or Hamman's sign ('crunching' sound of air in the mediastinum).
  — CXR will confirm the clinical diagnosis.
- If the pneumothorax is expanding under tension the clinical signs are more dramatic, because mediastinal compression by the expanding mass decreases venous return, impairs ventricular function and reduces cardiac output.
  — Dyspnoea, tachypnoea and eventual cyanosis.
  — Tachycardia, hypotension and eventual cardiac arrest.
  — There may be tracheal deviation and subcutaneous emphysema.
  — Tension pneumothorax may be bilateral.

Diagnosis of pneumothorax in the anaesthetised patient

- Predisposing clinical conditions as above.
- Initial signs may be non-specific, with hypotension and tachycardia, others include:
  — Diminished unilateral chest movement, wheeze, hyperresonance, diminished breath sounds, increased airway pressure.

— Tracheal deviation.
— Elevated CVP (if being monitored).
— Cyanosis, arrythmias and circulatory collapse.
— If the diagnosis is suspected confirmation should never await CXR. It is a vital clinical diagnosis.

Management

- Discontinue N_2O and give O_2 100%.
- Decompression via needle thoracocentesis followed by definitive chest drain (iv cannulae are too small to provide continued decompression).
- Underwater seal drain. Air from the pneumothorax drains underwater via a submerged tube in a sealed bottle and is then vented to atmosphere. The depth of water is important: if it is too shallow air may be entrained back into the drainage tube, if it is too deep the pressure may be too great to blow off the pneumothorax gas. Typical depth is 3–5 cm.

Marking points: Pneumothorax may be a life-threatening complication. You must be able to give a good account of the clinical features and explain the practical details of its management. As in any of these questions which relate to patient safety, if your overall management is suboptimal and would lead to harm then you are likely to receive a '1'.

For what reasons may a central venous catheter be inserted? Describe the normal pressure waveform and outline the value of central venous pressure monitoring. List the factors that may decrease and increase central venous pressure.

CVP monitoring can only properly be interpreted if the basic underlying principles are understood. This question is a mixture of the clinical and the scientific which aims to test precisely that.

Introduction
Central venous catheters are used widely in anaesthesia and in intensive care, and although the commonest indication for their use is direct pressure monitoring, there are other indications which are outlined below.

Reasons for insertion
- Monitoring of central venous pressure.
- Insertion of pulmonary artery catheter.
- Access for haemofiltration.
- Transvenous pacing for conduction abnormalities.
- Infusion port for drugs that cannot be given peripherally (some inotropes).
- Infusion port for total parenteral nutrition.
- Infusion port for chemotherapy.
- Aspiration of air from right heart after venous air embolism.

The normal pressure waveform
- Comprises three upstrokes (the 'a', 'c' and 'v' waves) and two descents (the 'x' and 'y') that relate to the cardiac cycle.
- 'a' wave: due to increased atrial pressure as atrium contracts (occurs at end-diastole).
- 'x' (or 'x'') descent: is the fall in atrial pressure as atrium relaxes.
- 'c' wave: supervenes before full atrial relaxation and is due to the bulging of the closed tricuspid valve into the atrium at the start of isovolumetric right ventricular contraction.
- 'x' descent: a continuation of the 'x' descent (interrupted by the 'c' wave) and represents the pressure drop as the ventricle and valve 'screw' downwards at the end of systole.
- 'v' wave: is the increase in right atrial pressure as it is filled by the venous return against a closed tricuspid valve.
- 'y' descent: is the drop in pressure as the right ventricle relaxes, the tricuspid valve opens, and the atrium empties into the ventricle.
- Any event that alters the normal relationship between the events above, will alter the wave form morphology: in atrial fibrillation e.g. the 'a' wave is lost, in tricuspid incompetence there is a giant 'V' wave which replaces the 'c' wave, the 'x' descent and the 'v' wave.

Value of CVP monitoring
- CVP is the hydrostatic pressure generated by the blood within the right atrium (RA) or the great veins of the thorax.
- It provides an indication of volaemic status (the large veins of thorax, abdomen and proximal extremities form a large compliant reservoir for sizeable percentage of blood volume). This may be actual or effective hypovolaemia, in which a loss of venoconstrictor tone decreases venous return.
- It provides an indication of right ventricular (RV function. RV dysfunction is reflected in higher filling pressures to maintain the same stroke volume (SV).

- RA pressure reflects RV end diastolic pressure (RVEDP) and frequently this is assumed to reflect LVEDP. This is not true, even in health, because the normal RV function curve is steeper and to the left of the LV curve (it ejects into a lower pressure system). For a given fluid load the SV of each is identical but the pressure rise in LV is > RV because of shallower slope of curve. In presence of RV or LV impairment only a PA catheter can provide sufficiently accurate diagnostic information.
- The commonest application of CVP measurement is the assessment of volaemic status. A single reading is unhelpful: trends are more useful, particularly when combined with fluid challenges. CVP is said to fall during haemorrhage by ~0.7 cmH$_2$O for every 100 ml lost (meanwhile the arterial BP may remain unchanged).

Decreases in CVP
- Hypovolaemia.
- Effective hypovolaemia (vasodilatation).
- Dehydration.
- Artefact: transducer is raised inadvertently.

Increases in CVP
- Volume overload.
- Right ventricular failure.
- Pulmonary embolus.
- Cardiac tamponade.
- Tension pneumothorax.
- SVC obstruction (if catheter tip is proximal).
- Portal hypertension (IVC back pressure).
- Artefact: transducer is lowered inadvertently.

Marking points: There is probably information for more than one question here, although in a paper you could draw the waveform and save yourself time. In an oral you might be expected to explain it step by step, hence the format in which it is described above. You must understand why the CVP does not reflect LV function, and that it measures not only volaemic status but also RV function.

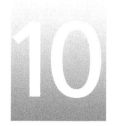

Anatomy, applied anatomy and regional anaesthesia

Describe the anatomy of the coeliac plexus. What are the indications for its therapeutic blockade?

This question comes as a surprise for many candidates, but the anatomy of the area is important and coeliac plexus block is very effective for malignant pain.

Introduction

The coeliac plexus is most commonly the target for anaesthetists who are treating malignant visceral pain. The anatomy may be described as follows:

- The coeliac plexus is the largest sympathetic plexus and lies anterior to the abdominal aorta where as a dense network of nerve fibres it surrounds the root of the coeliac artery at the level of L1 .
- There are two ganglia, right and left, which are closely related to the crura of the diaphragm.
- The plexus receives the greater splanchnic nerve (fibres from T5 to T9 or 10) and the lesser splanchnic nerve (fibres from T9/10 or T10/11).
- The plexus also receives some filaments from both the vagus and the phrenic nerves bilaterally.
- Superiorly lie the crura of the diaphragm; posteriorly is the abdominal aorta; laterally are the adrenal glands in the superior poles of left and right kidneys; the important anterior relation is the pancreas.
- **Therapeutic block.** The plexus can be blocked in conjunction with intercostal nerves in order to provide analgesia for intra-abdominal surgery. This technique does not have many enthusiasts. More commonly it is used for the relief of malignant pain, typically that due to carcinoma of the pancreas. Neurolytic blocks give good analgesia in up to 90% of patients, although the effect may only last for a number of months.
- **Non-malignant pain** such as chronic pancreatitis. Many clinicians are reluctant because of risks of paraplegia (1-2 per 1000 due to acute ischaemia at the watershed area of the cord), and limited duration of effect.
- **Diagnostic block.** Coeliac plexus block using local anaesthetic alone can be used for diagnostic purposes and for attempting to break a sympathetically mediated acute pain cycle.

Marking points: Anatomy questions are not all or nothing. If you omit some of the lesser details you will not fail, although your broad knowledge of the area must be sound. This is a specialised block of which you are unlikely to have direct experience and the marking is likely to acknowledge that your information will lack depth.

Describe the innervation of the larynx. What are the clinical consequences of damage to motor nerves?

The importance of this topic is self-evident, both in routine anaesthetic practice as well in areas of specialised neck surgery in which the recurrent laryngeal nerves may be vulnerable.

Introduction
Laryngeal reflexes which act to protect the integrity of the airway are as powerful as any in the body and are responsible for some of the more dramatic moments in anaesthetic practice. The sensory and motor innervation is outlined below.

Sensory innervation
- Innervation is via the vagus (10th cranial nerve) which divides into the superior and the recurrent laryngeal nerves. The superior branch divides into internal and external laryngeal nerves.
- The internal laryngeal nerve innervates the inferior surface of the epiglottis and the supraglottic region as far as the mucous membrane above the vocal folds.
- Below the vocal cords the sensory supply to the laryngeal mucosa is from the recurrent laryngeal nerve.

Motor innervation
- All the intrinsic muscles of the larynx (apart from the cricothyroid muscle which is supplied from the external branch of the superior laryngeal nerve) are supplied by the recurrent laryngeal nerves.
- The right recurrent laryngeal nerve leaves the vagus and loops beneath the subclavian artery to ascend to the larynx in the groove between oespophagus and trachea.
- The left recurrent laryngeal nerve passes beneath the arch of the aorta and again ascends in the groove between oesophagus and trachea.

Injuries to the laryngeal nerves
- The external branch of the superior laryngeal nerve supplies the cricothyroid muscle. This tenses the vocal cords. Damage will be followed by hoarseness. If it is unilateral this will be temporary (the other cricothyroid will compensate); if it is bilateral the hoarseness will be permanent.
- The recurrent laryngeal nerve supplies all those muscles which control the opening and closing of the laryngeal inlet.
- Partial paralysis affects the abductor muscles more than the adductors and so with unilateral injury the corresponding vocal cord is paralysed. This results in hoarseness.
- If both nerves are damaged then both cords oppose or even overlap each other in the midline. This leads to inspiratory stridor and has the potential to cause total obstruction.
- If one or both nerves are transected the vocal cord(s) adopt the cadaveric position in which they are partially abducted and through which airflow is much less compromised. Phonation, however, may be reduced to a whisper.

> **Marking points:** This is a straightforward and predictable question. Because this anatomical area is central to anaesthetic practice an accurate account will be expected.

Describe the arterial blood supply of the myocardium. What are the consequences of occlusion in the main parts of this arterial supply?

Coronary artery disease is common, and during every anaesthetic in which ECG monitoring is employed the perfusion of the myocardium is being monitored, albeit crudely. The anaesthetists' claim to be perioperative physicians is enhanced by knowledge of the functional anatomy of this important structure.

Introduction

Every anaesthetic which includes ECG monitoring is examining, albeit crudely, the state of myocardial oxygenation and, by extension, the state of the arterial supply whose anatomy is outlined below.

Anatomy

- The heart is supplied by the right and left coronary arteries: these originate from the ascending aorta (anterior and posterior aortic sinuses).
- The right coronary artery passes between the pulmonary trunk and the right atrial appendage to descend in the anterior atrioventricular groove.
- It gives off atrial and ventricular short branches to supply those structures.
- At the inferior border of the heart it effectively divides into the marginal branch which travels along the right ventricle towards the apex and the inferior interventricular artery which continues in the groove of the same name to anastomose with the circumflex artery (the corresponding branch of the left coronary artery). This anastomosis is variable.
- The left coronary artery is larger than the right, and after arising from the posterior aortic sinus, passes between the left atrial appendage and the pulmonary trunk.
- Divides shortly into the anterior interventricular (also known as left anterior descending) artery which passes down the interventricular groove giving off anterior ventricular branches, and into the circumflex artery which continues in the AV groove to anastomose with the inferior interventricular artery as above.

Consequences of occlusion

There are variations in the arterial supply to various areas of the myocardium, but in general the consequences of interruption to this supply can be summarised as follows:

- **Right main coronary or its branches.** Right ventricle, right atrium, part of the interventricular septum, sino-atrial node (in 65%), bundle of His, atrioventricular node (80%) and conducting system (80%) Also supplies a small diaphragmatic part of the left ventricle.
- **Left coronary artery or its branches.** Left ventricle , left atrium, part of the interventricular septum, sino-atrial node (in 35%), atrioventricular node (20%) and conducting system (20%).

> **Marking points:** There is overlap in distribution which means that it is impossible to attribute, for example, sino-atrial node dysfunction to right coronary ischaemia. These details are less important, therefore, than a broad knowledge of the basic anatomy.

Describe the anatomy of the nerves at the ankle which supply the foot. List the techniques that can be used to provide analgesia for surgery on the forefoot.

This is a question about ankle block. Details of this block are requested because it requires a more detailed answer than say for sciatic nerve block at the hip, which would be too short an answer for this paper.

Introduction
Forefoot surgery can be extremely painful and the ankle block is an effective means of providing prolonged analgesia. Its main disadvantage lies in the fact that five nerves need to be blocked before local anaesthesia is complete.

Anatomy of the nerves
- **Saphenous nerve.** This supplies a variable portion of the medial border of the foot and ankle. It is a terminal branch of the femoral nerve and is anaesthetised immediately anterior to the medial malleolus where it lies superficially, close to the saphenous vein.
- **Posterior tibial nerve.** This supplies the plantar surface of the foot. This is a branch of the sciatic nerve (which divides into tibial and common peroneal branches in the popliteal fossa) and is blocked behind the medial malleolus where it lies posterior to the posterior tibial artery.
- **Deep peroneal nerve.** Supplies only a small area of skin on the dorsum of the foot between first and second toes. It passes beneath the extensor retinaculum at the front of the ankle joint and is most readily blocked between the tendons of extensor hallucis and extensor digitorum longus where it lies lateral to the dorsalis pedis artery.
- **Sural nerve.** Supplies sensation to the fifth toe and the lateral border of the foot. It is a branch of the tibial nerve: at the level of the ankle it lies superficially behind the lateral malleolus.
- **Superficial peroneal nerve.** Supplies much of the dorsum of the foot (excepting the small area supplied by the deep peroneal and the lateral foot supplied by the sural nerve). It is a branch of the common peroneal nerve which further divides into terminal branches at the level of the malleoli. It is blocked with a wide ring of superficial infiltration between medial and lateral malleoli.

Local anaesthesia for the forefoot
- Possible techniques include:
  — Subarachnoid block.
  — Lumbar extradural block.
  — Sacral extradural block.
  — Sciatic nerve block at the hip.
  — Sciatic nerve block in the popliteal fossa.
  — Tibial nerve block in the popliteal fossa and common peroneal nerve block.
  — Ankle block.
  — Intraosseous nerve bock (for distal foot procedures).
  — Local infiltration.

Marking points: Foot surgery is common and its postoperative pain is underestimated. The ankle block is a predictable question about applied anatomy, while the list of possible techniques allows you to demonstrate that you are aware of the several other options which anaesthetists may favour.

Anatomy, applied anatomy and regional anaesthesia

Describe the anatomy of the femoral nerve relevant for the performance of a femoral nerve block. What is a 'three-in-one' block and for what may it be used?

It is common for anaesthetists to assume that the femoral nerve is a straightforward block to perform and that the 'three-in-one' block provides useful analgesia for hip surgery. Neither is true: the anatomy of the femoral nerve is quite complex and can be variable, and the benefits of 'three-in-one' block are unreliable. The question seeks an informed account which demonstrates that you understand this.

Introduction
The variable anatomy of the femoral nerve in the groin can make it difficult to perform a nerve block successfully if the practitioner relies on anatomical landmarks alone. Success rates are much higher if the nerve is located with a peripheral nerve stimulator, but their effective use still depends upon anatomical knowledge about the femoral nerve, relevant aspects of which are described below.

Anatomy
- The femoral nerve originates from the anterior primary rami of L2, L3 and L4 and enters the anterior thigh beneath the inguinal ligament.
- The femoral sheath is formed from an extension of the extraperitoneal fascia and contains the femoral vein (medially) and artery (laterally). It does not contain the femoral nerve.
- The nerve is invested in the fascia of the iliacus muscle (fascia iliacus) which separates it from the femoral sheath. Above this is the fascia of tensor fascia lata.
- The distance by which it is separated is variable. It may bear a close relation to the pulsation of the femoral artery or may be 1–2 cm or even more lateral to it. It can also be separated from the femoral sheath by a small part of the psoas muscle.
- The nerve usually starts to divide into its terminal branches at the base of the femoral triangle. In some subjects this division can start above the inguinal ligament.

'Three-in-one' block
- A 'three-in-one' block is the name given to a single injection which aims to block the femoral nerve, the obturator nerve and the lateral cutaneous nerve of the thigh.
- It is performed at the same site as that used for a femoral nerve block, but with two main differences: a larger volume of local anaesthetic solution is used (commonly 25–30 ml), and during injection firm distal pressure is applied.
- The larger volume and the pressure aim to spread the local anaesthetic rostrally back up into the psoas compartment so that all three nerves are blocked.
- The femoral nerve supplies the shaft of the femur, and the muscle and skin of the anterior part of the thigh.
- The obturator nerve supplies the adductor muscles of the hip, part of the hip joint, skin on the medial side of the thigh and part of the knee joint.
- The lateral cutaneous nerve supplies skin over the anterolateral thigh as far as the knee, and the lateral thigh from about the greater trochanter down to mid-thigh level.
- The block is performed commonly to provide perioperative analgesia following surgery on the hip. It occasionally seems to be effective, but as the anatomy demonstrates, in most cases this nerve block will not provide reliable analgesia for cutaneous sensation above the level of the greater trochanter, which is where many incisions for hip surgery are made. For this reason some anaesthetists describe it as 'block in search of an operation'.

> **Marking points:** The question expects you to demonstrate that via a knowledge of anatomy you appreciate the potential difficulties in femoral nerve block, and can explain the shortcomings of the 'three-in-1' block by reference to the areas which those nerves innervate.

Describe, with reference to the anatomical landmarks, the different approaches which are used commonly for local anaesthetic block of the sciatic nerve. Why is this block performed?

The sciatic nerve is the largest peripheral nerve in the body and it is accessible from a number of sites. For this reason, if no other, it makes an appropriate question in applied anatomy. It will help the credibility of your answer if you can convince the examiner that you have some experience in the performance of some of these blocks, by stressing, for example, the importance of always using a peripheral nerve stimulator.

Introduction
The sciatic nerve is the largest peripheral nerve in the body and is accessible from a number of different sites. As it supplies much of the lower leg it is a versatile nerve block which can be used to provide prolonged analgesia for a range of surgical procedures.

Approaches to the sciatic nerve

Posterior
- Patient lies supine position with upper leg flexed to 90° at hip and knee.
- A line is drawn from the greater trochanter to the ischial tuberosity. The nerve can be located just medial to the mid-point of this line at a depth of ~6 cm.

Posterior (classic approach of Labat)
- Patient lies in decubitus position with upper leg flexed to 90° at hip and knee.
- A line is drawn from the greater trochanter to the posterior superior iliac spine. From the mid-point of this line a perpendicular is dropped 3-5 cm. Insert the needle vertical to the skin and seek the nerve at ~6-8 cm.
- Alternatively a line can be drawn from the greater trochanter to the sacral hiatus and the injection made at its mid-point.

Anterior
- The nerve emerges from the greater sciatic foramen and lies between the ischial tuberosity and the greater trochanter of the femur. Before it passes down behind the femur it is accessible medial to the femur and just below the lesser trochanter.
- Patient lies supine and a line is drawn from the anterior superior iliac spine to the pubic tubercle.
- A line parallel is drawn from the greater trochanter.
- At the junction of the medial third and lateral two-thirds of the upper line a perpendicular is dropped to meet the lower.
- At this junction a long (150 mm) needle is inserted vertical to the skin until it contacts the medial shaft of femur. It is then redirected medially to slide off the femur before advancing another 5 cm or so to encounter the nerve in the region of the lesser trochanter.
- It is worth noting that in a proportion of patients the sciatic nerve lies immediately posterior to the femur at this point and is inaccessible to the anterior approach.

Lateral
- The patient lies supine. A long needle is inserted 3 cm distal to the most prominent part of the greater trochanter and seeks the nerve as it descends behind the femur.

Popliteal fossa block

- The sciatic nerve can be blocked in the popliteal fossa before it divides into its tibial and common peroneal branches.
- Patient lies lateral or prone and the proximal flexor skin crease of the knee is identified.
- A line is drawn vertically for about 7 cm from the mid-point of the skin crease.
- The injection is made ~1 cm lateral to this point.

Reasons for blockade

- The sciatic nerve provides a sensory supply to much of the lower leg via its main terminal branches, the tibial and the common peroneal nerves.
- It supplies the knee joint (via articular branches), and almost all of the structures below the knee.
- It does not supply a variable, but extensive cutaneous area over the medial side of the knee, lower leg and ankle, and medial side of the foot around the medial malleolus. This is supplied by the saphenous nerve (from the femoral).
- Sciatic nerve block alone will provide reliable analgesia for surgical procedures which involve the forefoot, the sole of the foot and the lateral side of the foot and ankle.
- In conjunction with femoral and with obturator nerve block it provides good analgesia for major knee surgery.

Marking points: Sciatic nerve block is very useful in orthopaedic surgery and the variety of approaches allows you to demonstrate your grasp of applied anatomy. It is likely that you are more familiar with, and experienced in, one or two approaches rather than the entire range. If you give some credible sense that you can perform these safely and accurately you will not be penalised too heavily for a less detailed knowledge of the others.

Describe how the main nerves which innervate the upper limb are formed from the brachial plexus. List the common approaches to local anaesthetic block of the plexus together with the main indications for their use.

An understanding of the anatomy of the brachial plexus is the key to successful regional anaesthesia of the upper limb. The anatomy is detailed, but is not so complex that it cannot be incorporated into a short answer question. It is a clinically important area of anatomy and is asked frequently.

Introduction
The accessibility of the brachial plexus at various sites ensures that, in theory at least, it is possible to perform all surgery on the upper limb under regional anaesthesia. Athough this is not always practical, it is frequently desirable to provide good peri-operative analgesia of long duration, and for this brachial plexus block excels.

Anatomy
- The plexus forms in the neck from the anterior primary rami of C5, C6, 7, C8 and T1.
- These five roots merge in the posterior triangle of the neck to form three trunks.
- C5 and C6 form the upper, and C7 the middle trunk (above the subclavian artery). C8 and T1 form the lower trunk (posterior to the subclavian artery).
- At the lateral border of the first rib the three trunks each divide into anterior and posterior divisions.
- The three posterior divisions form the posterior cord (described according to its relationship with the axillary artery) from which derives the radial nerve. (Also the axillary, thoracodorsal and upper and lower subscapular nerves.)
- The anterior divisions of upper and middle trunks form the lateral cord from which derive the median nerve (lateral head) and the musculocutaneous nerve. (Also the lateral pectoral nerve.)
- The anterior division of the lower trunk continues as the medial cord from which derive the ulnar nerve and the median nerve (medial head). (Also the medial cutaneous nerves of arm and forearm and the medial pectoral nerve.)

Approaches to the brachial plexus
- Interscalene
  — This block is particularly useful for shoulder surgery. It can be used to provide analgesia for more distal structures in the upper limb, but the ulnar nerve is frequently spared.
- Supraclavicular
  — This block provides reliable analgesia for most of the upper limb. It can be used for shoulder surgery, although the interscalene approach is usually preferred.
- Subclavian perivascular (several variations have been described)
  — Provides analgesia similar to that offered by the supraclavicular approach.
- Axillary
  — Provides good analgesia for surgery below the elbow. The musculocutaneous nerve may be spared, in which event supplemental analgesia may be needed by blocking the nerve between brachioradialis and the lateral epicondyle at the elbow.

Marking points: The key to good analgesia of the upper limb is an adequate knowledge of the brachial plexus. Anatomical minutiae are not required but this is a question about the applied anatomy of an important area, and you should convince the examiner that you would be able to produce a successful block.

Describe the anatomy of the internal jugular vein. List the complications of cannulation of this vessel and outline how each may be avoided.

This is an important structure in the practice of anaesthesia and intensive care medicine and an ability to cannulate the internal jugular vein is a core skill.

Introduction
The accessibility of the vessel and a complication rate that is lower than with many other approaches makes the internal jugular vein (usually the right) the site of choice for central venous cannulation for many anaesthetists.

Anatomy
- The internal jugular vein originates at the jugular foramen in the skull (which drains the sigmoid sinus).
- It follows a relatively straight course in the neck to terminate behind the sternoclavicular joint where it joins the subclavian vein.
- It lies together with the carotid artery and the vagus nerve within the carotid sheath throughout its course but changes its position in relation to the artery. Initially it lies posteriorly before moving laterally and then anterolaterally.
- It is superficial in the upper part of the neck before descending deep to sternocleidomastoid. In the neck the structures through which a cannulating needle passes are skin and subcutaneous tissue, the platysma muscle, sternocleidomastoid (lower neck) and the loose fascia of the caroid sheath.
- Anterior to the vein at the top of its course lie: internal carotid artery and vagus nerve.
- Posterior to the vein are (from above downwards): lateral part of C1, prevertebral fascia and vertebral muscles, cervical transverse processes, the sympathetic chain, and at the root of the neck, the dome of the pleura. On the left side it lies anterior to the thoracic duct.
- Medial to the vein are: carotid arteries (internal and common), cranial nerves IX, X, XI and XII.

Complications
Many of these can be avoided by the use of a needle which is guided by ultrasound.
- **Pneumothorax (and haemothorax)**
  — Risk is minimised by using a high approach which avoids the dome of the pleura.
- **Intrapleural placement**
  — Risk is minimised by using a high approach which avoids the dome of the pleura.
  — CXR will prevent inadvertent intrapleural infusion.
- **Air embolism**
  — Position patient head down during insertion.
- **Cardiac arrhythmias**
  — May occur if the guidewire or catheter is inserted as far as the heart.
- **Carotid artery puncture or cannulation**
  — Continue to palpate the artery medially throughout cannulation. Use ultrasound-guided needle.
- **Thoracic duct injury (chylothorax)**
  — Risk is minimised by using a high approach and by avoiding the left internal jugular.
- **Infection**
  — Central line infection can be disastrous. Avoid by aseptic technique and meticulous aftercare.

Marking points: Internal jugular cannulation is a core skill and your answer must demonstrate your knowledge of the major landmarks, and how your application of that knowledge allows you to minimise the risk of the listed complications.

Prior to subarachnoid or extradural block what landmarks are guides to the vertebral level? What are the main determinants of block height following subarachnoid injection of local anaesthetic solution?

This is a straightforward question relating to the practical anatomy and relevant pharmacology of an important anesthetic procedure. You cannot perform spinals safely or effectively unless you are able to answer these main points accurately.

Introduction
The spinal cord in the adult ends at the level of the intervertebral disc at L1/L2. There is some variation and in up to 10% the cord may end as high as T12/L1 or as low as L2/L3. (In the neonate the cord ends at the lower border of L3.)

Surface anatomy
- A line drawn between the highest points of the iliac crests (the intercristal or Touffier's line) passes across either the spinous process of L4 or the L4/L5 interspace.
- The lowest rib (palpable only in very thin subjects) is at the level of T12.
- The first spinous process which is clearly palpable is C7, the vertebra prominens (although T1 below it is actually more prominent still).
- The inferior angle of the scapula in the neutral position is at the level of T7 or T8.

Determinants of block height: significant factors
- **Drug dose**
  - The greater the mass of drug the higher and more prolonged the block. Probably the most important factor.
  - Volume is of minimal importance. Bupivacaine 15 mg in 15 mg ml (0.1%) achieves the same block height as bupivacaine 15 mg in 3 mg ml (0.5%).
- **Level of injection**
  - In the supine patient with a normal spine the maximum height of the lumbar lordosis is at L2/L3. Less local anaesthetic will move rostrally if the injection is made below that level.
- **Baricity of drug**
  - Plain solutions of local anaesthetic are isobaric relative to CSF at room temperature (CSF specific density 1.0003).
  - At body temperature they become slightly hypobaric.
  - Hyperbaric ('heavy') solutions are made so by the addition of glucose ('Heavy' bupivacaine contains glucose 8%).
  - In the supine patient with a normal spine hyperbaric solutions tend to pool in the thoracic kyphosis at T5/6, and produce blocks which generally are higher but more predictable than those produced by isobaric solutions.
- **Patient position**
  - Is linked to 'baricity' above: if the patient is in the decubitus position the curves of the spine have no influence.
  - Trendelenburg positioning will increase the rostral spread of a hyperbaric solution.
- **Patient height**
  - There may be reduced cephalad spread in taller subjects: the relationship is not reliable enough to allow any prediction.
- **Patient age**
  - There may be increased cephalad spread with advancing age, although again the block height cannot reliably be predicted.
- **Pregnancy (and multiple pregnancy)**
  - Term pregnancy is said to be associated with greater block height, which is

made higher still with multiple pregnancy. Mechanism may relate to relative smaller volume of dural sheath because of encroachment by engorged venous plexus.

- **Needle direction and speed of injection**
  — Rostral facing injection or forceful injection shortens the onset time but does not influence the final height of block.
- **Barbotage, weight of patient, gender of patient, adjuvant drugs, vasoconstrictors**
  — None has any significant effect on block height.

Marking points: Every individual taking this examination will have performed spinal anaesthesia, at least in obstetric practice. Unsound practice based on ignorance of the main points described above could potentially cause a patient grave harm. The answer will be marked accordingly.

Describe the anatomy of the sacrum. What are the clinical differences between sacral extradural (caudal) block in adults and in children?

The sacrum ('sacred bone') was believed by the ancients to be the site of the soul, the bone which was the last to decompose, and thus the one around which the new body would form. Attitudes are now less exalted. Caudal anaesthesia is a popular technique, particularly in children in whom it can provide analgesia similar to that provided by a low lumbar epidural. In contrast to other neuraxial blocks it requires no equipment other than a needle, syringe and/or intravenous cannula, and is simple to perform. This has been known to engender an inappropriately casual approach which belies the potential complications. This is another core area of anatomy.

Introduction

The anatomy of the sacrum can vary, and this normal variation is frequently (and probably unfairly) blamed for failures of caudal anaesthesia. The variation is largely confined to the dorsal wall and the typical anatomy can be described as follows.

- The sacrum is a triangular bone that articulates superiorly with the fifth lumbar vertebra, inferiorly with the coccyx and laterally with the ilia.
- The dorsal roof comprises the fused laminae of the five sacral vertebrae and is convex dorsally (the curve is variable between sexes and races).
- In the midline there is a median crest which represent the sacral spinous processes.
- Lateral to this is the intermediate sacral crest with a row of four tubercles which represent the articular processes. The S5 processes are remnants only and form the cornua which are the main landmarks for identifying the sacral hiatus.
- Along the lateral border are anterior and posterior foramina which are the sacral equivalent of intervertebral foramina of higher levels and through which the sacral nerve roots pass.
- Access to the canal is via the sacral hiatus at the level of the fifth sacral vertebra which represents a failure of development of the spinous process and the lamina. It is covered by the sacro-coccygeal membrane. In up to 7% of subjects fusion has taken place and so access is impossible. (Some authorities believe this to be an overestimate.)
- In addition to the dura superiorly the canal contains areolar connective tissue, fat, the sacral nerves, lymphatics, the filum terminale and a rich venous plexus.

Differences between adults and children

Anatomy

- The dura usually ends at the level of S2 in adults (although it can descend to within ~5 cm of the hiatus in some subjects). At birth the dura is as low as S4, but by ~2 years of age it ascends to adult levels.
- The sacral hiatus is easier to locate in children because it is not overlaid by the sacral fat pad that develops in adults.

Spread of solution

- Influenced in adults by total volume, speed of injection and posture (higher levels are reached if patient is 15° head up.
- There is good correlation in children between spread of a given dose and age. There is poor correlation between spread and weight and/or height.
- The sacral extradural space offers lower resistance to longitudinal spread than the adult. Epidural fat in children has a loose and wide-meshed texture, whereas in adults it becomes more densely packed and fibrous. There is less fibrous connective tissue per se in the sacral epidural space than in adults and the

combination of facts means that local anaesthetic spread is greater.

- In children it is possible to direct a 20 g 51 mm cannula directed rostrally to escape the sacral space altogether and allow what is in effect a lower lumbar epidural block. Generous volumes can be employed, therefore, if a high block is required. High blocks are much more difficult to achieve in adults.
- Complications such as intrathecal injection are more likely in children less than 2 years of age, otherwise the incidence of this and intravascular injection do not differ from those in adults.

Pharmacology

- Children up to and beyond the age of 6 years show cardiovascular stability in the face of blocks that would cause sympathetic blockade and hypotension in adults. This is probably due to some delay in maturation of the autonomic nervous system.

Marking points: If you wish to start your answer with an etymological flourish then you will certainly gain the examiner's attention, but it is not necessary. What is necessary is that you demonstrate very clearly knowledge of the core anatomy and the important reasons why caudals may behave differently in children and in adults.

Describe the anatomy of the epidural space at the level of the fourth lumbar vertebra. What are the main complications of extradural analgesia?

The increasing popularity of extradural analgesia for many types of surgery as well as for the pain of labour makes this a key subject for anaesthetists. Detailed knowledge will be expected.

Introduction

Interest in good analgesia and accelerated discharge after major surgery means that in some hospitals as many extradural catheters are provided for postoperative pain relief as for pain in labour. The technique is increasingly popular despite a long list of reported complications.

Anatomy

- The extradural (epidural) space is the area surrounding the dural sheath as it lies within the vertebral canal.
- It is traversed by the dural sheath (thickness in the lumbar region ~0.3–0.5 mm) comprising the membranes of the dura and arachnoid maters, the subarachnoid space containing CSF, the spinal nerves of the cauda equina and the filum terminale.
- Anteriorly the space is bounded by the body of the vertebra and the intervertebral disc, over which lies the posterior longitudinal ligament.
- Laterally it is bounded by the pedicles and the intervertebral foramina.
- Posteriorly it is bounded by the laminae of the neural arch.
- Ligamenta flava. There are two which meet in the midline and which connect the laminae of adjacent vertebrae. Each extends from the lower part of the anterior surface of the lamina above to the posterior surface of and upper margin of the lamina below. Their fibres run in a perpendicular direction, but when viewed in the sagittal plane the ligaments are triangular in shape with the apex of the triangle formed at the upper lamina.
- At the level of L4 the space contains the spinal nerves, each invested with a cuff of dura, loosely packed fat, areolar connective tissue, lymphatics and blood vessels, which include the rich valveless vertebral venous plexus of Batson.
- The depth of the posterior epidural space (between ligamenta flava and dura) is ~0.5 cm in the lumbar region. The greatest depth is at the L2 interspace in males, in whom it is ~6 mm.

Complications

Associated with the procedure

- Inadvertent dural puncture and subsequent postdural puncture headache (0.5%).
- Intravascular injection.
- Retained catheter or needle fragment.
- Inadvertent subdural block (may be as high as 0.1%).
- Failure (~1%).
- Unilateral or patchy block (~5–10%).
- Neurological sequelae (usually minor: 1 in 10 000).
- Epidural haematoma.
- Backache: local trauma but no evidence of sustained problem.

Associated with drugs that are injected

- Hypotension: due to limited sympathectomy (less with low dose/opioid mixtures).
- Total spinal or high spinal block.
- Systemic toxicity of local anaesthetic.

- Urinary retention.
- Pruritus, nausea, vomiting associated with extradural opioid.
- Respiratory depression: very unusual in puerperium.
- Injection of the wrong solution: many substances have been reported, including thiopental.
- Influence on labour and labour outcome: contentious, no firm supportive evidence.

Marking points: This is a very important area of anaesthetic practice and you will be expected to demonstrate a good three-dimensional grasp of the anatomy as well as being aware of all the material complications.

Describe the anatomy of the stellate ganglion and outline how you would perform a block. What are the indications for stellate ganglion block? List the main complications.

Stellate ganglion block is a common procedure in the chronic pain clinic, is simple to perform, and has significant potential complications. It is one of several procedures in the neck undertaken by anaesthetists (others include interscalene block, deep cervical plexus block and internal jugular cannulation) and this is an anatomical area with which you should be familiar.

Introduction
The evidence base for the therapeutic use of stellate ganglion blocks is not strong, but the technique is simple and it is a common chronic pain procedure. It also has significant potential complications which can be minimised by an understanding of the anatomy.

Anatomy
- The cervical sympathetic chain lies either side of the vertebral column in the fascial space: posterior is the fascia over prevertebral muscles, anterior is the carotid sheath.
- The area where the inferior cervical and the first thoracic ganglia meet either in close proximity or fusion is referred to as the stellate ganglion.
- It extends from the neck of the first rib where its lower part is covered anteriorly by the dome of the pleura to the transverse process of C7 where anterior lies the vertebral artery. By the level of C6 the vertebral artery has moved posteriorly into the foramen transversarium pending its ascent into the skull.
- Much of the sympathetic nerve supply to the head and neck as well as to the upper extremity synapses in or near the stellate ganglion.
- Sympathetic preganglionic fibres leave the cord from segments as widely separated as T1–T6 and although many converge in or around the stellate ganglion, some may bypass it.
- Hence large volumes may be needed to fill the space in front of the prevertebral fascia down to T4, but will produce reliable sympathetic blockade of head, neck and upper limb. It is more accurately described as a 'cervicothoracic block'.

Technique
There are two approaches that are commonly described: the anterior (sometimes called the 'paratracheal' anterior) approach, and the paratracheal.

Anterior
- The trachea and carotid pulse are gently retracted to allow identification of the most prominent cervical transverse process (the Chassaignac tubercle) at C6, the level of the cricoid cartilage.
- A lower approach to the ganglion's actual location at C7 risks both pneumothorax and vertebral artery puncture.
- The carotid sheath is moved laterally and the trachea medially before a 25–30 mm × 23–25G needle is directed perpendicularly down on to the tubercle.
- Once it has encountered bone the needle is withdrawn 4-5 mm. If this is not done there is a higher incidence of upper limb somatic blockade.
- Local anaesthetic in low concentration and high volume is injected (e.g. lidocaine (lignocaine) 0.5% or bupivacaine 0.125% × 15–20 ml).

Paratracheal
- Needle insertion is two finger-breadths lateral to the suprasternal notch and two finger-breadths superior to the clavicle. This identifies the transverse process of C7, immediately below Chassaignac's tubercle at C6, at the level of the cricoid cartilage.

- The sternocleidomastoid and carotid sheath are moved laterally before the needle is directed perpendicularly down on to the transverse process.
- Once it has encountered bone the needle is withdrawn 0.5–1.0 cm.
- Local anaesthetic in low concentration and high volume is injected (e.g. lidocaine 0.5% or bupivacaine 0.125% × 15–20 ml).
- This lower approach to the ganglion's actual location at C7 risks both pneumothorax and vertebral artery puncture.

Indications
- Indications for the block include any condition requiring sympathetic block of the head, neck and upper limb. These include:
  - **Neuropathic pain conditions:** Complex Regional Pain Syndromes Types I and II, post-herpetic neuralgia of head and neck, shoulder-hand syndrome (following CVA or ischaemia), phantom limb pain, pain associated with upper limb denervation.
  - **Ischaemic conditions:** thrombosis or microembolism, inadvertent intra-arterial injection, vasospastic disorders (e.g. Raynaud's), scleroderma, frostbite.
  - **Angina pectoris:** severe refractory chest pain due to coronary ischaemia.
  - **Miscellaneous:** hyperhidrosis and pain associated with Paget's disease of bone.

Complications
- Local trauma and haematoma (may compress airway if severe).
- Recurrent laryngeal nerve block – causes hoarseness.
- Brachial plexus block – via the anterior approach only a layer of fascia separates the plexus and the ganglion which is anterior to it.
- Carotid or vertebral arterial puncture +/– injection.
- Intrathecal injection.
- Pneumothorax (if approach is too low).
- Deep cervical plexus block (if approach is too high).

Marking points: A smaller list than the above of indications and the main complications will be enough, but knowledge of anatomy sufficient to allow the safe performance of the block will be expected. Describe one technique only, but justify it.

Describe how you would perform an interscalene block. What are the main indications and advantages? What are its disadvantages and specific complications?

Interscalene block is the only one of the three very useful approaches to the brachial plexus (the others being the supraclavicular and the axillary) which provides dense and reliable anaesthesia for shoulder surgery. The block is performed in an anatomical region that is full of significant structures and has the potential for more dramatic side effects than the others. It is therefore an area that you are expected to know.

Introduction

Interscalene local anaesthesia blocks the anterior primary rami of the nerves of C5, C6, 7, C8 and T1, before they merge in the posterior triangle to form the trunks of the brachial plexus.

Interscalene block

- The cervical nerves leave the intervertebral foramina and pass caudad and laterally between the scalenus anterior and the scalenus medius muscles. They are enclosed within a fascial compartment composed of the posterior fascia of the anterior scalene muscle, and the anterior fascia of the middle scalene muscle.
- The patient should be supine with the head turned slightly away from the side of injection and the arm by the side (gently pulled down if necessary to depress the shoulder).
- After requisite skin cleansing and draping, the interscalene groove between scalenus anterior and medius should be identified at the level of the cricoid cartilage C6.
- If the awake patient is asked to lift the head off the pillow (which tenses the sternocleidomastoid muscles) or to give a sniff, the groove becomes more evident. In the anaesthetised patient identification is helped by the fact that in >90% of subjects the external jugular vein overlies the groove at this level.
- The groove and the roots beyond are superficial and in most cases a stimulating needle no longer than 30 mm is needed. The needle should be held perpendicular to the skin in all planes as it is directed medial, posterior and caudad (inwards, backwards and downwards) towards the transverse process of C6 (Chaisssaignac's tubercle).
- Once muscle stimulation is apparent in the required distribution (usually shoulder movements mediated by C5,6) 20–30 ml of solution may be injected after aspiration and with all due precautions. In common with most plexus blocks into fascial compartments, large volumes of appropriately dilute solutions may be needed to obtain adequate analgesia of all the nerves involved.

Indications

- Interscalene block provides dense and reliable analgesia particularly of the upper roots of the brachial plexus, and there is usually some upwards spread to include the cervical plexus (C2,3,4), and so it is useful for all surgery on the shoulder (including shoulder replacement), and for procedures involving the upper arm.

Advantages

- The arm does not have to be moved before the block is performed (is therefore suitable following trauma.)
- Landmarks are consistent and are more readily appreciated in obese patients than they may be for other approaches.
- Pneumothorax risk is small compared with the supraclavicular approach (which can be used for upper arm and shoulder surgery).

Disadvantages

- Has several potential major complications that are not associated with other approaches.
- Does not provide reliable block of C8 and T1 and so ulnar sparing is frequent (some quote 30–40%).
- Blocks the phrenic nerve and so should be used cautiously in those with respiratory disease, and never bilaterally.

Specific complications

There are many important anatomical structures in the root of the neck, and the block in addition carries all of the complications associated with a paravertebral technique.

- Inadvertent extradural or intrathecal anaesthesia (total spinal) injection.
- Intra-arterial injection (vertebral artery).
- Phrenic nerve block. The phrenic nerve lies on scalenus anterior and is almost invariably affected by successful interscalene block.
- Vagal and recurrent laryngeal nerve block. May cause hoarseness of voice, but is usually a benign complication.
- Horner's syndrome is common, but this is innocuous, although the patient should be warned.
- Pneumothorax (risk is low with a high approach).
- Failure.

Marking points: This question requires a lot of information, much of which can be presented in list form. The important points are to emphasise the specific indications and to identify the specific (and not the generic) complications of the block.

A patient requires open reduction and internal fixation (ORIF) of a fractured radius and ulna, but refuses general anaesthesia. Compare the local anaesthetic blocks that might be considered suitable for this procedure.

This question tests your knowledge of the applied anatomy of the upper limb. This situation does arise and you need confidence in the technique that you choose. None is ideal and you should offer strategies for coping with partial failure.

Introduction
The forearm is innervated by nerves which originate from all three cords of the brachial plexus, and because an ORIF of radius and ulna involves both aspects of the forearm, effective anaesthesia requires moderately extensive block. The application of an upper arm tourniquet in awake patients may also require sensory block.

Innervation
- Surgery is likely to involve nerves which include:
  — Radial nerve (from the posterior cord).
  — Musculocutaneous (from the lateral cord).
  — Medial cutaneous nerve of the forearm (from the medial cord).
  — Ulnar nerve (from the medial cord).
- An arterial tourniquet may be tolerated for 30 minutes or so, beyond which time many patients find it unacceptable. Analgesia is provided by block of the:
  — Axillary nerve (posterior cord).
  — Medial cutaneous nerve of the arm (medial cord).
  — Intercostobrachial branches (from T2).

Regional anaesthetic options
- **Intravenous regional anaesthesia (Bier's block)**
  — Technically simple to perform with minimal complications.
  — Unlikely to provide anaesthesia dense enough for this type of surgery.
  — Exsanguination of affected limb using Esmarch bandage or air exsanguinator is likely to be very painful.
- **Interscalene brachial plexus block**
  — Can be performed without moving the damaged arm.
  — Some potentially serious complications: particularly central neuraxial spread and intra-arterial injection.
  — May not provide adequate analgesia in the ulnar distribution, even with the use of large volumes of local anaesthetic solution.
- **Supraclavicular brachial plexus block**
  — Can be performed without moving the damaged arm.
  — Risk of pneumothorax is ~1%, and onset is often delayed by up to 24 hours.
  — Provides the most reliable analgesia for all the nerves in the hand and forearm.
- **Infraclavicular and subclavian perivascular brachial plexus blocks**
  — Can be performed without moving the damaged arm.
  — Lower risk of pleural trauma.
  — Provides similar analgesia as the supraclavicular approach.
  — Neither are practised nor taught widely in the UK.
- **Axillary brachial plexus block**
  — Requires abduction of the damaged arm.
  — Lower risk of significant complications (apart from intravascular injection).
  — May not provide adequate analgesia in the distribution of the musculocutaneous (lateral cutaneous nerve of the forearm) nerve, which can leave the sheath high in the axilla. This nerve can be blocked with a

supplemental injection between brachioradialis and the lateral epicondyle at the elbow.

- **Mid-humeral block**
  — Requires abduction of the damaged arm.
  — In this approach the radial, median and ulnar nerves are blocked individually at the level of the humerus before they pass down into the forearm.
  — Minimal complication risk.
  — Provides good analgesia, but attempted block of two or three nerves increases the likely failure rate and the blocks are technically more difficult than some of the other approaches.
  — Not widely used nor taught in the UK.
- **Local infiltration**
  — Inadequate for this type of surgery.
  — May be useful as supplementation should the definitive block be suboptimal.

Marking points: Nerve blockade sufficient to allow surgery under local anaesthesia alone (as opposed to using it for postoperative analgesia) requires accurate knowledge of the innervation of the relevant areas and understanding of the potential deficiencies of the various blocks. In this type of question it always helps if your answer can convey some sense that you have clinical experience of the procedures that you are discussing.

What are the advantages of subarachnoid (spinal) anaesthesia compared with general anaesthesia? Outline the contraindications and list the main complications.

Spinal anaesthesia has become the technique of choice for elective caesarean section and its popularity for other forms of surgery is once more increasing after many years during which concerns about neurological sequelae and other complications restricted its use. Its use in obstetric anaesthesia alone makes this a core topic and apprehensive mothers frequently use lay language to ask the very questions above. You should be able to give them an informed and comprehensive answer.

Introduction

Many years of disuse followed the famous Woolley and Roe cases, in which two men were paralysed after spinal anaesthesia, but subarachnoid block is now undergoing resurgence, particularly in obstetric anaesthesia, to the point at which it has become a core skill. It is not uncommon for patients and even surgical colleagues to seek justification of the technique, the advantages of which may be summarised as follows.

Advantages compared with general anaesthesia

- Avoidance of the generic potential problems of GA: polypharmacy (a caesarean section e.g. will require up to eight different drugs); intubation problems; IPPV risks.
- Statistically is a safer form of anaesthesia (which is not the same as claiming it to be safer in the high risk patient, which it is not).
- Reduction in risk of venous thromboembolism (by up to ~50% in some orthopaedic procedures).
- Technique of choice in obstetric operative delivery: no drug load to fetus, no maternal loss of contact with the baby, earlier establishment of breastfeeding, earlier mobilisation, decreased thromboembolic risk.
- Decreased blood loss. Contentious. Measured over days the blood loss following hip arthroplasty e.g. may be the same as after a GA. Intraoperative blood loss is reduced by 20–30% (orthopaedic data).
- Stress response to anaesthesia and surgery is deferred by subarachnoid block, but it is not abolished.
- Mortality and serious non-fatal morbidity. A large meta-analysis which examined trials of regional (spinal and epidural) versus general anaesthesia concluded that mortality and much serious non-fatal morbidity was significantly reduced in the groups allocated to receive RA. (CORTRA 1999).

Contraindications

- **Absolute**
  - Patient refusal.
  - Disseminated intravascular coagulation.
  - Profound hypovolaemia.
  - Raised intracranial pressure.
  - Severe fixed cardiac output state.
  - Bowel obstruction or perforation (contraction due to unopposed parasympathetic activity may increase intraperitoneal soiling).
  - Local sepsis.
- **Relative (require assessment of the risk : benefit ratio)**
  - Anticoagulation.
  - Chronic respiratory disease (loss of intercostal function and dyspnoea when flat).
  - Severe spinal deformity (technical difficulty – but may be worth attempting).

— Chronic CNS disease (contentious – is defensive, not evidence-based paractice).
— Severe ischaemic heart disease +/– hypertension.

Complications (due both to drugs injected and the technique itself)

- **Cardiovascular**
  — Hypotension: due to decreased SVR and reduced CO.
  — Bradycardia: with high block which reaches the cardiac accelerator fibres (in practice experienced anaesthetists who have managed high blocks or total spinals do not always report the theoretical bradycardia that should ensue).
- **Respiratory**
  — Dyspnoea as intercostal nerves are blocked.
  — Diaphragmatic impairment if an unpredictably high block develops (can happen with normal doses).
- **Gastrointestinal**
  — Nausea and vomiting (usually associated with hypotension).
  — Increased intraluminal pressures.
- **Neurological**
  — Postdural puncture headache (PDPH) and possible sequelae: tinnitus, diplopia, cranial nerve palsies, subdural haematoma (rare, but reported).
  — Meningitis: bacterial or chemical.
  — Direct nerve trauma.
  — Compressive haematoma or abscess formation.
  — 6th nerve palsy (also palsies of all nerves bar olfactory, glossopharyngeal and vagus).
  — Anterior spinal artery syndrome (ischaemia of cord at watershed area due to hypotension).
- **Miscellaneous**
  — Due to drugs injected.
  — Opioid side effects (diamorphine, etc.): nausea, pruritus, respiratory depression.
  — Alpha$_2$ agonist side effects (clonidine, etc.): Sedation, hypotension, dry mouth.
  — Local anaesthetic agent (+/– vasoconstrictor): has been blamed for radiculitis, myelitis (epinephrine (adrenaline)), arachnoiditis.

Marking points: Imagine yourself justifying spinal anaesthesia to a surgical colleague. If you are well informed you will be convincing. That will apply also to your answer to this question on a core subject.

Pharmacology and applied pharmacology

Compare and contrast Ametop (amethocaine gel) and EMLA cream. Are there any dangers associated with their use?

EMLA is a significant drug in paediatric practice, but it is commonly prescribed automatically on paediatric wards and applied by the nursing staff. Ametop is a more recent preparation which can be supplied without prescription. This question assesses both basic pharmacological and clinical knowledge of two useful drugs.

Introduction

The introduction of effective topical analgesia to ameliorate the pain of venepuncture has been a very important innovation in paediatric anaesthesia. There are two preparations available: EMLA, which has been available for over 15 years, and Ametop (amethocaine gel), which is a more recent introduction.

Chemistry

Amethocaine (tetracaine)
- Ester linked local anaesthetic.
- Ametop is a 4% formulation produced as a white opalescent gel, containing 40 mg ml^{-1} of tetracaine (amethocaine) base.
- Onset: application for 30 minutes allows venepuncture; for 45 minutes allows intravenous cannulation.
- Duration: analgesia persists for 4–6 hours after gel removal.
- Produces some vasodilatation.
- Amethocaine is toxic and maximum dose should not be exceeded.
- Is not a prescription only medicine (POM).

EMLA (eutectic mixture of local anaesthetic)
A eutectic (Gk *eutektos* – 'easily melting') mixture is one in which the mixing of two substances of the same consistency produces a mixture of different consistency. This is related to an alteration in the melting point of the mixture: an example is ice and salt, which when mixed produce water.

EMLA is a mixture of two powders: lidocaine (lignocaine) (melting point 37°C) and prilocaine (67°C) which when mixed becomes a liquid at room temperature. This is made into a cream by the addition of emulsifier and thickener. Each droplet is 80% local anaesthetic (compared with 20% in a simple emulsion) and a pH value of 9.4 means that a high percentage is non-ionised base form.

- Onset: slower than Ametop: application for at least 45–60 minutes is necessary before venepuncture, and longer still for cannulation.
- Duration: analgesia wanes quicker than Ametop.
- Produces blanching of skin suggestive of some vasoconstriction.
- Is a POM.

Dangers
These drugs are generally very safe in the doses prescribed, but there some potential problems.

- Prilocaine is associated with methaemoglobinaemia. Neonates and infants with high levels of HbF are at greater risk.
- Toxicity if the drugs are applied inadvertently to mucous membranes.
- Airway anaesthesia: there are case reports of children who have eaten the occlusive dressings and produced topical anaesthesia of oropharynx and upper airways.

Marking points: These are common drugs whose universal use should not prevent awareness of their rare dangers. A sound knowledge of their basic chemistry will be expected.

A patient with a history of depression requires a hemicolectomy for likely carcinoma. He is taking a monoamine oxidase inhibitor (MAOI). What is your anaesthetic management?

Monoamine oxidase inhibitors are reappearing as a treatment for depression and it is important that anaesthetists are aware of the implications. This is a question about applied pharmacology and an examination of your judgement in a potentially difficult area.

Introduction
Dangerous interactions meant that MAOIs fell out of favour as a treatment for refractory depressive illness. Recently, however, newer agents have been synthesised and this class of drugs has enjoyed resurgence.

- **MAO** is a non-specific group of enzymes which are subdivided into two main groups:
    — **MAO-A** (mainly intraneuronal) degrades dopamine, norepinephrine (noradrenaline) and 5-hydroxytryptamine. Inhibition increases levels of amine neurotransmitters.
    — **MAO-B** (predominantly extracellular) degrades other amines such as tyramine.
    — Have only a minor role in terminating norepinephrine actions at sympathetic nerve terminals (reuptake is more important) or those of exogenous direct acting sympathomimetics.
- **Non-selective and irreversible MAO inhibitors**
    — Phenelzine, tranylcypromine, isocarboxazid, pargyline (used as antihypertensive).
    — Potentiate effects of amines (especially tyramine) in foods: hypertensive crises.
    — Potentiate effects of indirectly acting sympathomimetics.
    — Interact with opioids: especially of the piperazine group: pethidine and fentanyl to produce hyperpyrexia, excitation, muscle rigidity, coma (in extreme cases).
- **Selective and reversible MAO-A inhibitor**
    — Moclobemide: less potentiation of amines and fewer dietary restrictions necessary.
    — Indirect sympathomimetics should still be avoided.
- **Selective MAO-B inhibitor**
    — Selegiline (main use is in Parkinson's disease).

Anaesthesia
- Identify the agent in light of the information above.
- Can the operation be deferred?
    — If so the patient should be advised to discontinue the drug at least 2 weeks before anaesthesia.
    — The range of interactions is wide and the response is unpredictable.
    — Moclobemide is shorter acting and treatment can continue nearer to the planned surgery. It should probably be stopped some days before, however, to minimise risk of residual drug interacting.
    — There is danger in discontinuing treatment in depressed patients: expert opinion should be sought. Other antidepressant drugs must not be prescribed.
- If the operation cannot be deferred.
    — Anaesthetic management must take into account any likely interactions.

— Caution with use of extradural analgesia (possible need for vasopressors).
— Caution with use of opioids.
— Given the surgical procedure analgesia cannot be denied: it must be administered with great care and with the means to treat cardiovascular instability immediately at hand.

Marking points: Anaesthesia in patients taking MAOIs is potentially very hazardous. Your answer must make clear that you are aware of the specific dangers.

Describe the advantages and disadvantages of nitrous oxide in modern anaesthetic practice.

It is sometimes assumed that nitrous oxide is little more than a simple carrier gas with some analgesic action. Its pharmacology is complex and as it is used in a large proportion of all general anaesthetics given, it is a topic about which you should be knowledgeable.

Introduction
Nitrous oxide is the oldest anaesthetic agent, but it is far from being simply the carrier gas with modest analgesic actions that frequently it is assumed to be. In fact it has a complex pharmacology and is associated with potential problems which would almost certainly probably prevent it from ever being introduced as a new drug were it to have been discovered today.

Advantages
- Carrier gas for more potent anaesthetic agents.
- Low blood/gas partition coefficient (0.47) means rapid onset and equilibration.
- Second gas effect accelerates onset of anaesthesia.
- Analgesia: potency is underestimated. Acts partly at opioid receptors and has transient potency of morphine.
- Analgesic and weak anaesthetic actions (MAC^{50} is 105%) decrease the MAC of other inhalational agents.

Disadvantages
- **Second gas effect:** diffusion hypoxia (of modest clinical relevance: lasts <10 minutes and can be overcome with supplemental oxygen).
- **Diffusing capacity relative to nitrogen is high (×25)**
  — In non-compliant air-filled spaces: pressure increases (middle ear, nasal sinuses, eye if filled with gas such as SF_6 after vitreo-retinal work).
  — Pressure change is related arithmetically to alveolar partial pressure of N_2O: so that 50% N_2O leads to pressure increase of 0.5 atmospheres.
  — In compliant air-filled spaces: volume increases (pneumothoraces, bullae, bowel, air embolus, cuffs of ETTs).
  — Volume change is related geometrically to alveolar partial pressure of N_2O: the % increase is given by the % N_2O divided by $(1.0 - F_IN_2O)$. So at 50% the final percentage volume increase is 50/0.5 = 100%. At 75% a pneumothorax will triple in size after 30 minutes' administration.
- **Emetic** (sympathomimetic; opioid effects; +/− bowel distension)
- **Respiratory depressant**
  — Increase in rate to offset decreased tidal volume.
- **Cardiovascular system**
  — Direct negative inotrope and chronotrope.
  — Contractility decreased if cardiac function already impaired: exacerbates ischaemic change in any situation in which myocardial O_2 supply is exceeded by demand.
  — Indirect stimulant (sympathomimetic).
  — Pulmonary vascular resistance increases if there is pre-existing pulmonary hypertension.
- **Bone marrow toxicity and neurotoxicity**
  — Biochemical lesion in the liver is demonstrable after only 40 minutes (methionine synthetase inhibition).
  — Oxidises cobalt atom in vitamin B_{12} (cyanocobalamin).
  — B_{12} is co-factor for enzyme methionine synthetase.
  — Two linked reactions are affected: methionine synthesis is impaired because

a methyl group is not transferred from CH_3-tetrahydrofolate, and formation of tetrahydrofolate is impaired.

— Methionine is a precursor of *s*-adenosyl methionine which is incorporated into myelin (hence subacute combined systems degeneration of the cord in B_{12} deficiency).

— Tetrahydrofolate is an important substrate involved in nucleotide and DNA synthesis (hence megaloblastic anaemia in folate and B_{12} deficiency).

- **Teratogenicity**
  — Mechanisms above plus other actions (sympathomimetic) believed to contribute to possible teratogenicity.
- **Greenhouse effect**
  — N_2O is a greenhouse gas: anaesthesia contributes ~1% of global N_2O.

Marking points: You will not have time to elaborate all of the above points in a written answer, but you will be expected to know about the majority of them and to give some sense of their priority.

Give an account of the mechanisms of action of nitrous oxide. Explain why it is a potentially toxic agent.

This is a much more complex question than the previous one and seeks basic science information that is now finding its way into the general domain. Nitrous oxide is one of the core anaesthetic agents in use and so it is not unreasonable to expect reasonably detailed knowledge. The information presented here might be of more use to you during a viva in which you are doing well.

Introduction
Nitrous oxide is the oldest anaesthetic agent, but is far from being simply a carrier gas with modest analgesic actions. It has a complex pharmacology and is associated with potential problems which would almost certainly probably prevent it from ever receiving a product licence were it to be introduced today.

Mechanisms of action
Some of the proposed mechanisms for analgesia and anaesthesia are described below.

Anaesthesia
- **$GABA_A$ (mainly inhibitory) and NMDA (mainly excitatory) receptors in the CNS**
  - N_2O appears to have no effect on $GABA_A$ but can significantly inhibit NMDA-activated currents.
  - There is concern that NMDA antagonists can be neurotoxic: a potential problem if N_2O is used alone under hyperbaric conditions. If $GABA_A$ agonist agents are used as well they may exert a protective effect to offset this damage.
- **Dopamine receptors**
  - N_2O is stimulatory to dopaminergic neurones: may mediate release of endogenous opioid peptides.
  - Effects are partly antagonised by naloxone.

Analgesia
- **Opioid peptide release**
  - In peri-aqueductal grey matter of mid-brain.
  - Stimulates descending noradrenergic pathways which modulate pain processing via norepinephrine (noradrenaline) release.
  - Noradrenaline acts at α_2 receptors in the dorsal horn.
- **Other theories**
  - Activation of supraspinal descending pain inhibition system with an increase in enkephalinergic interneurones in the substantia gelatinosa of the cord.
  - These endogenous enkephalins inhibit transmission via substance P dependent synapses.

Toxicity
- **Bone marrow toxicity and neurotoxicity**
  - Biochemical lesion in the liver is demonstrable after only 40 minutes (methionine synthetase inhibition).
  - Oxidises cobalt atom in vitamin B_{12} (cyanocobalamin).
  - B_{12} is co-factor for enzyme methionine synthetase.
  - Two linked reactions are affected: methionine synthesis is impaired because a methyl group is not transferred from CH_3-tetrahydrofolate, and formation of tetrahydrofolate is impaired.
  - Methionine is a precursor of s-adenosyl methionine which is incorporated into myelin (hence subacute combined systems degeneration of the cord in B_{12} deficiency).

— Tetrahydrofolate is an important substrate involved in nucleotide and DNA synthesis (hence megaloblastic anaemia in folate and B_{12} deficiency).

● **Teratogenicity**

— Mechanisms above plus other actions believed to contribute to possible teratogenicity: alpha$_1$ adrenoceptor agonism is associated with disorders of left/right body axis development (such as situs inversus).

> **Marking points:** This a potentially complex answer. Take heart from the fact that this is at the cutting edge and that a sensible brief account of the established facts will be sufficient.

What drugs are used to treat hypotension caused by subarachnoid block? What factors influence your choice of agent in this situation?

Spinal anaesthesia is popular, and safe management of its foremost immediate complication is vital. This question tests your knowledge of the main vasopressors and your judgement in their use.

Introduction
Hypotension is the main immediate complication of subarachnoid block using local anaesthetic. Systemic blood pressure is determined by cardiac output (heart rate and stroke volume) and systemic vascular resistance. Logical treatment of hypotension depends on the recognition of which part of this equation is affected.

Fluids
• Are not drugs, but can be mentioned for completeness. May help the effective hypovolaemia associated with sympathetic block by increasing SV and CO, but effects may be short lived in the compliant circulation of the young. May overload the non-compliant circulatory system of the elderly.

Ephedrine
• **Plant derivative** (from Chinese plant Ma Huang), synthesised for medical use.
• **Sympathomimetic.** Direct and indirect actions with both α and ß effects, also inhibits breakdown of norepinephrine (noradrenaline) by MAO.
  — Main influence on BP is via increase in CO.
  — $Alpha_1$ effects: vasoconstriction.
  —$Beta_1$ effects: positive inotrope and chronotrope.
  —$Beta_2$ effects: bronchodilatation (and vasodilatation).
  — Dose 3–5 mg titrated against response and repeated as necessary.
  — Rapid onset, duration of action ~1 hour.
• **Clinical usage**
  — Is traditionally favoured in obstetric anaesthesia because it does not cause $alpha_1$ mediated vasoconstriction in uteroplacental circulation (but fetal EEG shows excitation for 6 hours).
  — Increases myocardial oxygen demand: caution in patients with pre-existing tachycardia.
  — Bronchodilator effect may be of benefit in chest disease.
  — Is arrhythmogenic: caution in patients with pre-existing cardiac disease.
  — Norepinephrine (noradrenaline) depletion due to its indirect action leads to tachyphylaxis.

Phenylephrine
• **$Alpha_1$ agonist.** Mainly direct acting (weak beta effects)
  — Main influence on BP is via $alpha_1$ vasoconstriction and increase in peripheral resistance.
  — Dose 50–100 μg titrated against response and repeated as necessary.
  — Rapid onset, duration of action ~1 hour (often less).
• **Clinical usage**
  — Can be used in obstetric anaesthesia (despite traditional avoidance of all pressors save ephedrine). Has no more deleterious effect on neonatal cord pH than ephedrine and is a more efficient vasopressor.
  — Causes reflex bradycardia (may need atropine or glycopyrrolate), not arrhythmogenic.
  — Useful in those in whom tachycardia should be avoided.

Methoxamine

- **Alpha$_1$ agonist.** Mainly direct, some indirect acting and some beta-adrenoceptor blocking action.
  - — Main influence on BP is via alpha$_1$ vasoconstriction and increase in peripheral resistance.
  - — Dose 2–4 mg titrated against response and repeated as necessary.
  - — Rapid onset (1–2 minutes), duration of action ~1 hour (often less).
- **Clinical usage**
  - — As for phenylephrine although there is no research to support its use in obstetrics.
  - — Is an efficient vasopressor.
  - — Causes bradycardia due to peripheral beta-blockade > reflex via baroreceptors.
  - — Useful in those in whom tachycardia should be avoided.

Metaraminol

- **Sympathomimetic.** Direct and indirect actions with alpha and beta effects (alpha predominate).
  - — Influence on BP is via alpha$_1$ vasoconstriction and increase in cardiac ouput with increased coronary blood flow.
  - — Dose 1–5 mg titrated against response and repeated as necessary.
  - — Rapid onset (1–3 min), duration of action ~20–25 min.
- **Clinical usage**
  - — As for methoxamine although there is no research to support its use in obstetrics.
  - — An efficient vasopressor.

Norepinephrine (noradrenaline)

- **Exogenous and endogenous catecholamine.** Powerful alpha$_1$ agonist with weaker beta effects.
  - — Influence on BP is via alpha$_1$ vasoconstriction and increase in peripheral resistance.
  - — Used as intravenous infusion (0.05–0.2 μg kg^{-1} min^{-1}) and titrated against the desired level of arterial pressure.
  - — Rapid onset and offset of action.
- **Clinical usage**
  - — More common in intensive care medicine.
  - — Reflex bradycardia is common.
  - — Sudden discontinuation of infusion may be accompanied by rebound severe hypotension. Must decrease rate slowly.

Marking points: There is more detail in this answer than you would need, but what you must demonstrate is your ability to make a safe choice of agent for treating pharmacologically induced hypotension.

Compare the pharmacology of atropine, hyoscine and glycopyrrolate. Outline their main uses in anaesthetic practice.

A knowledge of the applied pharmacology of these anticholinergic drugs is of obvious importance given that they are in very common use (hyoscine excepted). The question aims to test whether you appreciate the differences between the drugs which dictate their suitability in a particular clinical situation.

Introduction
These drugs are all anticholinergic agents which, when given in clinical doses, are selective for muscarinic receptors. This makes them especially useful for counteracting the autonomic effects that are associated with anaesthesia and surgery.

Chemistry
- Atropine and hyoscine are naturally occurring tertiary amines which cross lipid membranes (blood–brain; placenta) readily. Atropine is chemically related to cocaine and has weak local anaesthetic actions. Glycopyrrolate is a synthetic quaternary amine with minimal ability to penetrate these barriers.
- Duration of action:
  - Atropine: antivagal 1–2 hours; antisialogogue 3–4 hours.
  - Glycopyrrolate: antivagal 2–3 hours; antisialogogue 6–7 hours.
  - Hyoscine: actions are shorter than either.

Effects on systems
- **CNS.** Atropine and hyoscine cross the blood–brain barrier. Atropine may cause stimulation and excitement. Hyoscine has more potent central effects and causes sedation and amnesia. Glycopyrrolate has no effect.
- **Autonomic nervous system.** Depress all secretory activity, including sweating (temperature may rise).
- **CVS.** All are vagal antagonists: atropine and hyoscine can act as partial agonists at low doses and can cause bradycardia (Bezold–Jarisch effect). Vagolytic actions: atropine > glycopyrrolate > hyoscine and has the most rapid onset.
- **Respiratory system.** All cause bronchodilation: atropine = glycopyrrolate > hyoscine; and reduce bronchial secretions: hyoscine > atropine = glycopyrrolate. Dead space is increased.
- **Gastrointestinal tract.** All are antisialogogues: hyoscine > glycopyrrolate > atropine; anti-emetics: hyoscine > atropine (glycopyrrolate has no effect); all decrease tone of lower oesophageal sphincter (hyoscine least).

Main uses
- Protect myocardium from vagal inhibition (surgical manouevres, etc.) and as pre-medication for children (brisk vagal reflexes) This is a less widespread practice now.
- Decrease salivary and bronchial secretions; particularly before fibreoptic bronchoscopy: glycopyrrolate is an effective antisialogogue at doses which cause minimal tachycardia.
- Sedation and amnesia (hyoscine).
- Antagonism of the muscarinic effects of anticholinesterases: duration of action of glycopyrrolate is better matched to neostigmine (than is atropine).
- Anti-emetic (mainly hyoscine).
- Antispasmodic, bronchodilatory.

Marking points: The basic pharmacology of these drugs is not complex and you will be expected to give an accurate account of the main clinical differences between them.

Outline the pathways which mediate nausea and vomiting. Which groups of patients are particularly at risk in the perioperative period? Where do the commonly used anti-emetic drugs exert their actions?

Postoperative nausea and vomiting (PONV) is a problem that is almost as great as perioperative pain and is a core area of anaesthetic practice. This question tests your understanding of the underlying physiological principles and your ability to identify (and by inference treat) those patients who particularly are at risk.

Introduction

In many hospitals the establishment of acute pain teams has improved greatly the management of perioperative pain, and anaesthetists now have the challenge of dealing with another problem which may be almost equally distressing for some patients, that of postoperative nausea and vomiting (PONV).

Neural pathways

- Nausea and vomiting (which are reflexes) have afferent and efferent pathways linked to a central integrator: the vomiting centre (VC).
- **The VC receives inputs from many sources:**
  - Cortex: pain, fear, anxiety, association and other psychological factors, visual, olfactory stimuli, etc. may all provoke nausea and vomiting.
  - Cortex: organic disturbance such raised ICP, hypoxia (nausea is a sensitive early sign), vascular derangement (classical migraine).
  - Viscera: stimuli mediated by vagal and sympathetic afferents such as peritoneal irritation, visceral, including cardiac pain, gastric stasis, gastric irritation.
  - Chemoreceptor trigger zone.
- **The chemoreceptor trigger zone (CTZ) also receives inputs from many sources:**
  - Vestibular apparatus via the cerebellum.
  - Drugs: direct action of opioids (also sensitize the vestibular apparatus to motion), cytotoxic drugs, cardiac glycosides and many other agents.

Patients at particular risk of PONV

- **Patient associated**
  - Female > Male (2–4×).
  - Obese > Lean.
  - Young > Older.
  - Positive history (3×).
  - Early ambulation.
- **Surgery associated**
  - Intra-abdominal, laparoscopic.
  - Intracranial, middle ear.
  - Squint surgery, hysterectomy.
  - Pain: moderate to severe.
- **Anaesthesia and drug related**
  - Opioid analgesics.
  - Sympathomimetics (ketamine, N_2O).
  - Inhalational agents: isoflurane > others.
- **Disease related**
  - Intestinal obstruction.
  - Metabolic: hypoglycaemia.
  - Hypoxia, uraemia.
  - Hypotension.

Site of actions

- Histamine (H$_1$) receptors
  — Mainly in vestibular labyrinth.
  — Drugs: cyclizine, some phenothiazines (mixed actions), butyrophenones (weak) act as antagonists.
- Dopamine (D$_2$) receptors
  — In CTZ and influence vagal afferents.
  — Drugs are antagonists.
  — Bytyrophenones (e.g. droperidol), metoclopramide (central and peripheral actions), some phenothiazines.
- Cholinergic (muscarinic) receptors
  — In vestibular labyrinth and in CTZ.
  — Drugs are antagonists.
  — Hyoscine, atropine, glycopyrrolate, some phenothiazines (mixed actions).
- Serotonin (5-hydroxytryptamine) 5HT$_3$ receptors
  — Predominantly in the gastrointestinal tract.
  — Drugs are antagonists.
  — Drugs: ondansetron, granisetron.
- NK$_1$ receptors
  — Abundant in brainstem where emetic afferents converge.
  — Research NK$_1$ antagonists show modest promise.
- Others
  — Dexamethasone (site of action unknown).
  — Cannabinoids (act at CB1 endogenous cannabinoid receptor and modulate neurotransmitter release).
  — Propofol (effective in low dose infusion 1 mg kg^{-1} hr^{-1}).
  — Diphenidol (acts at vestibular apparatus).

Marking points: PONV is a core problem in anaesthesia which may only be addressed by the use of 'balanced anti-emesis'. The effective prescription of anti-emetics requires some knowledge about their diverse sites of action.

Describe the effects of magnesium sulphate. What are its uses in the acutely ill?

Candidates have been taken by surprise by questions on magnesium because they have been unaware both of its physiological importance and of the wide range of clinical applications. Your answer should convey some appreciation of its significance.

Introduction

Magnesium is the fourth most important cation in the body as well as being the second most important intracellular cation. It activates at least three hundred enzyme systems and is a drug for which clinicians are finding increasing therapeutic uses.

Actions

Many processes are dependent on Mg^{2+} including the production and functioning of ATP (to which it is chelated) and the biosynthesis of DNA and RNA. It has an essential role in the regulation of most cellular functions and acts as a natural Ca^{2+} antagonist. High extracellular Mg^{2+} leads to an increase in intracellular Mg^{2+} which in turn inhibits Ca^{2+} influx through Ca^{2+} channels. It is this action which appears to mediate many of its effects. It has an anti-adrenergic action: release at all synaptic junctions is decreased, so it also inhibits the release of catecholamines. Therapeutic level is 4–8 mmol L^{-1}.

Effects on systems

- **CNS and PNS**
  - Penetrates blood–brain barrier poorly but depresses the CNS and sedates.
  - Acts as a cerebral vasodilator.
  - Interferes with release of neurotransmitters at all synaptic junctions.
  - Deep tendon reflexes are lost at 10 mmol L^{-1}.
- **Cardiovascular**
  - Mediates a reduction of vascular tone via direct vasodilatation.
  - There is sympathetic block and inhibition of catecholamine release.
  - Decreases cardiac conduction and decreases myocardial contractile force. This intrinsic slowing is partly opposed by vagolytic action.
- **Respiratory**
  - No effect on respiratory drive (but may weaken respiratory muscles). It is an effective bronchodilator used in severe refractory asthma.
  - Respiratory paralysis at 15 mmol L^{-1}.
- **Uterus**
  - Powerful tocolytic.
  - Crosses placenta rapidly and may exert similar effects in the newborn: hypotonia, apnoea.
- **Renal**
  - Vasodilator and diuretic.

Therapeutic uses

- **Pre-eclampsia and eclampsia.** $MgSO_4$ decreases systemic vascular resistance and is used to reduce CNS excitability. Use in UK to pre-empt eclamptic convulsions is not yet as widespread as in the USA.
- **Acute arrhythmias.** It is effective at abolishing tachyarrhythmias: particularly ventricular, adrenaline-, digitalis- and bupivacaine-induced. ECG shows widening QRS with prolonged P–Q interval. At blood levels of 15 mmol L^{-1} SA and AV block is complete and cardiac arrest will supervene at 25 mmol L^{-1}.
- **Hypomagnesaemia:** nutritional, endocrine, malabsorption, critical illness.
- **Tetanus:** rare in the UK, but $MgSO_4$ infusion is the primary treatment for the muscle spasm and autonomic instability caused by this condition.
- **Epilepsy:** can be used in status epilepticus.

Marking points: Ignorance of the all the uses of $MgSO_4$ will be excused as long as you can explain its main mechanism of action and its important common uses, particularly in obstetrics.

Describe the pharmacology of propofol.

Propofol is the most commonly used agent for induction of anaesthesia in the UK. It is used also for the maintenance of anaesthesia and for sedation in intensive care. The importance of a detailed knowledge of this agent is self-evident.

Introduction

Since its introduction in the late 1980s propofol has become the most commonly used agent for induction of anaesthesia in the UK. The popularity of total intravenous anaesthesia (TIVA) with propofol is also increasing and the drug is widely used to provide sedation in intensive care patients.

Chemistry

- Propofol is a substituted stable phenolic compound: 2,6 di-isopropylphenol. It is highly lipid soluble and water insoluble and is presented as either a 1% or 2% emulsion in soya bean oil. Other constituents include egg phosphatide and glycerol. It is a weak organic acid with a pK_a of 11.

Mechanism of action

- In common with many other drugs which produce general anaesthesia the mechanism of action is not wholly clear. It may enhance inhibitory synaptic transmission by activation of the Cl^- channel on the b_1 subunit of the GABA receptor. It also inhibits the NMDA subtype of glutamate receptor.

Uses

- Propofol is used for the induction of anaesthesia in adults and children, for the maintenance of anaesthesia, for sedation in intensive care, and for sedation during procedures under local or regional anaesthesia. It has an anti-emetic action and is sometimes given by very low dose infusion to chemotherapy patients.

Dose and routes of administration

- The drug is only used intravenously. A dose of 1–2 mg kg^{-1} will usually induce anaesthesia in adults. Children may require twice this dose.

Onset and duration of action

- An induction dose of propofol will lead to rapid loss of consciousness (within a minute). Rapid redistribution to peripheral tissues (distribution half-life is 1–2 minutes) leads to rapid awakening. The elimination half-life is quoted at between 5 and 12 hours.

Main effects and side-effects

- **Central nervous system.** CNS depression and induction of anaesthesia. May be associated with excitatory effects and dystonic movements, particularly in children. The EEG displays initial activation followed by dose-related depression. The data sheet states that it is contraindicated in patients with epilepsy, although this has been disputed.
- **Cardiovascular system.** Systemic vascular resistance falls and it is unusual to see compensatory tachycardia. A relative bradycardia is common and the blood pressure will fall. Propofol is a myocardial depressant.
- **Respiratory system.** Propofol is a respiratory depressant which also suppresses laryngeal reflexes. It was this attribute which allowed the use of the laryngeal mask airway to become widespread.
- **Gastrointestinal system.** The drug is anti-emetic.
- **Other effects.** Propofol causes pain on injection. It is not licensed for use in obstetric anaesthesia. There is a risk of hyperlipidaemia in intensive care patients who have received prolonged infusions.

Pharmacokinetics

- Propofol is highly protein bound (98%) and has a large volume of distribution (4 L kg^{-1}). Distribution half-life is 1–2 minutes and elimination half-life 5–12 hours. Metabolism is mainly hepatic with the production of inactive metabolites and conjugates which are excreted in urine.

Miscellaneous

- Propofol is not a trigger for malignant hyperpyrexia and it may also be used safely in patients with porphyria. It does not release histamine and adverse reactions are very rare.

Marking points: Propofol is a drug central to anaesthetic practice in the UK. You will be expected to know a good deal about it.

Describe the pharmacology of ketamine.

Ketamine is of interest because its pharmacology has been elucidated more clearly than with many other agents, and because investigation of the S(+) isomer as an agent with fewer side effects has renewed the drug's promise.

Introduction

Ketamine is unique amongst anaesthetic agents in that by causing 'dissociative anaesthesia' a single dose can produce profound analgesia, amnesia and anaesthesia. Its pharmacology has been elucidated more clearly than with other induction agents and is summarised below.

Chemistry

- Ketamine is a derivative of phencyclidine (PCP) which is an anaesthetic agent used in veterinary practice and which is also a drug of abuse known as 'angel dust'. It is water soluble and is presented in three different concentrations. It is an acidic solution of pH 3.5–5.5. All formulations now contain preservative which precludes its use in central neural blockade. It is presented as a racemic mixture of two enantiomers:

Mechanism of action

- Ketamine is an NMDA (*N*-methyl-D-aspartate) receptor antagonist. The NMDA receptor is a glutamate receptor in the CNS, glutamate being the major excitatory neurotransmitter in the brain. The receptor incorporates a cation channel to which ketamine binds. Ketamine also has effects on opioid receptors; acting as a partial μ antagonist and as a partial agonist at κ and δ receptors. (Note that the nomenclature of opioid receptors is undergoing change.) It may therefore exert its analgesic effects after intrathecal or extradural injection at spinal κ receptors.

Uses

- Ketamine can be used for the induction of anaesthesia in adults and children, for so-called 'field' anaesthesia as a single anaesthetic agent outside the hospital setting, for bronchodilatation in severe refractory asthma, and for sedo-analgesia during procedures performed under local or regional anaesthesia.

Dose and routes of administration

- The drug can be administered via intravenous, intramuscular, oral and rectal routes. It has been used in extradural and intrathecal doses. An intravenous dose of 1–2 mg kg^{-1} will usually induce anaesthesia. The intramuscular dose is 5–10 mg kg^{-1}. Subhypnotic doses are usually up to 0.5 mg kg^{-1}.

Onset and duration of action

- An induction dose of ketamine does not lead to hypnosis within one arm–brain circulation time. Consciousness will be lost after 1–2 minutes but the patient may continue to move and to make incoherent noises. Intramuscular administration will take 10–15 minutes to take effect. The duration of action is between 10 and 40 minutes.

Main effects and side effects

- **Central nervous system.** Dissociative anaesthesia. Afferent input is not affected but central processing at thalamocortical and limbic levels is distorted. Anecdortally it is reported that ketamine is much less effective in brain-damaged patients. The drug produces profound analgesia as well as amnesia. The drug increases intracranial pressure and CMRO$_2$.
- **Cardiovascular system.** Ketamine is sympathomimetic and increases levels of circulating catecholamines. On isolated myocardium it acts as a depressant.

Indirect effects result in tachycardia, increase in cardiac output and blood pressure, and an increase in myocardial oxygen consumption.

- **Respiratory system.** Ketamine is a respiratory stimulant. It is also said to preserve laryngeal reflexes and tone in the upper airway. It antagonises the effects of acetyl choline and 5-hydroxytryptamine on the bronchial tree and causes clinically useful bronchodilation.

- **Gastrointestinal system.** Salivation increases. As with most anaesthetic agents with sympathomimetic actions the incidence of nausea and vomiting is increased.

- **Other effects.** The use of ketamine has been limited by its CNS side effects. It is associated both with an emergence delirium and also with dysphoria and hallucinations. These can appear many hours after recovery from anaesthesia. Benzodiazepines may attenuate the problem.

Pharmacokinetics
- Ketamine is weakly protein bound (25%). Metabolism is hepatic: demethylation produces the active metabolite norketamine (0.3× as potent). Further metabolism produces conjugates which are excreted in urine.

Miscellaneous
- There is increasing interest in the use of the S(+) enantiomer which is 3–4× as potent as the R(–) enantiomer and which is associated with shorter recovery times and with fewer psychotomimetic reactions.

> **Marking points:** Ketamine is significant because it is unique and has a complex and interesting pharmacology. Examiners may use the subject to explore concepts such as the NMDA receptor and chirality.

What drugs may be used for the immediate control of acute hypertension or to induce deliberate hypotension? What is their mechanism of action?

This is a question which can appear in several guises. You may be asked about the treatment of hypertension in recovery or on ITU, you may be asked about the management of phaeochromocytoma, you may be asked to discuss induced hypertension or to outline the management of a patient with hypertensive disease of pregnancy. You should be able to take the information that is offered below and adapt it to the particular context.

Introduction

Systemic blood pressure is determined by cardiac output (heart rate and stroke volume) and systemic vascular resistance. Logical treatment of severe acute hypertension or the deliberate production of hypotension can be directed at different parts of this equation as appropriate for the clinical context. It is first important first to identify and to treat any underlying cause.

Identify any precipitating cause
* **Recovery and intensive care**
    — Pain or anxiety (analgesia and anxiolysis).
    — Bladder distension (urinary catheter).
    — MAO interaction.
    — Hypercapnia (intervene as appropriate).
    — Raised intracranial pressure (intervene as appropriate).
    — Essential hypertension.
    — Excess of vasopressor.
* **Obstetrics**
    — Hypertensive disease of pregnancy (treat as below).
    — Pain or anxiety (analgesia: avoid amnesic anxiolytics during labour).
    — Pre-existing essential hypertension.

Treatment
* **General points**
    — Choice of drug and route will depend upon how rapidly control is needed.
    — Precipitate falls in blood pressure can be associated with catastrophic drops in perfusion of essential areas, such as the retinal circulation, because the autoregulatory curve may be shifted to the right.

Alpha-adrenoceptor blockers

Phentolamine
* Non-selective alpha antagonist ($\alpha_1 : \alpha_2$ is 3 : 1) with weak beta sympathomimetic action.
    — Influence on BP is via block of alpha$_1$ vasoconstriction with decrease in peripheral resistance as well as mild beta sympathomimetic vasodilatation.
    —Alpha$_2$ blockade increases norepinephrine (noradrenaline) release.
    — Dose 1–5 mg titrated against response and repeated as necessary.
    — Rapid onset (1–2 min), duration ~ up to 15–20 min.

[Phenoxybenzamine, prazosin, doxazosin]
* These alpha-blockers are not usually used for rapid control of blood pressure.

Beta-adrenoceptor blockers
* There are many examples: all are competitive anatagonists, but their selectivity for receptors is variable. Selective beta$_1$ antagonism is useful. Influence on BP is

probably due to decreased cardiac output via decreased heart rate, plus some inhibition of the renin–angiotensin system. Unopposed alpha$_1$ vasoconstriction may compromise the peripheral circulation without causing hypertension.

— **Atenolol.** Selective beta$_1$ antagonist except in high doses. Long acting with $t_{1/2}$ of ~7 hours.
— **Esmolol.** Relatively selective beta$_1$ antagonist. Ultra short-acting with $t_{1/2}$ of ~9 minutes. Hydrolysed by non-specific esterases.
— **Labetalol.** Both an alpha and beta antagonist (ratio is 1 : 7), so get decrease in SVR without reflex tachycardia. Is a common agent in anaesthetic, obstetric anaesthetic and intensive therapy use. Elimination $t_{1/2}$: 4–6 hours.

Ganglion blockers

- Antagonists at nicotinic receptors at autonomic ganglia (sympathetic and parasympathetic) but no effect at nicotinic receptors of neuromuscular junction.
  — **Trimetaphan.**
  — Direct vasodilator effect in peripheral vessels.
  — Histamine releaser.
  — Antagonises hypoxic pulmonary vasoconstriction.
  — Reflex tachycardia is common.
  — No longer popular.

Direct vasodilators

- **Hydralazine**
  — Hypotension via direct vasodilatation plus weak alpha antagonist action.
  — Mediated via increase in cyclic GMP and decrease in available intracellular Ca^{2+}.
  — Arteriolar tone affected > venous.
  — Reflex tachycardia is common.
- **Glyceryl trinitrate (GTN) nitroglycerin**
  — Mediates hypotensive action via nitric oxide.
  — NO activates guanylate cyclase which increases cyclic GMP within cells which in turn decreases available intracellular Ca^{2+}.
  — Causes venous more than arteriolar vasodilatation, hence decreases venous return and preload. Decreased myocardial oxygen demand due to decrease in wall tension.
  — Rapid onset (1–2 min) and offset (3–5 min) allows good control of BP: no rebound hypertension on discontinuing infusion.
  — Increases cerebral blood flow and intracranial pressure.
  — Tolerance may develop: can be prevented by intermittent dosing.
- **Sodium nitroprusside (SNP)**
  — Mediates hypotensive action via nitric oxide as with GTN.
  — Arterial and venous dilatation: hypotension and reflex tachycardia.
  — Tachyphylaxis by uncertain mechanism in some patients.
  — Increases cerebral blood flow and intracranial pressure.
  — Rapid onset (1–2 minutes) and offset (3–5 minutes) allows good control of BP: but may see rebound hypertension when infusion is stopped.
  — Complex metabolism leads to production of free CN^- which is potentially very toxic (irreversible binding of cytochrome oxidase) at levels of > 8 μg ml^{-1}.
  — Giving set must be protected from light.

Alpha$_2$-adrenoceptor agonists

- **Clonidine**
  — Alpha agonist with α_2 affinity ~ 200×α_1.
  — Mediates hypotensive action via reduced central sympathetic outflow and

by stimulation of presynaptic receptors which inhibit norepinephrine (noradrenaline) release into the synaptic cleft.
— Has analgesic and sedative actions.
— Elimination $t_{1/2}$ is too long to allow its use for fine control of acutely raised blood pressure but it can be a useful adjunct in low doses.

Marking points: This is a question about the rational application of pharmacology to an acute anaesthetic problem. It will be assumed that you have had to use at least some of these drugs and that you should be able to justify their administration by an understanding of their actions. There is, of course, far more detail in the answer than you would have time for in a written question, but you might well have to explain some mechanisms of action in a viva.

What is meant by 'chirality'? What is its relevance for anaesthetic drugs?

You might count yourself unlucky were this to appear as a written question, or perhaps more likely in the orals. Were you, alas, to fail the exam, you might even travel home seething at the injustice of being asked a question such as this. The recent introduction of ropivacaine and levobupivacaine, however, has made it a possible examination topic, and so you may as well be prepared.

Introduction
'Chirality' is derived from the Greek, means 'having handedness', and defines a particular type of stereoisomerism. Right and left hands are mirror images of each other but cannot be superimposed when the palms are facing in the same direction. Similarly many drugs, including substances relevant to anaesthesia, exist as right- and left-handed forms that are mirror images but which cannot be superimposed. These particular isomers are known as 'enantiomers' (substances of opposite shape), and this form of stereo-isomerism is dependent on the presence of a chiral centre, which is typically a carbon atom with four groups attached.

Nomenclature
- Nomenclature can be very confusing because of differing conventions that have been used.
- One convention simply describes optical activity:
  — Enantiomers that rotate plane polarised light to the right: (+) = (dextro) = (d).
  — Enantiomers that rotate plane polarised light to the left: (−) = (laevo or levo) = (l).
- Another convention is based on a molecule's configuration in relation to (+) glturaldehyde which was arbitrarily assigned a 'D' (not 'd') configuration. Substances were denoted 'D' or 'L' according to comparison with the model substance, and the optical direction added.
- The currently accepted convention is that which assigns a sequence of priority to the four atoms or groups attached to the chiral centre.
- With the smallest group extending away from the viewer the arrangement of the largest to the smallest, if clockwise is designated 'R' for rectus, if anticlockwise 'S' for sinister. The optical direction is added to give, e.g. S(−) bupivacaine. (The pharmaceutical company confuses matters by calling it 'levobupivacaine', presumably because it sounds preferable to 'sinister bupivacaine'.)

Anaesthetic relevance
- Chiral drugs that are found in nature are usually single enantiomers, because they are synthesised enzymatically in reactions that are stereospecific.
- Such drugs include:
  — Atropine (laevo).
  — Cocaine (laevo).
  — Morphine (laevo).
  — Hyoscine (laevo).
  — Norepinephrine (noradrenaline) (laevo).
  — Ephedrine (laevo).
- Most synthetic chiral drugs are racemic mixtures, and in the case of the examples above, are less potent than the pure enantiomers because the d- forms are much less active.
- This is predictable because drug receptor sites are likely to contain chiral amino acids which are stereoselective.
- The clinical behaviour of the enantiomers, and in particular their toxicity, is related to the chiral form, and this is relevant to local anaesthetics.

— **Prilocaine.** S(+) enantiomer is a stronger vasoconstrictor and is metabolised more slowly than the R(−) form which therefore produces higher concentrations of *o*-toluidine and a greater risk of methaemoglobinaemia.

— **Ropivacaine.** This is the pure S(−) enantiomer of propivacaine and is associated with a safer cardiovascular profile in overdose.

— **Bupivacaine.** S(−) enantiomer has less affinity for, and dissociates quicker from, myocardial sodium channels. Reduced risk of CVS and CNS toxicity.

- There is also interest in ketamine enantiomers: the S(+) form is up to 4× as potent as the R(−) form and is associated with fewer emergence and psychotomimetic phenomena.

Marking points: Chirality is of some relevance to anaesthesia and has safety implications, particularly in relation to local anaesthetics. You will be heading for a '2+' and will impress the examiner greatly if you can unravel the nomeclature as above, but you must be at least aware of the concept in relation to the newer drugs ropivacaine and levobupivacaine.

Clinical measurement and equipment

Describe the physical principles of the pulse oximeter. What are the limitations of the technique?

Most anaesthetists believe that continuous measurement of oxygen saturation during anaesthesia is absolutely essential. Equally essential, therefore, is a broad understanding of how the technique works with particular reference to its limitations and potential sources of error.

Introduction
Pulse oximetry has been widely available for only about 12 years but very rapidly has become established as arguably the single most important form of monitoring in anaesthetic practice.

Physical principles
- Oxygenated haemoglobin (HbO_2) and deoxygenated haemoglobin (Hb) have differential absorption spectra.
- At a wavelength of 660 nm (red light) HbO_2 absorbs less than Hb, hence its red colour.
- At a wavelength of 940 nm (infra-red light) this is reversed and Hb absorbs more than HbO_2. At 800 nm – the isobestic point - the absorption coefficients are identical.
- The pulse oximeter uses two light emitting diodes which emit pulses of red (660 nm) and infra-red (980 nm) light every 5–10 μs from one side of the probe. The light is transmitted through tissue to be sensed by a photocell.
- The output is submitted to electronic processing during which the absorption of the blood at the two different wavelengths is converted to a ratio which is compared to an algorithm produced from experimental data.
- Oximetry aims to measure the saturation in arterial blood, and so the instrument detects the points of maximum and minimum absorption (during cardiac systole and diastole). It measures the pulsatile component and subtracts the non-arterial constant component before displaying a pulse waveform and the percentage oxygen saturation. Hence, strictly defined, it is measuring the S_pO_2 (plethysmographic) rather than the S_aO_2 (arterial).

Sources of errror and limitations
- Pulse oximetry is calibrated against volunteers and so calibration against dangerously hypoxic values is impossible. The instruments are less accurate at S_pO_2 values <70%.

- Interference for ambient light. Can occur if light is bright and direct, but the pulsed nature of the emissions is intended to allow detection of and compensation for any ambient light.
- Loss of the pulsatile component. Occurs in conditions of hypoperfusion, hypothermia, peripheral vasoconstriction, narrow pulse pressure, arrythmias which distort the points of maximum and minimum absorption, venous congestion.
- Movement artefact or electrical interference (neither are major problems).
- Infra-red absorption by other substances: nail varnish, staining from e.g. nicotine.
- More significant is absorption by abnormal haemoglobins and other substances:
  — Heavy smokers or CO poisoning: carboxyhaemoglobin (COHb) has a similar absorption coefficient to HbO_2 and will give abnormally high reading of ~96%.
  — Jaundiced patients: bilirubin has a similar absorption coefficient to Hb and will give abnormally low saturations.
  — Methaemoglobinaemia: MetHb has absorption similar at both wavelengths and gives a reading of ~84%.
  — Dyes such as methylene or disulphine blue give falsely low readings.

Problems in interpretation
- Pulse oximetry does not detect respiratory failure. A high F_IO_2 may mask ventilatory failure by ensuring high S_pO_2% readings.
- In very anaemic patients S_pO_2% readings may show high saturations although oxygen delivery to the tissues may be impaired.

Marking points: This is clearly a core topic and a clear understanding of the principles and limitations of pulse oximetry will be expected.

Describe the physical principles which underlie the function of a 'Rotameter' flowmeter. What factors may lead to inaccuracies in its use?

There are few anaesthetics given which do not involve the use of at least one 'Rotameter' flowmeter. ('Rotameter' is a tradename which continual use has given the status of a generic object.) It is important, therefore, to be aware of how they function as well as of potential sources of inaccuracy.

Introduction

It would be unusual to find many anaesthetics, either general or local, which do not involve the administration of at least oxygen via a 'Rotameter'. 'Rotameter' is the tradename for a variable-orifice, fixed-pressure-difference flowmeter, which gives a continuous indication of the rate of gas flow.

Physical principles

- A bobbin floats within a vertical conical glass tube, supported by the gas flow which is controlled by a needle valve.
- At low flows the orifice around the bobbin is an annular tube and the gas flow is laminar. Flow rate through a tube is related to the viscosity of the gas and the fourth power of the radius.
- At higher flows and further up the tube the area of the orifice is larger in relation to the bobbin and the flow is turbulent. Flow rate is related to the density of the gas and the square of the radius.
- These factors mean, therefore, that 'Rotameters' have to be calibrated for the specific gases that they are measuring and are not interchangeable for different gases.
- The pressure across the bobbin at any flow rate remains constant, because the force to which it gives rise is exactly balanced by the force of gravity acting on the bobbin.

Other features

- The bobbin is designed with small slots or fins in its upper part so that it will rotate centrally within the gas stream. This is to prevent it sticking to the side of the tube because of dirt or static electricity.
- To prevent the accumulation of static charge tubes have either a conductive coating or have a conductive strip at the back.
- The flowmeter blocks are designed to ensure that the bobbin remains visible at the top of the tubes.

Sources of inaccuracy

- Accumulation of dirt or static electricity not overcome by the design features above.
- Flowmeter block that is not vertical: the bobbin must not impinge on the sides of the tube.
- Back pressure on the gas flow may still be a problem on some anaesthetic machines.
- Cracked seals or tubes may provide a source of error.

> **Marking points:** This is a straightforward question which includes some physics and some practical application. It is a thin question and most of the points above would be expected.

How does a capnometer or capnograph measure CO$_2$ concentration? What useful information is conveyed by the capnogram (the graph of CO2 against time)?

Together with pulse oximetry, capnography is regarded by most anaesthetists to be indispensable. Some believe it to be more useful than oximetry because of the large amount of information that can be obtained from an end-tidal CO$_2$ reading and a capnograph trace. This question aims to explore whether you are aware of the clinical information that can be obtained during routine CO$_2$ monitoring.

Introduction
Capnography has the potential to convey a large amount of vital clinical information about both the respiratory and cardiovascular status of a patient, and for this reason there are many anaesthetists who believe it to be the single most useful form of monitoring in anaesthetic practice.

Physical principles
- Most capnographs measure CO$_2$ by means of infra-red absorption. A molecule will absorb infra-red radiation as long as it contains at least two different atoms.
- The system comprises an infra-red source, a filter to ensure that only radiation of the desired wavelength is transmitted, a crystal window (glass absorbs infra-red), sample chamber and photodetector.
- The fraction of radiation absorbed is compared with a reference gas (so regular calibration against zero and known CO$_2$ concentrations is essential) before the value is displayed.
- The infra-red wavelength absorbed varies with the gas, thereby allowing its identification. There is some overlap between CO$_2$ and N$_2$O for which modern instruments can compensate, collision broadening would otherwise elevate falsely the CO$_2$ readings.

Clinical information
- **No CO$_2$ trace:**
  — Oesophageal intubation. Its use is mandatory wherever tracheal intubation is used.
  — Disconnection of breathing system.
  — Tracheal tube displacement.
  — Cessation of CO$_2$ production due to circulatory arrest.
- **Low or falling end-tidal CO$_2$:**
  — Hyperventilation. May be due e.g. to pain or inadequate anaesthesia in a spontaneously breathing patient, or to over-ventilation in IPPV.
  — Pulmonary embolism (gas or thrombus). Sudden fall of CO$_2$ excretion due to compromise of the pulmonary circulation.
  — Decreased cardiac ouput, hypoperfusion, shock.
- **Normal end-tidal CO$_2$:**
  — Adequate ventilation.
- **High or rising end-tidal CO$_2$:**
  — Inadequate ventilation.
  — Rebreathing (this may just increase the baseline which does not return to zero).
  — Soda lime exhaustion.
  — Malignant hyperpyrexia or other hypermetabolic state in which CO$_2$ production increases.
- **Abnormal capnography wave forms:**
  — Slow upstroke and slowly rising plateau: indicates chronic or acute airway obstruction (this may be lower or upper airway as well as in the breathing system).

— Inspiratory dips in the wave form: indicates partial recovery from neuromuscular blockade.
— Raised baseline: rebreathing as above.

Marking points: This is another core topic which will be marked stringently. Capnography contributes greatly to anaesthetic safety by conveying significant cardiac and respiratory information. You will be expected to show that you understand why it does so.

How can jugular venous bulb oxygen saturation be measured? What is the purpose of this investigation? What factors cause it to increase or decrease?

This is an area of specialist practice which you may not have encountered. If you are struggling the answer is best developed from first principles.

Introduction

Jugular venous oxygen saturation ($S_{jv}O_2$) provides a measure of global cerebral oxygenation and finds uses in neurosurgery, in neurotrauma and in cerebral monitoring during cardiac surgery.

Measurement

- $S_{jv}O_2$ is usually measured via an intravascular catheter threaded retrogradely up the internal jugular vein as far as the jugular bulb. Normal value is 55–75%.
- A fibreoptic catheter uses reflectance oximetry (as in PA monitoring of mixed venous saturation) to provide continuous $S_{jv}O_2$ monitoring. As with pulse oximetry the apparatus uses the light absorption spectra of haemoglobin and deoxyhaemoglobin.
- Catheter placement can be facilitated by locating the vessel using ultrasound, and is verified by lateral skull X-ray which should confirm the tip lying at the level of, and medial to, the mastoid process.
- Alternatively a sample may be taken directly from the jugular bulb and the oxygen saturation measured by co-oximetry.

Factors which change $S_{jv}O_2$

- $S_{jv}O_2$ is an indirect indicator of cerebral oxygen utilisation: when O_2 demand exceeds supply then extraction increases and $S_{jv}O_2$ falls (desaturated at <50%), conversely when supply exceeds demand it rises (luxuriant at >75%). It is a specific measure of global cerebral oxygenation but is not sensitive to smaller focal areas of ischaemia.
- The difference in oxygen content between arterial and jugular venous blood ($A_{jv}DO_2$) is given by CMRO$_2$ (cerebral metabolic rate for O_2)/ CBF (cerebral blood flow). Normal is 4–8 ml O_2/100 ml of blood.
- If $A_{jv}DO_2$ is <4 supply is luxuriant: if >8 it suggests ischaemia
- Increased oxygen demand or decrease in supply (fall in $S_{jv}O_2$ and rise in $A_{jv}DO_2$) results from:
  — Raised ICP.
  — Systemic hypotension (severe).
  — Hypocapnia (<3.75 kPa).
  — Arterial hypoxia.
  — Cerebral vasospasm.
  — Increased metabolic demand: pyrexia, seizures.
- Decreased oxygen demand or increase in supply (rise in $S_{jv}O_2$ and fall in $A_{jv}DO_2$) results from:
  — Decreased metabolic demand (hypothermia; sedation).
  — Increased blood supply.
  — Hypercapnia.
  — Arterial hyperoxia.
  — Brain death (minimal demand).

Marking points: The question tests your understanding of the basic principle that while decreased oxygenation always indicates potential cerebral dysfunction, increased oxygenation may also be a herald of cerebral damage. A logical approach based on first principles will stand you in good stead.

Explain the basic principles of surgical diathermy. What are its potential problems?

Diathermy is used very widely in surgical practice but it does have implications for the anaesthetist, who will be blamed, unfair though it may seem, should a patient suffer a burn due to malpositioning of the plate. Diathermy may also interfere with monitors and can disrupt pacemaker function and so is a topic on which some basic knowledge is expected.

Introduction

Diathermy is used widely in surgical practice, both for coagulation and for cutting, and relies on the heating generated as an electric current passes through a resistance that is concentrated in the probe itself.

Principles of action

- Heat generation is proportional to the power that is developed: typically 50–400 W.
- A high frequency sine waveform is used for cutting: typically 0.5 MHz.
- A damped waveform is used for coagulation: typically 1.0–1.5 MHz.
- High frequency is necessary because muscle is very sensitive to direct current and to alternating current at frequencies less than ~10 kHz. This is particularly important in relation to myocardial muscle: low frequencies may precipitate fibrillation.
- Burning and heating effects can occur at all frequencies.

Types of diathermy

- **Unipolar.** There are two connections to the patient: the neutral (or indifferent) patient plate, and the active coagulation or cutting electrode. Current passes through both but the current density at the active electrode is very high and generates high temperatures. At the patient plate the current density is dispersed over a wide area and heating does not occur. The patient plate and hence the patient is kept at earth potential, which reduces the risks of capacitor linkage (in which diathermy current may flow in the absence of direct contact). Modern diathermy machines incorporate isolating capacitors to minimise the problem. An alternative is to use an earth free or floating circuit.
- **Bipolar.** Current is localised to the instrument: it passes only from one blade of the forceps to the other. Bipolar diathermy uses low power, and this limits its efficacy in the coagulation of all but small vessels. The circuit is not earthed.

Problems

- Thermal injury at the site of the indifferent electrode (the diathermy plate) which must be in close and even contact with a large area of skin, ideally an area that is well perfused and which will dissipate heat. Adhesive and conductive gels are useful. If the area of contact is small the current density increases to the point at which a burn is probable.
- Thermal injury at metal contact site if plate is detached or malpositioned. The diathermy current may flow to earth through any point at which the patient is touching metal (operating table, lithotomy poles, ECG electrodes, etc.) and cause a burn.
- Activation of instrument when it is not in contact with the tissue to be cut or coagulated.
- Circuit may be completed via a route that does not include the indifferent electrode: may result in a burn.
- Alcoholic skin preparation solutions have ignited after diathermy activation.
- Interference with pacemaker function (indifferent electrode should be sited as far distant as possible and bipolar should be used if possible).

- Diathermy may lead to ischaemia and infarction of structures supplied by fine end-arteries. Classic examples include the penis (hence unipolar must be avoided in circumcision) and the testis which has a vulnerable vascular pedicle.

> **Marking points:** You may be forgiven if you do not know the precise frequencies and wave forms associated with types of surgical diathermy, but you must be aware of the potential dangers to patients and how to maximise safety.

Outline ways of measuring humidity and evaluate the methods by which gases can be humidified in clinical practice. Why is this important?

Anaesthesia frequently involves bypassing sites in the upper airway that are responsible for the humidification of inspired gases. Artificial humidification is important in the context both of anaesthesia and intensive care, and so you will be expected to know about the different methods that are commonly used.

Introduction

The mass of water vapour that is present in a given volume of air (the absolute humidity) varies with temperature so that at 20°C fully saturated air contains 17 g m^{-3}. By the time that it reaches the alveoli at 37°C this air is fully saturated and contains 44 g m^{-3}. Anaesthetic and medical gases, however, are dry and may bypass the normal humidification mechanisms.

Measurement

- **Hair hygrometer.** The hair, which is linked to a spring and pointer, elongates as humidity increases. It is accurate between relative humidities of ~30% and 90%.
- **Wet and dry bulb hygrometer.** Cumbersome. Temperature difference between two thermometers relates to evaporation of water round the wet bulb which in turn relates to ambient humidity. Calculated from tables.
- **Regnault's hygrometer.** Accurate. Air is blown through ether within a silver tube. The temperature at which condensation appears on the outer surface is the dew point, the temperature at which ambient air is fully saturated. The ratio of the s.v.p. at the dew point to the s.v.p. at ambient temperature gives the relative humidity. Determined from tables.
- **Transducers.** As a substance absorbs atmospheric water there is a change either in capacitance or in electrical resistance.
- **Mass spectrometer.** Accurate. Expensive.

Methods of humidification

- **HME (heat and moisture exchange) filter.** This is a widely used method, which is passive, and which cannot, therefore, attain 100% efficiency, but which may reach 70–80%. The HME contains a hygroscopic material within a sealed unit. As the warm expired gas cools so the water vapour condenses on the element, which is warmed both by the specific heat of the exhaled gas and the latent heat of the water. Inhaled, dry and cool gas is thus warmed during inspiration, during which process the element cools down prior to the next exhalation. Problems include moderate inefficiency in prolonged use, increased dead space, infection risk.
- **Water bath (cold).** Passive, in that dry gases bubble through water at room temperature. The system is inefficient (~30%) and becomes more so as the loss of latent heat of vaporisation cools the water further.
- **Water bath (warm).** Active. Dry gases bubble through water which is heated, usually to 60°C (to inhibit microbial contamination). Very efficient >90%. More complex and risk of thermal injury to patient (minimised by thermostats).
- **Nebulisers.** Active. Gas driven and ultrasonic. Not in common use. Can deliver gas with >100% relative humidity and may overload pulmonary tree with fluid.

Consequences of failure to humidify gases

- Drying and keratinisation of parts of the tracheobronchial tree.
- Reduction of ciliary activity and impairment of the mucociliary escalator.
- Inflammatory change in the ciliated pulmonary epithelium, drying and crusting of secretions.
- Mucus plugging, atelectasis, superimposed chest infection, impaired gas exchange.

Patients at risk

- Those undergoing prolonged anaesthesia.
- Those with pre-existing respiratory disease in whom the impairment of important pulmonary defence functions will be more significant.
- Those at the extremes of age: neonates, infants and the elderly.
- All intensive care patients.

Marking points: Detailed information about methods of measuring humidity is much less important than an awareness of the advantages and limitations of the devices that are in use. Commonsense alone should help you to identify which patients are particularly at risk and you will be expected to do so.

Describe the features of a modern anaesthetic machine that contribute to the safety of a patient undergoing general anaesthesia.

This is a core topic. Your answer can readily be arranged by following the gas flow through from cylinder or pipeline to the fresh gas outlet. The features are numerous and you will have little time to do more than list them.

Introduction
The modern anaesthetic machine delivers accurate mixtures of anaesthetic gases and inhalational agents at variable, controlled flow rates and at low pressure. It accomplishes this via a number of features that are best described by tracing the gas flow through the system from the cylinder or pipeline to the fresh gas outlet.

Gas cylinders
- Colour coded for the UK (but no international consistency).
- Molybdenum steel: robust construction and rigorous regular hydraulic testing (which also applies to the cylinder outlet valve).
- Pin-index system (unique to each gas) prevents connection to the wrong yoke, and side guards on each yoke ensure that the cylinders are vertical.
- Bourdon pressure gauge indicates cylinder pressure.
- Pressure regulator/reducing valve reduces pressure to 4 bar, and a relief valve is located downstream in case of regulator failure.

Gas pipelines
- Colour coded for the UK (but no international consistency).
- Reducing valves lower pressures to 4 bar.
- Schrader coupling system ensures that connections are non-interchangeable.
- The hose connection to the anaesthetic machine should be permanent, the threads are gas specific (NIST – non-interchangeable screw thread) and a one-way valve ensures unidirectional flow.

Flow restrictors
- Placed upstream of the flowmeter block and protect the low-pressure part of the system from damaging surges in gas pressure from the piped supply.
- May sometimes be used downstream of vaporiser back bar to minimise back pressure associated with IPPV.

Oxygen failure devices
- Systems vary. In one example a pressure sensitive valve closes when O_2 pressure falls below 3 bar, and the gas mixture is vented, activating an audible warning tone. The same valve opens an air-entrainment valve so that the patient cannot be exposed to a hypoxic mixture resulting from failure of O_2 delivery.

Flow control valves
- These govern the transition from the high to the low pressure system. Reduce the pressure from 4 bar to just above atmospheric as gas enters the flow meter block.
- An interlock system between O_2 and N_2O control valves prevents N_2O administration of >75%.

Flowmeters
- Constant pressure variable orifice flowmeters, calibrated for specific gas.
- Antistatic coating to prevent sticking, vanes in bobbin to ensure rotation.
- Oxygen knob in UK is always on the left, is larger, is hexagonal in profile and is more prominent than the others (this position risks hypoxic mixture if there is damage to a downstream flow meter tube).

- CO_2 has disappeared from many machines: where it is still delivered it is usually governed to prevent a flow >500 ml min^{-1}.

Vaporisers and back bar
- Most common is temperature-compensated variable bypass device to allow accurate delivery of dialled concentrations.
- Locking mechanism on back bar prevents more than one vaporiser use at a time.
- Non-return valve on back bar prevents retrograde flow (the pumping effect of IPPV).
- Pressure relief valve on downstream end of back bar protects against increases in the pressure within the circuit.

Emergency oxygen flush
- O_2 is supplied direct from the high pressure circuit upstream of the vaporiser block and provides 35–75 L min^{-1} (if the O_2 flowmeter needle valve is opened fully it delivers ~ 40 L min^{-1}).
- Both methods may cause barotrauma in vulnerable patients.

Common gas outlet
- Receives gases from the back bar and from the emergency O_2 flush.
- Swivel outlet with standard 15 mm female connection.

Marking points: A logical approach which follows the path of delivered gas should ensure that you do not miss the important features. You will not have time to do much more than complete a list, but your answer will greatly be improved if you add a bit more detail in one or two key areas (for example the O_2 failure device and the flowmeter block and position of control knobs).

Classify the common types of hypoxia. What are the features of an anaesthetic machine which are designed to minimise the risk of delivering hypoxic gas mixtures?

The importance of these topics is obvious. The concept of oxygenation is fundamental to anaesthetic practice, and machine safety is another core subject (is similar to the previous question)

Introduction
The whole practice of anaesthesia itself is based on the avoidance of hypoxia, the causes of which are classified as follows.

Causes of hypoxia
- **Hypoxaemic hypoxia.** P_aO_2 is low because of hypoxic inspired gas mixture, severe alveolar hypoventilation or apnoea, ventilation/perfusion mismatch (endobronchial intubation, lung disease etc).
- **Stagnant hypoxia.** P_aO_2 and haemoglobin oxygen-carrying capacity are normal but the blood supply to tissues is inadequate due to diminished cardiac output or occlusion of the peripheral vascular system.
- **Anaemic hypoxia.** P_aO_2 is normal but low haemoglobin reduces O_2 carriage and delivery to tissues.
- **Cytotoxic hypoxia.** P_aO_2 and haemoglobin oxygen-carrying capacity are normal but cellular poisons inhibit O_2 utilisation. Examples are CN or CO which poison cytochrome systems.

Anaesthetic machine features
- Gas cylinders
  - These are colour coded for the UK (but no international consistency).
  - Pin-index system (unique to each gas) prevents connection to the wrong yoke, and side guards on each yoke ensure that the cylinders are vertical.
  - Bourdon pressure gauge indicates cylinder pressure.
- Gas pipelines
  - Colour coded for the UK (but no international consistency).
  - Schrader coupling system ensures that connections are non-interchangeable.
  - The hose connection to the anaesthetic machine should be permanent, the threads are gas specific (NIST – non-interchangeable screw thread) and a one-way valve ensures unidirectional flow.
- Oxygen failure devices
  - Systems vary. In one example a pressure sensitive valve closes when O_2 pressure falls below 3 bar, and the gas mixture is vented, activating an audible warning tone. The same valve opens an air-entrainment valve so that the patient cannot be exposed to a hypoxic mixture resulting from failure of O_2 delivery.
- Flow control valves
  - An interlock system between O_2 and N_2O control valves prevents N_2O administration of >75%.
- Flowmeters
  - Constant pressure variable orifice flowmeters, calibrated for specific gas.
  - Antistatic coating to prevent sticking, vanes in bobbin to ensure rotation.
  - Oxygen control knob in UK is always on the left, is larger, is hexagonal and is more prominent than the others (however this position risks hypoxic mixture if there is damage to a downstream flowmeter tube).
- Oxygen analyser
  - Should be placed as near to the patient as possible, typically at the common fresh gas outlet.

Marking points: There are two topics in one question here, although they are clearly linked and could appear together in an oral question. Understanding of the important fundamentals of both will be expected.

What factors associated with the anaesthetic machine and patient breathing system may cause barotrauma? How is the risk reduced? Why is a high airway pressure alarm system important during general anaesthesia?

This is another variant on the machine safety theme but with a different emphasis. You will see that familiarity with the basic features of the modern anaesthetic machine can be very useful.

Introduction

High airway pressure (P_{aw}) may indicate a direct problem with the patient or a problem with the machine and breathing system that imminently may damage a patient. High P_{aw} alarms alert the anaesthetist to either possibility without distinguishing between the two.

Equipment features

- **Gas cylinders and pipelines**
  - Deliver very high and potentially lethal pressures.
  - Pressure regulator/reducing valve reduces pressure to 4 bar, and a relief valve is located downstream in case of regulator failure.
  - Reducing valves on pipelines lower pressures to 4 bar.
- **Flow restrictors**
  - Placed upstream of the flowmeter block and protect the low-pressure part of the system from damaging surges in gas pressure from the piped supply.
- **Flow control valves**
  - These govern the transition from the high to the low pressure system. Reduce the pressure from 4 bar to just above atmospheric as gas enters the flowmeter block.
  - Needle valves restrict flow.
- **Vaporisers and back bar**
  - Pressure relief valve on downstream end of back bar protects against increases in the pressure within the circuit.
- **Emergency oxygen flush**
  - O_2 is supplied direct from the high-pressure circuit upstream of the vaporiser block and can provides 35–75 L min^{-1} (if the O_2 flowmeter needle valve is opened fully it delivers ~40 min^{-1}).
  - O_2 flush may be jammed or held open. It should not be lockable.
  - Both methods may cause barotrauma in vulnerable patients.
- **Ventilator pressure relief valve**
  - Closes during inspiratory phase of IPPV and vents gas after bellows refills. Should it stick in the closed position the P_{aw} will increase.
- **Scavenging system**
  - A pressure relief valve in system vents excess gas in reservoir to atmosphere. If this valve fails then pressure is transmitted back to the breathing system.
- **Breathing system and airway**
  - Kinks or obstruction in breathing system hoses will increase P_{aw}.
  - One-way PEEP valve will obstruct flow if placed in the inspiratory limb and will obstruct expiratory flow if incorrectly orientated in the expiratory limb.
  - APL (adjustable pressure-limiting valve) will vent gas into the scavenging system; if it is screwed shut the bag will distend with an increase in pressure.
  - Anaesthesia breathing bags are designed so that pressure will not exceed ~50–60 mmHg (behave according to the law of Laplace: $P = 2T/R$). Problematic only in patients with lung disease (e.g. emphysema).
  - ETT (or LMA) may kink or obstruct, may get cuff herniation.

Value of high airway pressure alarm

- Should be placed so that it senses pressure on the patient side of the inspiratory and expiratory valves, not the machine side, so is as close to the airway as possible.
- Warns of danger to the patient of barotrauma (factors described above).
- Warns of problems with the patient in whom high airway pressure may be caused by:
  — Bronchoconstriction.
  — Pneumothorax.
  — Expiratory efforts against ventilator (as muscle relaxants wear off).

Marking points: It is important not to confuse a machine airway pressure with a patient airway pressure and to recognise those parts of the system which risk causing barotrauma. Even if there is insuffucient time to provide all the details your answer should emphasise aspects of safe practice.

Cardiac and thoracic anaesthesia

What are the main postoperative problems which occur in the first 24 hours following a coronary artery bypass graft? Outline their management.

Coronary artery bypass grafting (CABG) is a common procedure in the developed world, but although it has become routine there remain a large number of potential complications, many of them related to cardiopulmonary bypass (CPB), which can affect every organ system. The question is testing your appreciation of the main principles rather than specifics. If you are struggling then it may help to consider the worse case scenarios, given the huge array of complications of CPB that have been described.

Introduction
Surgery for coronary artery disease involves the insertion of a vascular graft in an organ which may have precarious function. The surgery may be prolonged and is enabled by the use of cardiopulmonary bypass, which as a non-physiological process has been associated with a large number of complications. There are, therefore, several problems which may occur in the first postoperative day.

Cardiovascular
- **Cardiac failure.** Cardiac output may be compromised because of pre-existing ischaemic damage or because the myocardium is stunned after CPB and prolonged surgery.
  - Deterioration is prevented by optimising oxygen supply in face of demand.
  - Monitor function (PA catheter) and manage accordingly: inotropic support and vasodilators may suffice. May need intra-aortic ballon pump counter-pulsation or assist devices (depending on the centre).
- **Tamponade.** Cardiac output may be compromised by tamponade.
  - High index of suspicion and early decompression.
- **Arrhythmias.** Cardiac output may be compromised by arrhythmias.
  - Seek cause (e.g. K^+ derangement) treat with anti-arrhythmics or pacing as required.
- **Bleeding.** Cardiac output may be compromised by surgical bleeding or coagulation problems.
  - Check coagulation; discontinue drugs which may be contributing, coagulation factors and platelets if indicated. Re-operation if bleeding continues.

Systems problems

Many relate to CPB and potential effect of hypoperfusion and emboli on end-organs.

- **Central nervous system.** Failure to recover full consciousness.
  — Persistent drug effects? (particularly if hypothermic).
  — Micro-emboli during / after CPB: air, silicon, debris, fat, platelet aggregates.
  — Cerebral hypoperfusion.
  — Manage by maintaining cerebral perfusion pressure and oxygenation (but beware stressing the graft by elevated systemic pressures).
- **Renal.** CPB reduces blood flow and GFR by 30%.
  — Hypoperfusion and emboli may lead to acute renal failure.
  — Appropriate renal support according to impairment.
- **Pulmonary.** May get 'pump lung': oedema due to overload with subsequent ARDS-like picture.
  — Supportive ventilatory and circulatory management.
- **Gastrointestinal.** Organ impairment may follow hypoperfusion and emboli.
  — Pancreatitis, bowel ischaemia leading to acute abdomen.
  — May need surgical intervention.

Marking points: Details of subspecialty practice are not required and you will pass this question as long as you can give a logical overview of the important possible postoperative complications. You can predict these by thinking about the procedure. Why is it done? For ischaemic heart disease and associated features. How is it done? Using CPB with all its attendant problems.

What are the principles of cardiopulmonary bypass in the adult? What are the main complications of this technique?

Cardiopulmonary bypass (CPB) provides a substitute intact circulation while the heart is isolated. It may make sense, therefore, for you to consider how the normal circulation functions, because CPB is analogous. The technique is complex and invasive and so there are complications associated with the mechanics. It is non-physiological and yet perfuses every organ and system in the body Many of the complications, therefore, are predictable, even if your acquaintance with cardiac anaesthesia is slight.

Introduction
A patient who is on CPB has the temporary equivalent of an intact circulation. The differences are that the heart is isolated, the flow is (usually) non-pulsatile, and the circulation is exteriorised. Bypass is non-physiological and although it enables complex cardiac surgery it has been associated with numerous complications.

Principles of cardiopulmonary bypass
- CPB replaces the functions of the intact circulation by ensuring organ perfusion with oxygen-enriched blood from which CO_2 has been removed.
- Components include:
  - **Venous line** (usually from vena cavae) drains into a reservoir for gas exchange in which blood is oxygenated and CO_2 is removed.
  - **Bubble oxygenator** in which O_2 is bubbled through the perfusate (cheap, simple, but requires defoaming to reduce air emboli and damages formed blood components).
  - **Membrane oxygenator** in which gas exchange takes place across a semi-permeable membrane (fewer emboli form and less damage to RBCs).
  - **Arterial line** (usually to ascending aorta) via a pump (roller or centrifugal): flow may be non-pulsatile or pulsatile (no proven benefit).
  - **Pump** for cold cardioplegic solution (contains potassium for EMD arrest, energy substrate for metabolism).
  - **Ventricular drain** to vent heart: may get some aortic regurgitation if not prevented by aortic cross-clamp, or flow through bronchial and thebesian veins. May overdistend LV and cause critical ischaemia and post-bypass dysfunction.
  - **Filters (27 micron)** on both sides of the circulation to remove air and blood micro-emboli (also reduce platelets).
  - **Heat exchanger** is crucial part of the system to allow temperature control (hypothermia reduces oxygen demand by 6–9% per °C fall in core temperature).
  - **Priming:** the system (volume 1.5–2.5 L) is primed either with crystalloid or colloid/crystalloid. Acute haemodilution is inevitable as soon as bypass is established. Can prime with blood if necessary to maintain haematocrit at 20–25%.
  - **Anti-coagulation.** Crucial. Coagulation within any part of the circuit (pump or patient) is lethal. Synthetic surfaces of circuit cause diffuse thrombosis and oxygenator failure if anticoagulation is inadequate.
- Complications of circuit
  - Arterial side: cannula may kink, block or fail to deliver adequate flow.
  - Venous side: low return: bleeding, obstruction, air lock, aortic dissection.
  - Oxygenator failure.
  - Pump may cause aortic dissection.
  - Coagulation may be inadequate.
  - May react to protamine reversal (anaphylactoid, histamine release, hypotension, pulmonary hypertension).

— Inadequate LV venting: cardiac distension.
— Embolism: air, silicon, fat, platelet aggregates.

Complications associated with perfusion

- **Hypothermia:** coagulopathy, hyperglycaemia, drug metabolism reduced.
- **Fluid overload** (common).
- **Coagulopathy:** is related to CPB time (>2 hours is deleterious); decrease in platelet number and function may deplete Factors V and VIII.
- **Myocardial stunning** after cardioplegia (temperature is crucial).
- **Complement activation:** may get 'post-perfusion lung' (ARDS).
- **Central nervous system:** potential ischaemia due to hypoperfusion, problems with emboli: air, thrombus, debris, silicon (subtle post-bypass deficits are common).
- **Renal function:** bypass decreases renal blood flow and GFR by 30% (worse if bypass time is prolonged).
- **Gastrointestinal:** hypoperfusion of splanchnic bed and potential for critical gut ischaemia, pancreatic and liver dysfunction.

Marking points: If you can convey the basic principles of an artificial circulation you should be able to outline the major complications which follow. The complete list will not be expected.

What are the anaesthetic implications of mitral stenosis?

Rheumatic heart disease is the commonest cause of mitral stenosis, but both problems are increasingly rare. Valvular disease is of interest to anaesthetists because of the risk that anaesthesia and surgery will cause perioperative decompensation. It is a popular exam topic because it allows discussion of physiology and pharmacology applied to a fixed cardiac output state.

Introduction
Mitral stenosis is almost always rheumatic in origin and is increasingly rare. It is a progressive disease that leads to a fixed output state which is maintained by compensatory mechanisms, and it is the propensity for anaesthesia to disrupt these mechanisms that makes it such a significant condition.

Pathophysiology
- Narrowing (almost always rheumatic in origin) is slowly progressive and symptoms appear relatively early. May suddenly deteriorate if there is an increased demand for cardiac output as in pregnancy, or if atrial fibrillation supervenes.
- Determination of the pressure gradient across the valve (LA : LV) is less reliable than estimations of valvular area, which is the key factor which determines flow. Normal mitral valve area is 4–6 cm^2 and stenosis may be graded as severe (<1 cm^2), moderate (1.1–1.5 cm^2) and mild (1.6–2.5 cm^2) (There is a gap between 2.5 and 4 cm^2, which would be classified, presumably, as 'very mild' or 'insignificant'.)
- As narrowing progresses the contribution of atrial contraction to left ventricular filling increases from 15% to 40%. This is why the onset of atrial fibrillation may be so catastrophic. Atrial dilatation and hypertrophy results from this compensation. In time the increased left atrial pressure (LAP) is reflected in pulmonary hypertension and right ventricular overload.
- Relative bradycardia allows sufficient time for diastolic flow across the stenosis.

Anaesthesia implications
- The main aim is to prevent decompensation.
- **Bradycardia** may allow an increased stroke volume but the cardiac output may drop unacceptably as a result. **Tachycardia** may diminish stroke volume to the point that cardiac output is even more impaired.
- Sudden onset of **atrial fibrillation** must be treated aggressively, with DC cardioversion if necessary, otherwise pulmonary oedema may supervene. If atrial fibrillation is already present the ventricular response rate must be controlled. Patients may also be on oral anticoagulants which will need to be changed to parenteral heparin during the perioperative period.
- **Normovolaemia** must be maintained. If LAP falls then cardiac output will drop. Volume must be sufficient to allow flow across the stenotic valve. Patients may also be very sensitive to any increase in venous return (as can occur with the use of an arterial tourniquet or placing the patient in lithotomy, as well as with infusions of fluid) which may precipitate pulmonary oedema. Cardiac output cannot increase in response to enhanced venous return.
- **Effective myocardial** contractility is important for the maintenance of cardiac output in mitral stenosis (as in most valvular lesions), and undue depression must be avoided.
- Must avoid increasing **pulmonary vascular resistance** (hypercapnia, hypoxia, acidosis, nitrous oxide). Right heart failure, should it supervene, must also be treated aggressively.
- **Systemic vascular resistance** must be maintained in order to allow adequate coronary perfusion during diastole.

- **Infective bacterial endocarditis** potentially affects any abnormal valve and antibiotic prophylaxis should be given.

> **Marking points:** Anaesthesia in patients with mitral stenosis risks interference with their normal mechanisms of compensation. Successful management rests on an understanding of how those mechanisms may be affected. Your answer should reflect this.

What are the anaesthetic implications of aortic stenosis?

Aortic stenosis may be caused by rheumatic heart disease, but also occurs as a consequence of degeneration and calcification in a congenitally abnormal (usually bicuspid) valve. Anaesthetic management is based upon the need to avoid perioperative decompensation. Like mitral stenosis, it is a popular exam topic because it allows discussion of physiology and pharmacology applied to a fixed cardiac output state.

Introduction

Unlike mitral stenosis aortic stenosis may progress without symptoms so that sudden death may even be the first presenting feature. Like mitral stenosis it leads to a fixed output state which is maintained by compensatory mechanisms, and it is the propensity for anaesthesia to disrupt these mechanisms that makes it a significant condition. Decompensated mitral stenosis manifests as heart failure; decompensated aortic stenosis may be fatal.

Pathophysiology

- Determination of the pressure gradient across the valve (left ventricle : ascending aorta) is less reliable than estimations of valvular area, which is the key factor that determines flow. Normal aortic valve area is 2.5–3.5 cm^2 and an area <1 cm^2 is an indication for immediate surgical valve replacement. At areas <0.7 cm^2 any demand for increased cardiac output (exercise, pyrexia, pregnancy, etc.) is associated with angina pectoris, syncope and sudden death. Clinical signs include narrowed pulse pressure (<30 mmHg suggests severe disease). Systolic blood pressure may be lower than expected because of the reduced cardiac output (SBP = CO × SVR).
- As narrowing progresses there is increased pressure loading on the LV, which undergoes concentric hypertrophy. The less compliant hypertrophic LV has increased O$_2$ demand and reduced O$_2$ supply (systole through the stenosed valve is prolonged and so diastolic time during the cardiac cycle is proportionately reduced).
- Atrial contraction makes a significant contribution to left ventricular filling, which must be maintained. Atrial fibrillation may lead to decompensation.

Anaesthesia implications

- The main aim is to prevent decompensation, in particular by maintaining coronary perfusion during diastole.
- **Effective myocardial contractility** is important for maintenance of cardiac output in aortic stenosis (as in most valvular lesions), and undue depression must be avoided. Increasing myocardial drive will increase myocardial work and O$_2$ demand, and may precipitate subendocardial ischaemia.
- **Systemic diastolic blood pressure** must be maintained. If SVR falls then coronary diastolic perfusion may fail with disastrous consequences. Vasodilatation must be avoided and preload maintained to allow flow across the stenotic valve. This has obvious implications for the use of the many anaesthetic agents which decrease SVR, including local anaesthetics used in subarachnoid and extradural block. Cardiopulmonary resuscitation in the presence of aortic stenosis and LV hypertrophy is rarely successful.
- **Bradycardia** will decrease cardiac output but **tachycardia** is even more detrimental because it limits diastolic coronary perfusion. Arrhythmias, including atrial fibrillation, require urgent treatment, but myocardial depressants such as beta-adrenoceptor blockers are better avoided.
- **Infective bacterial endocarditis** potentially affects any abnormal valve and antibiotic prophylaxis should be given.
- These patients can be very difficult to manage. Anaesthesia should include invasive monitoring of intra-arterial and central venous pressure, and it may be

necessary to run a continuous infusion of vasopressor such as norepinephrine (noradrenaline) to ensure that SVR is maintained.

Marking points: Anaesthesia in patients with aortic stenosis risks fatal interference with the normal mechanisms of compensation. As with other valvular lesions their successful management rests on an understanding of how those mechanisms may be affected. If any part of your suggested management is likely to prove disastrous you will fail this question with a '1'.

How do you confirm that a double-lumen endobronchial tube has been placed correctly? Outline the possible complications associated with this procedure.

Some argue that clinical confimation of double-lumen tube placement should largely be historical, although clinical assessment may have a place in conjunction with other techniques. Most of the complications are linked to malposition and this is the area on which your answer should concentrate.

Introduction
Double-lumen bronchial tubes, which allow separation and isolation of the lungs, have an important role in thoracic, aortic, spinal and gastro-oesophageal surgery. The surgical procedures are generally complex and prolonged and the hazards of one-lung anaesthesia itself mandate that tube positioning must be optimal.

Clinical confirmation
- Double-lumen endobronchial tubes (DLEBT) are bulky when compared to a conventional tracheal tube, and are more complex to insert. Different tubes require different insertion techniques but in all cases there is rotation within the airway of between 90° and 180°.
- **Length of tube.** Correct insertion defines the situation in which the upper surface of the bronchial cuff is immediately distal to the bifurcation of the carina. The distance can be measured. The average depth of insertion for a patient of height 170 cm is 29 cm, and the distance alters by 1 cm for every 10 cm change in height. This distance from the incisors can therefore be used as a guide.
- **Auscultation (both lung fields).** With both tracheal and endobronchial cuffs inflated, check bilateral and equal air entry (allowing for pulmonary pathology).
- **Auscultation (alternate lung fields).** Clamp one side and check that breath sounds disappear on the ipsilateral, and remain on the contralateral side. Reverse the process.
- **Palpation.** During all three stages above, manual ventilation using the reservoir bag will reveal whether it has normal compliance (again allowing for pulmonary pathology).
- **Monitoring:** oximetry and, particularly, capnography when compared from both lumina, may indicate placement problems.
- **Malpositioning.** If the above signs indicate that the tube is in the wrong place a combination of manoeuvres (unilateral clamping and bronchial cuff inflation-deflation with repeated auscultation) can in theory identify the site and nature of malposition. In practice this can be difficult, particularly if the tube moves during surgery when access to the chest wall is limited.

Fibreoptic bronchoscopy
- It is evident, however, that clinical confirmation is insufficient. NCEPOD's 1998 examination of oesophagogastrectomy implicated problems with double lumen tubes in 30% of deaths. Studies have confirmed that critical malpositioning occurs in over 25% of cases and general misplacements complicate over 80% of uses.
- Variations in anatomy are common, particularly if distorted by tumour or effusion.
- Routine use of fibreoptic bronchoscopy is the only way of avoiding these problems and ensuring accurate positioning as well as intraoperative checking if indicated. It also minimises the complications of DLEBT placement as outlined below.

Complications of double-lumen tubes

- Malposition
  — Occlusion of major bronchus with lobar collapse and secondary infection.
  — Failure to achieve adequate lung separation and one-lung ventilation. This may necessitate prolonged surgical retraction with associated trauma.
  — Failure to protect dependent lung from infected secretions from non-dependent lung (catastrophic in e.g. case of bronchopleural fistula).
- Trauma during insertion and rotation
  — Disruption of the tracheobronchial tree, may be associated with excessive endobronchial cuff pressures.
  — Trauma to larynx and supraglottic structures.

Marking points: Fibreoptic confirmation of tube placement is not the gold standard but probably should be the accepted standard. Your answer should emphasise the inferior nature of clinical tests, and concentrate on the advantages of bronchoscopy. You will then be able to avoid detailed description of all the clamping and unclamping manouevres which are becoming historical.

What physiological changes are associated with one-lung anaesthesia? Describe the management of a patient in this situation who becomes hypoxic.

One lung anaesthesia is a technique that is used for complex and specialist procedures, but the physiological changes that ensue are of particular anaesthetic relevance and so make it an attractive science-based clinical topic. You will be expected to understand the basic principles rather than (as used to be the case) details of the many and varied double lumen devices and bronchial blockers that historically were used.

Indications
The indications for anaesthesia during which one lung is deliberately collapsed to facilitate surgical exposure include pulmonary, aortic, spinal and oesophageal surgery. Patients undergoing such procedures are commonly high risk and the physiological changes imposed by one lung anaesthesia can present a significant challenge.

Physiological changes
- The surgical side is uppermost and the non-ventilated upper lung is usually described as the non-dependent lung.
- When ventilation is interrupted the remaining blood flow takes no part in gas exchange and this shunt contributes to hypoxia.
- The shunt is reduced because gravity favours flow to the dependent lung, and because surgical compression and lung retraction may further decrease blood flow.
- Surgical ligation of non-dependent vessels (in their entirety if a pneumonectomy is being performed) will also reduce shunt.
- Hypoxic vasoconstriction decreases flow by ~50% to the non-dependent lung and may reduce shunt from ~50% down to 30% (which is still significant).
- The dependent lung loses volume because of compression, and hypoxic vasoconstriction, should it occur, may divert some blood to the non-dependent lung.
- Secretions may pool in the dependent lung and suction removal via a double-lumen tube may be difficult.

Ventilatory management
- Ventilator settings: same as for double-lung ventilation with tidal volume of ~10 ml kg^{-1}: higher volumes increase P_{aw} and vascular resistance so more blood may flow to the non-ventilated lung and increase shunt. Lower volumes may cause atelectasis.
- Although shunt is not substantially improved by supplemental O_2 the F_1O_2 is usually increased to 0.8–1.0.
- The respiratory rate is adjusted to keep P_aCO_2 at ~40 mmHg (5.3 kPa).

Management of hypoxia
- Check F_1O_2 and increase if necessary (but may not help if substantial shunt is the problem).
- Check tidal volume and ventilator indices.
- Check double-lumen tube position with fibreoptic bronchoscope (displacement to a suboptimal position is common).
- Maintain P_aCO_2 at ~5.3 kPa as hypocapnia may decrease hypoxic pulmonary vasoconstriction.
- Add CPAP to upper lung (~5 cmH$_2$O) and warn surgeon that lung may partially re-expand.

- Add PEEP to lower lung (~5 cmH$_2$O) to increase volume in potentially atelectatic areas – but note that this may increase vascular resistance and divert blood to upper lung.
- Increase both CPAP and PEEP in small increments.
- If none of these manoeuvres works it may be necessary to revert to full double-lung ventilation (with retraction to allow surgery to continue).

Marking points: You must demonstrate an effective strategy for dealing with an episode of hypoxia, because this will demonstrate that you understand the underlying principles of one-lung anaesthesia.

Index

A

Acute Lung Injury, see 'Acute Respiratory Distress Syndrome'
Acute Respiratory Distress Syndrome 147–148
ARDS, see 'Acute Respiratory Distress Syndrome' 38
Air embolism, recognition and diagnosis 39–40
Air embolism, recognition and management
Alcohol abuse, chronic, anaesthetic implications 128–129
ALI, see 'Acute Respiratory Distress Syndrome'
'Ametop' (amethocaine gel) 273–274
Amniotic fluid embolism 161–162
Amputation, post-operative pain 222
Anaemia, anaesthetic implications 116–117
Anaesthetic machine, prevention of hypoxia 309–310
Anaesthetic machine, safety features 307–308
Analgesia, influence on recovery 228–229
Ankle block, anatomy of 251
Aortic stenosis, anaesthetic implications 319–320
Aspiration, see 'Pulmonary aspiration'
Asthma, see 'status asthmaticus'
Atopine 283
Atrial fibrillation 77–78
Autonomic neuropathy, anaesthetic considerations 102
Awake fibreoptic intubation, see 'Fibreoptic intubation'
Awareness, causes of 29
Awareness, detection of 28

B

Barotrauma, anaesthetic machine and 311–312
Bleeding, post-tonsillectomy 180–181
Blood transfusion, immunological consequences 51
Brachial plexus, anatomy 255

Bradycardia 20
Brain injury, secondary damage 210
Bronchoscopy, paediatric 193–194
Burns, paediatric, management of 191–192
Bypass, see 'Cardiopulmonary bypass'

C

Cancer pain, principles of management 226–227
Capnography 300–301
Cardiopulmonary bypass, principles of 315–316
Cardiopulmonary bypass, complications of 315–316
Carotid endarterectomy 54–55
Caudal, see 'Sacral extradural'
Causalgia, see 'Complex Regional Pain Syndrome'
Cerebral blood flow, regulation 214
Cerebral blood flow, influence of anaesthesia 214
Cervical spine, acute injury 223–224
Chair dental anaesthesia 73–74
Chirality 295–296
Chronic obstructive pulmonary disease 109, 118–119
Chronic renal failure, see 'Renal failure, chronic'
Circulatory changes at birth 196–197
Coagulation, peri-operative 19
Coeliac plexus, anatomy 247–248
Common cold and anaesthesia 200–201
Complex Regional Pain Syndrome 224–225
Congenital heart disease, anaesthetic implications 196–197
Cord prolapse, anaesthetic management 175–176
Coronary artery by-pass graft, post-operative problems 313–314
Corticosteroids, response to surgery 56–57
Corticosteroids, replacement regimens 56–57
Coryza, see 'Common cold'
Cricothyroidotomy 153
CVP (central venous pressure) 245–246

D

Dantrolene 36
Day case surgery, anaesthetic arrangements for 41
Day case surgery, discharge criteria 82–83
Day case surgery, selection criteria 71–72
Desaturation, during failed intubation 64
Diabetes Mellitus 94–95
Diathermy, surgical, principles and problems 303–304
Difficult intubation, see 'Tracheal intubation'
Double-lumen endobronchial tubes 321–322
Down syndrome, anaesthetic considerations 183
Drug addict, anaesthesia for 110–111
Dural puncture, inadvertent, management of 158
Dystrophia myotonica, anaesthetic implications 101

E

ECT, physiological consequences 75–76
Elderly, see 'old age'
Elective surgery, reasons for cancellation 15
EMLA 273–274
Epidural for labour, reasons for failure 165–166
Epidural, mobile 160
Epiglottitis, diagnosis and management 187–188
Extradural analgesia, complications 262–263
Extradural space, anatomy 262
Eye injury, penetrating 235–236

F

Feeding, see 'Nutrition'
Femoral nerve, anatomy for nerve block 252
Fibreoptic intubation, awake 86–87
Fluids, for resuscitation 231–232

G

Glycopyrrolate 283
Guillain-Barré Syndrome, diagnosis and management 131–132

H

Haemofiltration 139–140
Haemorrhage, major obstetric 173–174
Haemorrhage, massive 238–239
Haemorrhage, physiological response 240–241
Heat loss, mechanisms of 43–44
HELLP syndrome 171–172
HIV, risks to staff 105
Headache, after regional anaesthesia 155–156
Headache, postpartum, differential diagnosis 155–156
Head-down position, hazards of 46
Head injury, anaesthesia following 205
Head injury, closed, ITU management 210
Head injury, secondary damage, see 'Brain injury'
Head injury, indications for intubation and ventilation 206–207
Head injury, transfer 208–209

Heart block, classification and management 136–137
Heart transplant, anaesthetic considerations 99–100
Herniorrhaphy, analgesia for 195
High airway pressure 311–312
High spinal, recognition and management 167–168
Humidification 305–306
Hyoscine 283
Hypercapnia, causes and effects 69–70
Hypertension, acute treatment of 292–294
Hypertension, pre-operative assessment 126–127
Hypotension, causes of during TURP 22
Hypotension, following subarachnoid block, see 'Vasopressors'
Hypotension, induced 79–81
Hypothermia, effects of 43–44
Hypoventilation, post-anaesthesia 16
Hypoxia, classification 309–310
Hysterectomy, abdominal, post-operative analgesia 215–216

I

Induced hypotension, see 'Hypotension, induced'
Infant, anatomical differences 179
Infant, physiological differences 177–178
Inhalational injury, see 'Smoke inhalation injury'
Internal jugular vein, anatomy 256–257
Internal jugular venous cannulation, complications 256–257
Interscalene block 266–267
Intra-arterial drug injection 88–89
Intracranial pressure (ICP) 203–204
Intraocular pressure (IOP) 96
Intubation, see 'Tracheal intubation'

J

Jehovah's Witness, anaesthesia in 13–14
Jugular venous bulb, oxygen saturation 302

K

Ketamine, pharmacology of 290–291

L

Laparoscopy, complications of 33
Laryngeal Mask Airway, in difficult intubation 26
Larynx, innervation 249
Latex allergy 42
Lithotomy position, hazards of 45–46
Local anaesthetic drugs, toxicity 32

M

Magnesium Sulphate 286–287
Magnetic Resonance Imaging, anaesthetic implications 17
Magnetic Resonance Imaging, monitoring problems 18
Malignant hyperthermia, diagnosis and management 34–35

Malignant hyperthermia, pathophysiology and investigation 36–37
Mechanical ventilation, weaning 141–142
Mitral stenosis, anaesthetic implications 317–318
Monoamine oxidase inhibitors, anaesthesia and 275–276
Multiple sclerosis 108
Muscle weakness in ICU patients 138
Myasthenia gravis 112–113
Myocardial infarction, perioperative risk factors 24–25
Myocardium, arterial supply of 250
Myxoedema, see 'Thyroid disease'

N

Near drowning 189–190
Neuropathic pain, symptoms and causes 217
Neuropathic pain, causes and management 218–219
Nitrous oxide, advantages and disadvantages 277–278
Nitrous oxide, mechanisms and toxicity 279–280
Nutrition, parenteral and enteral 143–144

O

Obesity, anaesthetic problems of 27
Obstetric haemorrhage, see 'Haemorrhage, major obstetric'
Old age, anaesthetic implications 52–53
One lung anaesthesia 323–324
Oxygen delivery, optimisation 149–150
Oxygen toxicity 151–152

P

Pacemakers 60–61
Paediatric bronchoscopy 193–194
Paediatric life support 184–185
Pain relief, see 'Analgesia'
Patient controlled analgesia (PCA), safety features 65–66
Penetrating eye injury, see 'Eye injury, penetrating
Percutaneous tracheostomy, see 'Tracheostomy, percutaneous'
Phaeochromocytoma 103–104
Pneumothorax, causative mechanisms 242
Pneumothorax, diagnosis and management 243–244
Porphyria, anaesthetic significance 114–115
Post-dural puncture headache, management 159
Post-herpetic neuralgia, clinical features and treatment 220–221
Post-operative cognitive deficits, factors in the elderly 49–50
Post-operative nausea and vomiting 284–285
Pre-eclampsia, aetiology and anaesthetic implications 163–164
Premature neonate, anaesthetic risks 198–199
Premedication 84–85
Prone position 58–59
Propofol, pharmacology of 288–289
Pulmonary artery catheters 145–146
Pulmonary aspiration of gastric contents 47–48

Pulse oximetry, principles and limitations 297–298
Pyloric stenosis, management in infants 182

R

Reflex sympathetic dystrophy, see 'Complex regional pain syndrome'
Renal failure, chronic, anaesthetic implications of 122–123
Retained placenta, anaesthesia for 157
'Rotameter' flowmeter 299

S

Sacral extradural block, adults and children 260–261
Sacrum, anatomy 260
Sciatic nerve block, approaches and indications 253–254
Sedation, definition and techniques 67–68
Sickle cell disease 106–107
Smoke inhalation injury, diagnosis and assessment 237
Smoking, anaesthetic implications 120–121
Spinal anaesthesia, see 'Subarachnoid anaesthesia'
Spinal cord injury, anaesthesia following 212–213
Status asthmaticus, emergency management 133–134
Stellate ganglion, anatomy, blockade and complications 264–265
Steroids, see 'Corticosteroids'
Stress response to surgery 30–31
Stridor in children, differential diagnosis 180
Subarachnoid anaesthesia, high block, see 'High spinal'
Subarachnoid anaesthesia for caesarean section, pain during 169–170
Subarachnoid anaesthesia block height 258–259
Subarachnoid versus General Anaesthesia
Swan-Ganz catheter, see 'Pulmonary artery catheter'

T

Tachycardia 21
'Three-in-one' block 252
Thromboembolism, deep venous, prevention of 23
Thyroid disease, anaesthetic implications 124–125
Thyroid surgery, anaesthesia for 92–93
Thyrotoxicosis, see 'Thyroid disease'
Tracheal intubation, complications 90–91
Tracheal intubation, difficult 62–63
Tracheostomy, indications 135
Tracheostomy, percutaneous 153–154
Trigeminal neuralgia, presentation, pathogenesis and treatment 223

U

Upper limb, local anaesthetic blocks 268–269

V

Vasopressors, in spinal anaesthesia 281–282